T0337878

Markers
in Cardiology

A CASE-ORIENTED
APPROACH

Markers in Cardiology

A CASE-ORIENTED APPROACH

EDITED BY

Jesse E. Adams, MD, FACC
University of Louisville
Division of Cardiology
100 Mallard Creek
Louisville, KY 40202
USA

Fred Apple, PhD
Department of Laboratory Medicine and Pathology
Hennepin County Medical Center and University
of Minnesota School of Medicine
Minneapolis, MN
USA

Allan S. Jaffe, MD
Cardiovascular Division and Cardiovascular Research
Institute and Division of Laboratory Medicine
Mayo Clinic and Medical School
Rochester, Minnesota
USA

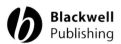
Blackwell
Publishing

© 2007 by Blackwell Publishing
Blackwell Futura is an imprint of Blackwell Publishing

Blackwell Publishing, Inc., 350 Main Street, Malden, Massachusetts 02148-5020, USA
Blackwell Publishing Ltd, 9600 Garsington Road, Oxford OX4 2DQ, UK
Blackwell Science Asia Pty Ltd, 550 Swanston Street, Carlton, Victoria 3053, Australia

First published 2007

1   2007

ISBN: 978-1-4051-3418-7

Library of Congress Cataloging-in-Publication Data

Markers in cardiology : a case-oriented approach / edited by Jesse E. Adams, Allan S. Jaffe,
Fred Apple.
    p. ; cm.
    Includes bibliographical references and index.
    ISBN 978-1-4051-3418-7 (alk. paper)
    1. Myocardium–Diseases–Diagnosis.   2. Biochemical markers.   I. Adams, Jesse E.
    II. Apple, Fred S.   III. Jaffe, Allan, M.D.
    [DNLM: 1. Biological Markers–Case Reports.   2. Heart Diseases–diagnosis–Case Reports.
    3. Troponin–diagnostic use–Case Reports.
    WG 141 M345 2007]

    RC385.M9.M364 2007
    616.1'24–dc22

                                                                                    2007000191

A catalogue record for this title is available from the British Library

Commissioning Editor: Steve Korn
Development Editor: Fiona Pattison
Editorial Assistant: Victoria Pitman

Set in 9.5/12pt Palatino by Aptara Inc., New Delhi, India
Printed and bound in Singapore by COS Printers Pte Ltd

For further information on Blackwell Publishing, visit our website:
www.blackwellcardiology.com

The publisher's policy is to use permanent paper from mills that operate a sustainable forestry
policy, and which has been manufactured from pulp processed using acid-free and elementary
chlorine-free practices. Furthermore, the publisher ensures that the text paper and cover board
used have met acceptable environmental accreditation standards.

Contents

Contributors

Jesse E. Adams, MD FACC
University of Louisville
Division of Cardiology
100 Mallard Creek
Louisville, KY 40202
USA

Fred Apple, PhD
Department of Laboratory Medicine and
Pathology
Hennepin County Medical Center and University
of Minnesota School of Medicine
Minneapolis, MN
USA

Luciano Babuin, MD, PhD
Cardiovascular Division and Cardiovascular
Research Institute and Division of Laboratory
Medicine
Mayo Clinic and Medical School
Rochester, Minnesota
USA

Aaron L. Baggish, MD
Massachusetts General Hospital
Harvard Medical School
Boston, MA
USA

Harold E. Bays, MD
L-MARC Research Center
3288 Illinois Avenue
Louisville, Kentucky
USA

William C. Cromwell, MD
Medical Director
Division of Lipoprotein Disorders
Presbyterian Center for Preventive Cardiology
Charlotte
North Carolina, *and;*
Hypertension and Vascular Disease Center
Wake Forest University School of Medicine
Winston-Salem, North Carolina
USA

Christopher deFilippi, MD
Department of Medicine
University of Maryland
Baltimore, Maryland
USA

Evangelos Giannitsis,
Medizinische Universitätsklinik Heidelberg
Department of Cardiology
Im Neuenheimer Feld 410
69120 Heidelberg
Germany

Allan S. Jaffe, MD
Cardiovascular Division and Cardiovascular
Research Institute and Division of Laboratory
Medicine
Mayo Clinic and Medical School
Rochester, Minnesota
USA

James L. Januzzi, MD
Massachusetts General Hospital
Harvard Medical School
Boston, MA
USA

Hugo A. Katus, MD
Medizinische Universitätsklinik Heidelberg
Department of Cardiology
Im Neuenheimer Feld 410
69120 Heidelberg
Germany

Susanne Korff,
Medizinische Universitätsklinik Heidelberg
Department of Cardiology
Im Neuenheimer Feld 410
69120 Heidelberg
Germany

Johannes Mair, MD
Universitaetsklinik fuer Innere Medizin
Klinische Abteilung fuer Kardiologie
Anichstrasse 35
A-6020 Innsbruck
Austria

Alan Maisel, MD
Professor of Medicine
University of California
Director, CCU and Heart Failure Program
San Diego VA Healthcare System
San Diego, CA
USA

Peter A. McCullough, MD, MPH
Department of Medicine
Divisions of Cardiology, Nutrition, and
Preventive Medicine
William Beaumont Hospital
Royal Oak, MI
USA

W. Frank Peacock, MD, FACEP
Vice Chief
Emergency Cardiology Research
Medical Director of Event Medicine
Emergency Department
The Cleveland Clinic
Cleveland, OH
USA

Jose Antonio Perez, MD
Cardiovascular Division and Cardiovascular
Research Institute and Division
of Laboratory Medicine
Mayo Clinic and Medical School
Rochester, Minnesota
USA

Suresh Pothuru, MD
Department of Medicine
University of Maryland
Baltimore, Maryland
USA

Peter P. Toth, MD, PhD
Director of Preventive Cardiology
Sterling Rock Falls Clinic
Sterling
Illinois, *and;*
University of Illinois College of Medicine
Peoria, Illinois
USA

Alan H.B. Wu, PhD
Department of Laboratory Medicine
University of California, San Francisco
Clinical Chemistry Laboratory
San Francisco General Hospital
San Francisco
USA

Preface

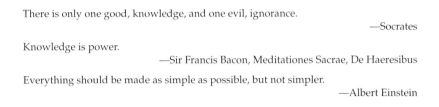

There is only one good, knowledge, and one evil, ignorance.
                                                        —Socrates

Knowledge is power.
            —Sir Francis Bacon, Meditationes Sacrae, De Haeresibus

Everything should be made as simple as possible, but not simpler.
                                                  —Albert Einstein

The application of biomarkers has revolutionized the practice of cardiology, allowing more facile and accurate diagnoses. Increasingly sensitive assays and utilization of markers in combination have furthered the file in the last decade, but with this increased sophistication has also come increased frustration on the part of some clinicians. Some feel that low levels of troponins, for example, that do not appear to correlate with anatomic data obtained during cardiac catheterization, for example, represent "trash" troponin results. This point of view is indicative of the frustrations that many clinicians find in attempting to properly interpret biomarker values. It is necessary to properly understand these assays and how they intercalate with other diagnostic modalities to properly facilitate patient care. Although clinicians would prefer easy answers, the reality is that biomarker values are only as good as those interpreting them in the context of the clinical situation. Elevations can be associated with acute disease or more chronic abnormalities and there are substantial issues with how the markers are measured and differences related to patient presentation and underlying demographics that often can explain elevations or their lack. The idea of not chasing biomarker abnormalities when we know they most often have prognostic implications is unwise. The real question is how to do these evaluations in the best way so we can provide the appropriate care for our patients and not waste our valuable time and resources inappropriately. Thus, perhaps the term "the smart chasing of biomarker abnormalities" might be considered.

In thinking about how we might best help with this, we decided that developing a book of cases that would represent real world patient problems with potential explanations for values of troponins, natriuretic peptides, and other analytes might be a helpful adjunct to clinicians who are often busy and find it difficult to stay up with all the details of the literature. The cases by a highly distinguished group of clinician investigators are presented as an attempt to provide a roadmap with which to consider the various clinical presentations in which BNP and troponin may be useful. Obviously, every nuance cannot be covered. On the other hand, if we can provide guidance and help only a small percentage of clinicians who use the book to learn how best to treat patients, we believe we will have made a contribution.

We would like to know if this approach is useful. Therefore, we would very much appreciate your feedback and cases from those of you who are interested so that when and if we redo this book, it will become even more helpful to those of you who smartly chase these biomarker abnormalities. In the long run, it is our goal to help translate the science of our field into practical patient care.

Jesse Adams, MD, FACC
Fred Apple, PhD
Allan Jaffe, MD, FACC

PART 1

Cardiac troponins

Basics of cardiac troponin: practical aspects of assays, potential analytical confounders, and clinical interpretation

Fred S. Apple

Case 1

Following an episode of shortness of breath and fainting, a 79-year-old woman is driven to the emergency department by her family. She has a history of rheumatoid arthritis and coronary artery disease, with limited physical activity. Her initial electrocardiogram (ECG) showed mild, nonspecific changes, including T waves. To assist in her differential, serial cardiac troponin (cTn) values were obtained. While the clinician did not expect the patient to have a myocardial infarction (MI), her substantial increase in cTnI (based on a first-generation assay that is no longer on the marketplace) was at odds with (a) neither a rising or falling pattern found on subsequent values and (b) normal and unchanging total creatine kinase (CK) and creatine kinase-MB (CK-MB) values. Following clinician contact with the laboratory, reanalysis of the specimens using a second-generation cTnI assay by the same manufacturer and a third-generation cTnT assay demonstrated no detectable cTn, and the laboratory results were corrected in the medical record. Follow-up studies by the laboratory revealed the presence of a heterophile-interfering antibody, which once removed (Scantibody tubes) resulted in normal cTnI values by the original assay.

Time (h)	Total CK	CK-MB	cTnI 1st	cTnI 2nd	cTnT
0	25	1.5	20.8	< 0.025	< 0.01
6	29	1.4	23.0	< 0.25	< 0.01
15	28	1.3	24.8	< 0.025	< 0.01

All units ng/mL.
1st, initial, first-generation assay; 2nd, second-generation assay.

Case 2

The patient presents with a chief complaint of "I have a pain in my chest that hurts very bad." He is a diabetic with a history of atypical chest pain over the past 3 months. He now presents with ischemic symptoms, chest pain, shoulder pain, aching jaw, and nausea. His ECG demonstrates an ST-segment elevation acute MI. His initial cTnT value is increased above the 99th percentile reference cutoff (>0.01 ng/mL) at 0.013 ng/mL and increases to 0.073 ng/mL over the next 4 hours. He is immediately transferred, following medical therapy, to the catherization laboratory, where a stent is successfully placed.

Time (h)	Initial cTnT	Serum cTnT	Plasma cTnT
0, presentation	0.013	0.013	0.010
4	0.073	0.073	0.022
8	0.025	0.133	0.025
12	0.293	0.763	0.293

All units ng/mL.

However, the laboratory findings after the initial rising cTnT over the first two samples (0h and 4h), followed by a subsequent decrease on the 8h sample, were quite perplexing to both the attending cardiologist and the pathologist in the laboratory, since the patient was diagnosed with an acute, evolving ST-segment elevation MI. At 12 hours, the cTnT value again demonstrated an increasing value. An astute laboratory medicine resident reviewing the case recollected a paper that demonstrated the potential of lower cTnT results in heparin-plasma specimens (green top tubes) versus serum (red top tubes). Further investigation did reveal that the 0h and 4h specimens were serum and that the 8h and 12h specimens were heparin plasma, and both plasma samples had analytically false low values. When waste serum specimens, drawn for other chemistries, were located in the laboratory refrigerator for the same 8h and 12h draw times and reanalyzed, both showed substantially higher and rising cTnT concentrations at 0.133 and 0.763 ng/mL as expected. Since July 2006, the cTnT assay by Roche, now a fourth-generation assay, has been reformulated and currently does not show any significant difference between serum and heparin plasma, allowing for a laboratory to use mix and matched specimen types. However, as cTnI assays have also been shown to demonstrate either a constant or random lower heparin-plasma cTnT lower bias, it is recommended to use only one specimen type for an individual patient when ruling in or out an acute MI.

Case 3

A 64-year-old male is found unresponsive at home by his wife while he was sitting and apparently watching a football game on a Sunday afternoon at 2:30 p.m. 911 was called after she was unable to arose him. Emergency medical services arrive within 15 minutes and upon examination his ECG demonstrates an ST-segment depression and T waves. He is transported on 100% oxygen to the hospital, and is now awake but disoriented, but complaining of severe chest pain and left shoulder pain. His ECG remains unchanged and his 0h presenting cTnI concentration performed at the bedside using a point-of-care (POC) assay (15-min turnaround time) is within normal limits: less than the 99th percentile cutoff of 0.04 ng/mL. During the course of the patient's treatment in the emergency department, a second POC cTnI at 3 hours is also normal. However, a call from the central laboratory at this time reports that the initial plasma sample (0h) when reanalyzed per protocol in the central laboratory reflects an increased value of 0.07 ng/mL (central laboratory 99th percentile cutoff 0.025 ng/mL). Based on this discrepant finding, the patient is immediately transferred to a telemetry unit and the diagnosis of a non-ST-segment elevation MI is made. Further investigation of two additional serial cTnI samples shows a rising pattern by both the POC and central laboratory assays, but reveals that the POC assay's poor low-end analytical sensitivity was not able to detect the early increase in cTnI until 8h versus 0h for the second-generation central laboratory cTnI assay. Further it was found that there was a poor correlation between the two different assays. This case demonstrates the importance of understanding the limitations of first-generation versus second-generation assays, irrespective of whether they are POC or central laboratory platforms. The first-generation assays are not as analytically sensitive nor as precise as the newer generation troponin assays. Therefore, different clinical impressions based on the troponin assay used can confuse the clinician caring for a patient. One needs to know the assay and understand that not all assays are created equal.

Time (h)	POC cTnI	Central laboratory cTnI
0, presentation	< 0.04	0.07
3	< 0.04	0.18
8	0.09	0.37
12	0.33	1.05

All units ng/mL.

Discussion of Cases 1, 2, and 3

A European Society of Cardiology/American College of Cardiology (ESC/ACC) consensus conference along with the AHA (American Heart Association)/ACC guidelines for differentiating acute MI and unstable angina codified the role of cTn monitoring by advocating that (a) the diagnosis of MI and (b) establishing a high-risk profile (evidence of myocardial injury) are based on increases of cTnI or cTnT in the appropriate clinical setting [1–3]. These guidelines are also supported by parallel statements by the IFCC Committee on Standardization of Markers of Cardiac Damage (C-SMCD) [4]. The guidelines recognized the reality that neither the clinical presentation nor the ECG had adequate clinical sensitivity and specificity for detecting MI without the use of biomarkers. The guidelines do not suggest that all increases of these biomarkers should elicit a diagnosis of acute MI or high-risk profile—only those associated with the appropriate clinical and ECG findings. When cTn increases not due to acute ischemia, the clinician is obligated to search for another etiology for the elevation (see Chapter 8). Overall, the goal of both laboratorians and clinicians is to establish acceptable, uniform criteria for all cTn assays so that they can be objectively evaluated for their analytical qualities [5] and clinical performance [2, 3].

The first investigators to develop an assay (radioimmunoassay) to measure cTn using polyclonal anti-cTnI antibodies were Cummins *et al.* [6]. While the assay showed approximately 2% cross-reactivity with skeletal TnI, it still had excellent clinical specificity for cardiac muscle injury. However, the assay was never developed for commercial use. The first monoclonal, anti-cTnI antibody-based immunoassay was described by Bodor *et al.* [7]. This assay has <0.1% cross-reactivity with skeletal TnI, but it was not suited for clinical use because of the lengthy assay time. Over the past 15 years, numerous manufacturers have described the development of monoclonal antibody-based diagnostic immunoassays for the measurement of cTnI and cTnT in serum [8, 9]. Assay times range from 5 to 30 minutes. Table 1.1 shows that over a dozen assays have been cleared by the Food and Drug Administration (FDA) for patient testing within the United States on central laboratory and POC-testing platforms.

Table 1.1 FDA-cleared cTn assays.

Assay	LLD	99th	WHO-ROC	10% CV*
Abbott ARCH	0.009	0.012	0.3	0.032
Abbott AxSYM ADV	0.02	0.04	0.4	0.16
Abbott i-STAT[†]	0.02	0.08 (WB)	ND	0.1
Bayer Centaur	0.02	0.1	1.0	0.35
Bayer Ultra	0.006	0.04	0.9	0.03
Beckman Accu	0.01	0.04	0.5	0.06
Biosite Triage[†]	0.05	<0.05	0.4	NA
bioMerieux Vds	0.001	0.01	0.16	0.11
Dade RxL	0.04	0.07	0.6–1.5	0.14
Dade CS[†]	0.03	0.07	0.6–1.5	0.06
DPC Immulite	0.1	0.2	1.0	0.6
MKI Pathfast	0.006	0.01	0.06	0.06
Ortho Vitros ES	0.012	0.032	0.12	0.053
Response[†]	0.03	<0.03 (WB)	ND	0.21
Roche Elecsys	0.01	<0.01	0.03	0.03
Roche Reader[†]	0.05	<0.05 (WB)	0.1	ND
Tosoh AIA	0.06	0.06	0.31–0.64	0.06

LLD, lower limit of detection; 99th, percentile reference limit; ROC, receiver operator characteristic curve optimized cutoff; 10% CV, lowest concentration to provide a total imprecision of 10%.
*Per manufacturer.
[†]POC assay. Adapted from Ref. [8].

In addition to these quantitative assays, several assays have been FDA cleared for the qualitative determination of cTnI and cTnT. Over 50% of the assays are newer second-, third-, or fourth-generation assays that have improved low-end analytical sensitivity, without analytical interferences that have plagued first-generation assays.

Two major hurdles are present that limit the ease for switching from one cTnI assay to another. Assay concentrations fail to agree because (1) there is currently no primary reference cTnI material available for manufacturers to use for standardizing their assays and (2) different epitopes are recognized by the different antibodies used on individual platforms. An effort has been underway for the past 3 years by the AACC Subcommittee on Standardization of Cardiac Troponin I to prepare a primary reference material [10, 11]. In collaboration with the National Institute for Standards and Technology (NIST), a reference material, a cTnT–cTnI–cTnC ternary complex, has been identified (SRM 2921). Working with NIST and the in vitro diagnostic industries, preliminary round-robin studies have demonstrated that while standardization of assays remains elusive, harmonization of cTnI concentrations by different assays has been narrowed from a 20-fold difference to a 2- to 3-fold difference [11].

cTnI is present in the circulation in three forms: (1) free, (2) bound as a two-unit binary complex (cTnI–cTnC), and (3) bound as a three-unit ternary complex (cTnT–cTnI–cTnC). In addition, there are potentially several additional forms that also exist for these three forms, representing N- and C-terminal degradation forms, oxidation and reduction forms, and phosphorylated forms [12]. Therefore, different assays do not produce equivalent concentration results, and comparisons of absolute cTnI and cTnT concentrations in clinical studies cannot and should not be made because not all assays measure the different forms with equal molarity (Case 3). Comparisons between assay systems must view changes as relative to each assay's respective upper reference limit. Users must understand the analytical characteristics of each troponin assay prior to clinical implementation.

There is only one cTnT assay in the marketplace, currently a fourth generation, due to intellectual property rights owned by Roche. Several adaptations of the cTnT immunoassay kit marketed by Roche Diagnostics (Indianapolis, IN) have been described. Two monoclonal anti-cTnT antibodies are used in the second- through fourth-generation assays. Skeletal muscle TnT is no longer a potential interferent, as was found in the first-generation ELISA cTnT assay [13]. In contrast to cTnI, no standardization bias exists for cTnT because the same antibodies (M11, M7) are used in both the central laboratory and POC quantitative and POC qualitative assay systems. The fourth-generation assay is no longer prone to interference due to heparin, as found in green top sample collection tubes, which previously was shown to cause assay-decreased cTnT and assay-dependent cTnI values when compared to serum [14].

Surveys on cTn use have been carried out, but the data in the peer-reviewed literature are minimal. The distribution of cTn assays used as reported over the

Table 1.2 Quality specifications—cTn assays.

A.	Analytical factors
1.	Antibody specificity—recognize epitopes in stable part of molecule and equimolar for all forms
2.	Influence of anticoagulants
3.	Calibrate against natural form of molecule
4.	Define type of material useful for dilutions
5.	Demonstrate recovery and linearity of method
6.	Describe detection limit and imprecision (10% CV)
7.	Address inferents, i.e., rheumatoid factors, heterophile antibodies
B.	Preanalytical factors
1.	Storage time and temperature conditions
2.	Centrifugation effects—gel separators
3.	Serum-plasma–WB correlations

past several years by the College of American Pathologists surveys accounted for approximately 85% of cTnI assays (11 vendors) and 15% cTnT assays (1 vendor). Approximately 10–15% of all users utilize POC-testing assays.

In 2001, the IFCC C-SMCD established recommended quality specifications for cTn assays [5]. The objectives were intended for use by the manufacturers of commercial assays and by clinical laboratories utilizing troponin assays. The overall goal was to attempt to establish uniform criteria in order that all assays could objectively be evaluated for their analytical qualities and clinical performance. Both analytical and preanalytical factors were addressed as shown in Table 1.2. First, an adequate description of the analytical principles, method design, and assay components needs to be made. This includes the following recommendations. Antibody specificity as to what epitope locations are identified needs to be delineated. Epitopes located on the stable part of the cTnI molecule should be a priority. Further, assays need to clarify whether different cTn forms (i.e., binary versus ternary complex) are recognized in an equimolar fashion by the antibodies used in the assay. Specific relative responses need to be described for the following cTnI forms: free cTnI, the cTnI–cTnC binary complex, the cTnT–cTnI–cTnC ternary complex, and oxidized, reduced, and phosphorylated isoforms of the three cTnI forms [15]. Further, the effects of different anticoagulants on binding of cTnI need to be addressed (Case 2) [14]. Second, the source of material used to calibrate cTn assays, specifically for cTnI, should be reported. Currently, a cTnI standardization subcommittee of the AACC is recommending the use of SRD 2921 as a primary reference material that will assist in at least harmonizing cTnI concentrations across different assays, providing traceability [11]. Because antibody differences will always be present in different assays, complete standardization will never be possible for cTnI. For cTnT however, as there is only one assay manufacturer (Roche Diagnostics), standardizing between assay generations has been consistent. Third, assays need to describe minimal detection limits and total imprecision at the 99th percentile reference cutoff, as well as potential interferent, such as rheumatoid factors, heterophile antibodies, human antimouse antibodies (Case 1). Preanalytical factors that should be described include effect of storage time and temperature, effect of glass versus plastic tubes and gel separator tubes, and influence of anticoagulants and whole blood measurements. As more assay systems are devised for POC testing, the same rigors applied to the central laboratory methodologies need to be adhered to by the POC-testing systems.

While clinicians and laboratorians continue to publish guidelines supporting TATs of <60 minutes for cardiac biomarkers, the largest TAT study published to date has demonstrated that TAT expectations are not being met in a large proportion of hospitals. A CAP Q-probe survey study of 7020 cTn and 4368 CK-MB determinations in 159 hospitals demonstrated that the median and 90th percentile TAT for troponin and CK-MB were as follows: 74.5, 129, 82, 131 minutes, respectively [16]. Less than 25% of the hospitals were able to meet the <60-minute TAT, representing the biomarker order-to-report time. Unfortunately, a separate subanalysis of just POC-testing systems was not reported. However, preliminary data have shown that implementation of POC cTn testing can decrease TATs to <30 minutes in cardiology critical care and short-stay units [17]. These data highlight the continued need for laboratory services and health-care providers to work together to develop better processes to meet a <60-minute TAT as requested by physicians.

Defining the 99th percentile of a reference group for cTn assays should be determined in each local laboratory by internal studies using the specific assay used in clinical practice or accept the validation provided in the peer-reviewed literature [18]. Further, acceptable imprecision (coefficient of variation, % CV) of each cTn assay has been defined as ≤10% CV at the 99th percentile reference limit [19]. Unfortunately, the majority of laboratories do not have the resources to perform adequately powered reference-range studies nor the ability to carry out National Committee for Clinical Laboratory Standards (NCCLS) protocols to establish total imprecision criteria for every cTn assay in the marketplace. However, newer generation assays are now starting to meet these imprecision goals. Therefore, clinical laboratories need to rely upon the peer-reviewed published literature to assist in establishing local reference limits. Numerous reference studies have been carried out for specific cTn assays. When reviewing these studies, caution must be taken when comparing the findings reported in the manufacturer's FDA-cleared package inserts, with the findings reported in journals because of differences in total sample size, distributions by gender and ethnicity, age ranges, and the statistic used to calculate the 99th percentile given. To date, very few in vitro diagnostic companies have published their 99th percentile cutoffs in their package inserts. There is no established guideline set by the FDA to mandate a consistent evaluation of the 99th percentile reference limit for cTn. The largest and most diverse reported reference range study to date shows plasma (heparin) 99th percentile reference limits for eight cTn assays (seven cTnI and one cTnT; [18]. These studies were performed in 696 healthy adults (age range 18–84 yr) stratified by gender and ethnicity.

The data, while generally in agreement with information provided by personal communication by the manufacturer, demonstrate several issues. First, two cTnI assays show a 1.2- to 2.5-fold higher 99th percentile for males versus females. Second, two cTnI assays demonstrated a 1.1- to 2.8-fold higher 99th percentile for African Americans versus Caucasians. Third, there was a 13-fold difference between the lowest versus the highest measured cTnI 99th percentile limit. The lack of cTn assay standardization (there is no primary reference material available) and the differences in antibody epitope recognition between assays (different assays use different antibodies) give rise to substantially discrepant concentrations. What is generally recognized, though, as long as one understands the characteristics of an individual assay and does not attempt to compare absolute concentrations between different assays, clinical interpretation should be acceptable for all assays.

Operationalizing the 2000 ESC/ACC redefinition of MI consensus document, which is predicated on cTn monitoring, has already substantially impacted the rate of defining MI in day-to-day clinical practice, in the emergency department, in epidemiology, in clinical trials, in society, and in public policy [3]. To quote Harvey D. White, DSc (cardiologist from New Zealand), "Things ain't what they used to be" [20]. Characteristics used to define a disease in one county may be interpreted differently by clinicians in another nation, thus possibly rendering comparison of cardiac disease between countries difficult but not impossible. In this light, a statement cosponsored by the AHA, the World Heart Federation Councils on Epidemiology and Prevention, the Center for Disease Control and Prevention, and the National Heart, Lung, and Blood Institute recently published a case definition for acute coronary heart disease (CHD) in epidemiology and clinical research studies [3]. This statement was based on a systematic review of evolving diagnostic strategies, with the goal of developing standards for population studies of CHD. The definition of CHD cases was deemed dependent on symptoms, signs, ECG, and/or autopsy findings and biomarkers. Cardiac biomarkers, measures of myocardial necrosis, were prioritized for use as follows: cTn > CK-MB mass > CK-MB activity > CK. An adequate set of biomarkers was determined to be at least two measurements of the same biomarker at least 6 hours apart (similar to the preestablished ESC/ACC consensus [2]). A diagnostic biomarker was, at least, one positive biomarker in an adequate set showing a rising or falling pattern in the setting of clinical ischemia and the absence of noncardiac causes of biomarker elevation. An equivocal biomarker was when only one available measurement was positive, but not in the clinical setting of ischemia or in the presence of nonischemia causes. A positive biomarker was defined as exceeding the 99th percentile or the lowest concentration at which a 10% CV can be demonstrated.

For clinical trials, to avoid the confusion of multiple centers using multiple assays, several approaches are recommended for utilizing cTn testing [8, 21]. First, analyze all samples from trial centers in a core, central laboratory with a precise, well-defined assay. Second, provide all trial centers with the same well-defined assays. Third, uniformly define each center's assays by using the 10% CV concentration (assay dependent), thus not relying on local laboratory criteria and troponin cutoffs. Fourth, use a multiple (two- to threefold) of the 10% CV cutoff value. Fifth, if trials decide to use cutoff values defined in earlier studies, the degree of variability should be reported. However, since these earlier recommendations, the Global Task Force for defining MI has superseded the 10% CV value, and now, along with laboratory and emergency medicine organizations, 100% endorse the use of the 99th percentile reference cutoff. The revision from the 10% CV to the 99th percentile cutoff was supported by two studies that showed that imprecision at the 99th percentile did not significantly impact the diagnostic use or risk stratification assessment of patients presenting with clinical symptoms suggestive of acute coronary syndrome (ACS) [22, 23].

The advances in diagnostic technology in the development of improved low-end analytical detection of cTn have begun to impact the prevalence of acute MI detection. Accumulating data suggest that the more sensitive cTn tests result in greater rates of MI diagnosis and greater rates of cTn positivity compared to other markers [3, 24]. Milder and smaller degrees of myocardial injury will be detected. Clinical cases that were earlier classified as unstable angina will be given a diagnosis of MI (due to an increased cTn), and now procedure-related troponin increases, i.e., following angioplasty, will be labeled as an MI. The importance of small troponin increases even within the 99th percentile reference range has been confirmed by their association with a poor prognosis [24, 25]. Based on several studies that compared CK-MB and cTn assays in ACS patients, a substantial increase in rate of MIs ranging from 12 to 127% was detected [3]. In one of the studies by Lin *et al.*, a subset (5%) of cTnI-negative, but CK-MB-positive patients revealed the potentially underlying false-positive MI rate when using CK-MB as a standard for MI detection [24]. This was likely due to release of CK-MB from skeletal muscle in the absence of myocardial injury. Further, a subset (12%) of cTnI-positive, CK-MB-negative patients demonstrated a subset of patients diagnosed as having had an MI that would not have been detected without cTn monitoring. These data support the implementation of cTn in place of, not in combination with, CK-MB.

Thus, the quality of cTn assays is improving with release of second-, third-, and fourth-generation immunoassays. Manufacturers are working more closely with clinical and laboratory investigators to appropriately validate the analytical qualities of new assays. Implementation of these new assays into clinical trials will be crucial for establishing an appropriate evidence-based literature. As cTn assay implementation grows and lower analytical cutoffs are implemented for detection of myocardial injury, diagnosis of MI, and risk stratification, patient care and management will be impacted across society.

Several factors have been identified for being responsible for both analytical false-positive cTn findings without the presence of myocardial injury [26] and false-negative findings when myocardial injury was present [27]. Common causes of false-positive cTn findings have been due to heterophile antibodies, such as rheumatoid factors, human antianimal antibodies, fibrin clots, microparticles in specimens, and analyzer malfunctions. Heterophile antibodies, for example, are antibodies produced against poorly defined antigens with weak affinities. Patients with autoimmune disease often have rheumatoid factors. Immunoglobulins reacting with other immunoglobulins induce nonspecific cross-reactivity in some troponin assays. Human antimouse antibodies develop as a result of treatments with mouse (animal) immunoglobulins and are antibodies with strong affinities. These present a problem when immunoglobulins from the same species (mouse anti-cTn antibodies) are used in the test (cTn) assay. In both cases, their presence can be demonstrated following absorption with immunoglobulin additives tested following processing with either scantibody tubes or the Immunomedics product. While the majority of cTn assays incorporate sufficient amounts of animal immunoglobulins in their reagents and are able to eliminate these potential interferences, several first-generation assays have remained prone to falsely increased results because of these factors (Case 1). Typically, when an assay shows this type of interference, increased cTn concentrations do not demonstrate typical serial rising or falling patterns as expected in MI, but remain consistently increased over time. Typically, when an interferent is suspected, reanalyzing a "false-positive" specimen utilizing an alternative cTnI or cTnT assay will likely correct the inaccuracy.

One case report documented a false-negative immunoassay results for cTnI, probably resulting from the interference of circulating IgG-class autoantibodies with high affinity for cTnI in a 69-year-old man with an MI [27]. More recently, preliminary findings of "some yet unidentified, variable component, present in blood of healthy volunteers and ACS patients," that interferes with commercial assays of cTnI causing decreased concentrations in ACS particles have been reported [28]. Supplementation of N- and C-terminal affinity antibodies appeared to resolve the interference. Further studies are underway to clarify the mechanism of this interaction.

References

1 Braunwald E, Antman EM, Beasley JW et al. ACC/AHA guideline update for the management of patients with unstable angina and non-ST-segment elevation myocardial infarction—2002: summary article. A report of the American College of Cardiology/American Heart Association Task Force on Practice Guidelines (Committee on the Management of Patients With Unstable Angina). *Circulation* 2002;**106**:1893–2000.
2 Alpert JS, Thygesen K, Antman E et al. Myocardial infarction redefined—a consensus document of the Joint European Society of Cardiology/American College of Cardiology Committee for the redefinition of myocardial infarction. *J Am Coll Cardiol* 2000;**36**:959-969.
3 Luepker RV, Apple FS, Christenson RH et al. Case definitions for acute coronary heart disease in epidemiology and clinical research studies. *Circulation* 2003;**108**:2543–2549.
4 Panteghini M, Apple FS, Christenson RH, Dati F, Mair J, Wu AH. Proposals from IFCC committee on standardization of markers of cardiac damage (C-SMCD): recommendations on use of biochemical markers of damage in acute coronary syndrome. *Scand J Clin Lab Invest* 1999;**59**(suppl 230):103–112.

5 Panteghini M, Gerhardt W, Apple FS *et al.* Quality specifications for cardiac troponin assays. *Clin Chem Lab Med* 2001;**39**:174–178.

6 Cummins B, Auckland ML, Cummins P. Cardiac specific troponin-I radioimmunoassay in the diagnosis of acute myocardial infarction. *Am Heart J* 1987;**113**:1333–1344.

7 Bodor GS, Porter S, Landt Y *et al.* Development of monoclonal antibodies for an assay of cardiac troponin-I and preliminary results in suspected cases of myocardial infarction. *Clin Chem* 1992;**38**:2203–2214.

8 Apple FS, Wu AHB, Jaffe AS. European Society of Cardiology and American College of Cardiology guidelines for redefinition of myocardial infarction: how to use existing assays clinically and for clinical trials. *Am Heart J* 2002;**144**:981–986.

9 Collinson PO, Boa FG, Gaze DC. Measurement of cardiac troponins. *Ann Clin Biochem* 2001;**38**:423–449.

10 Christenson RH, Duh SH, Apple FS *et al.* Standardization of cardiac troponin I assays: round robin performance of ten candidate reference materials. *Clin Chem* 2001;**47**:431–437.

11 Christenson RH, Duh SH, Apple FS *et al.*, for the American Association for Clinical Chemistry Cardiac Troponin I Standardization Committee. Toward standardization of cardiac troponin I measurements. Part II: Assessing commutability of candidate reference materials and harmonization of cardiac troponin I assays. *Clin Chem* 2006;**52**:1685–1692.

12 Katrukha AG, Bereznikova AV, Esakova TV *et al.* Troponin I is released in bloodstream of patients with acute myocardial infarction not in free form but as complex. *Clin Chem* 1997;**43**:1379–1385.

13 Apple FS, Ricchiuti V, Voss EM, Ney A, Odland M, Anderson PAW. Expression of cardiac troponin T isoforms expressed in renal diseased skeletal muscle will not cause false positive results by the second generation cardiac troponin T assay by Boehringer Mannheim. *Clin Chem* 1998;**44**:1919–1924.

14 Gerhardt W, Nordin G, Herbert AK *et al.* Troponin T and I assays show decreased concentrations in heparin plasma compared to serum: lower recoveries in early than in late phases of myocardial injury. *Clin Chem* 2000;**46**:817–821.

15 Katrukha AG, Bereznikova AV, Esakova TV *et al.* Troponin I is released in bloodstream of patients with acute myocardial infarction not in free form but as complex. *Clin Chem* 1997;**43**:1379–1385.

16 Novis DA, Jones BA, Dale JC *et al.* Biochemical markers of myocardial injury test turnaround time: a College of American Pathologists Q-probe Study. *Arch Pathol Lab Med* 2004;**128**:158–164.

17 Apple FS, Chung AY, Kogut ME, Bubany S, Murakami MM. Decreased patient charges following implementation of point-of-care cardiac troponin monitoring in acute coronary syndrome patients in a community hospital cardiology unity. *Clin Chim Acta* 2006;**370**:191–195.

18 Apple FS, Quist HE, Doyle PJ *et al.* Plasma 99th percentile reference limits for cardiac troponin and creatine kinase MB mass for use with European Society of Cardiology/American College of Cardiology consensus recommendations. *Clin Chem* 2003;**49**: 1331–1336.

19 Panteghini M, Pagani F, Yeo KT *et al.* Evaluation of the imprecision at low range concentrations of the assays for cardiac troponin determination. *Clin Chem* 2004;**50**:327–332.

20 White HD. Things ain't what they used to be: impact of a new definition for myocardial infarction. *Am Heart J* 2002;**144**:933–937.

21 Newby LK, Alpert JS, Ohman EM *et al.* Changing the diagnosis of acute myocardial infarction: implications for practice and clinical investigations. *Am Heart J* 2002;**144**:957–980.

22 Apple FS, Parvin CA, Buechler KF, Christenson RH, Wu AHB, Jaffe AS. Validation of the 99th percentile cutoff independent of assay imprecision (% CV) for cardiac troponin monitoring for ruling out myocardial infarction. *Clin Chem* 2005;**51**:2198–2200.

23 Kupchak P, Wu AHB, Ghani F, Newby LK, Ohman EM, Christenson RH. Influence of imprecision on ROC curve analysis for cardiac markers. *Clin Chem* 2006;**52**:752–753.

24 Lin JC, Apple FS, Murakami MM *et al.* Rates of positive cardiac troponin I and creatine kinase MB among patients hospitalized for suspected acute coronary syndromes. *Clin Chem* 2004;**50**:333–338.

25 James S, Flodin M, Johnston N, Lindahl B, Venge P. The antibody configurations of cardiac troponin I assays may determine their clinical performance. *Clin Chem* 2006;**52**:832–837.

26 Fitzmaurice T, Brown C, Rifai N, Wu A, Yeo K. False increase of cardiac troponin I with heterophilic antibodies. *Clin Chem* 1998;**44**:2212–2214.

27 Bohner J, von Pape KW, Hannes W, Stegmann T. False negative immunoassay results for cardiac troponin I probably due to circulating troponin I autoantibodies. *Clin Chem* 1996;**42**:2046.

28 Eriksson S, Junikka M, Laitinen P *et al.* Negative interference in cardiac troponin I immunoassays from a frequently occurring serum and plasma component. *Clin Chem* 2003;**49**:1095–1104.

CHAPTER 2

Diagnostic use of cardiac troponins in ST-segment elevation myocardial infarction

Susanne Korff, Hugo Katus, Evangelos Giannitsis

Introduction

In patients with acute ST-segment elevation myocardial infarction (STEMI), the diagnosis and immediate initiation of reperfusion therapy is based on standard 12-lead electrocardiogram (ECG). Because cardiac markers appear in blood after a substantial time after onset of symptoms, cardiac markers are neither helpful for early diagnosis nor should results be awaited to initiate reperfusion treatment in patients with STEMI.

Nevertheless, the appearance of cardio-specific troponins in blood indicates myocardial necrosis and thus allows retrospective confirmation of acute myocardial infarction (MI), particularly when the ECG is poorly interpretable or confounded by preexisting ST-segment elevation because of ventricular aneurysm or by Q waves, pacemaker rhythm, or preexisting or newly developed bundle branch blocks (BBB). Other important reasons to determine cardiac troponins (cTn) in the setting of STEMI include monitoring the efficacy of reperfusion, assessment of short- and long-term risk, and estimation of infarct size. When and how often cTn should be measured in clinical practice in the setting of STEMI will be illustrated in a representative clinical case.

Representative clinical case

History

On October 15, 2005, at 2:00 a.m., a 61-year-old man was admitted to our emergency ward. He reported severe left thoracic chest pain at rest with radiation to the neck and left arm that began the day before at 10:30 p.m., i.e., 3 1/2 hours before admission and lasted for 2 hours. In the past weeks he experienced similar episodes of milder intensity during exertion. There were no concomitant vegetative symptoms or dyspnea. He had never suffered from palpitations, dizziness, or syncope. Cardiovascular risk factors were arterial hypertension, hypercholesterinemia, and insulin-dependent diabetes mellitus since 1984. The patient had quit smoking 2 years ago (20 packyears). Medications on admission were nifedipine 20-mg tablet and simvastatin 20-mg tablet once daily and metformin 850-mg tablet twice daily.

Electrocardiogram
Figure 2.1 depicts the ECG of the patient. The precordial leads showed monophasic ST-segment elevations in V1–V3. Besides, there were ST-segment elevations up to 0.1 mV in lead aVL. These ST-segment elevations were superimposed on an RBBB. In addition, there were ST-segment depressions in leads II, III, and avF and in the precordial leads V5 and V6. Besides, there was a first-degree atrioventricular block.

Cardiopulmonary examination
There were no findings of congestive heart failure, no third or fourth heart sound, no cardiac murmurs, and pulse rate 80 bpm—normal pulmonary findings.

Laboratory findings
Laboratory parameters on admission are shown below:

Sodium	139 (135–145 mmol/L)
Potassium	5.65 (3.5–4.8 mmol/L)
Creatinine	0.99 (<1.3 mg/dL)
Urea	85 (<45 mg/dL)
Creatine kinase	375 (<174 U/L)
cTnT	0.26 (<0.03 µg/L)
C-reactive protein	3.0 (<5 mg/L)
WBC	18.52 (4.0–10.0 cells/nL)
Hemoglobin	14.1 (13–17 g/dL)
Platelets	303 (150–440 cells/nL)

Medical treatment
Immediately after diagnosis of STEMI, the patient received 600 mg clopidogrel and 500 mg aspirin orally as well as 5000 units unfractionated heparin intravenously. In addition, the glycoprotein (GP) IIb/IIIa inhibitor tirofiban was administered in the emergency room before coronary angiography. After percutaneous coronary intervention (PCI), tirofiban was continued for 48 hours.

Coronary angiography
Coronary angiography was performed immediately, revealing a severe coronary three-vessel disease with a total occlusion of the proximal left anterior descending artery (LAD). The LAD could be successfully recanalized. On left ventricular angiography the left ventricular function was severely impaired. PCI resulted in an incomplete reperfusion of the infarct-related artery (thrombolysis in myocardial infarction (TIMI) flow grade 2). Figure 2.2 shows the occluded LAD before (a) and after (b) revascularization.

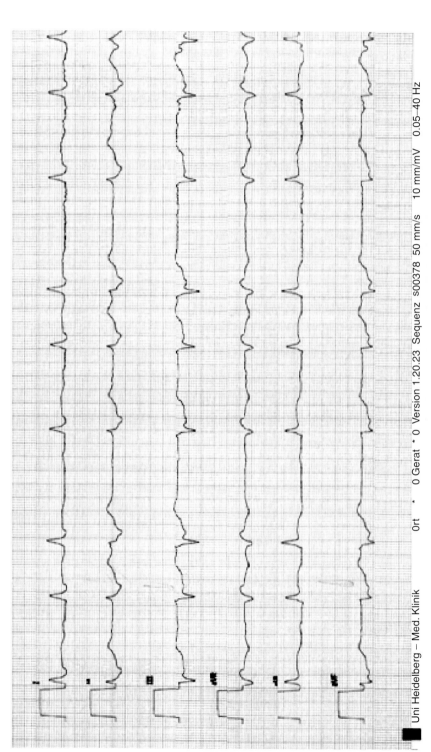

Figure 2.1 Admission ECG.

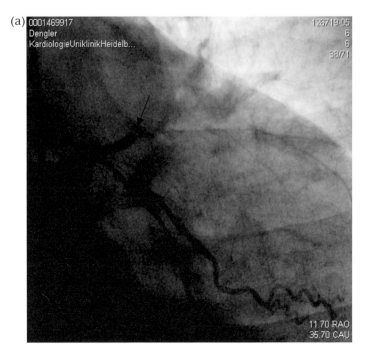

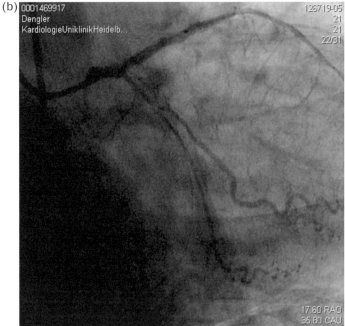

Figure 2.2 Coronary angiogram. (a) The left coronary system before PCI with the total occlusion of the proximal LAD (arrow). (b) Following balloon dilatation and placement of two stents blood flow in the LAD could be successfully restored.

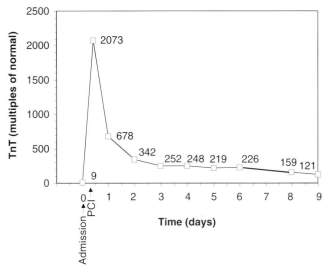

Figure 2.3 Time course of cTnT. There is a steep increase in cTnT following reopening of the infarct-related coronary artery, which represents the washout of cTnT from necrotic myocytes. The peak cTnT is of short duration, which reflects successful revascularization. In patients with no revascularization, there is no peak.

Inhospital course

During coronary angiography, the patient developed cardiogenic shock. After implantation of an intraaortal balloon pump he was monitored and had an uneventful stay on our intensive care unit. Troponin T values were determined immediately after PCI and every day until discharge. Figure 2.3 shows the kinetic of cTnT in our patient. On admission, cTnT level was 0.26 μg/L, which was nine times above the reference limit. Following coronary angiography, cTnT levels increased to 2073 times upper limit of normal and then declined rapidly. This release kinetic is typical for an early successful reperfusion of an occluded coronary artery. On Day 4, a gadolinium-enhanced magnetic resonance imaging (MRI) was done in order to assess left ventricular function and to estimate the infarct size. The infarct size was measured by addition of the volumes of late enhancement in contiguous short-axis slices of known thickness. Absolute infarct mass and relative infarct size was calculated. Figure 2.4 shows the cardiac MRI of this patient on Day 4 after the index event. The infarcted area was quantified to more than 140 g (Fig. 2.5).

Follow-up

The patient was discharged from our hospital after 10 days on October 25. On follow-up, he reported limited physical exercise capacity and shortness of breath at exercise classified as functional NYHA (New York Heart Association) class III. There was no evidence for recurrent myocardial ischemia or clinical restenosis. Transthoracic two-dimensional echocardiography demonstrated an

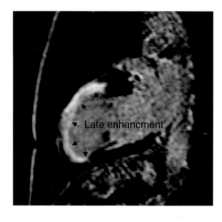

Figure 2.4 Cardiac MRI. Sagittal two-chamber view of the heart. The arrows indicate the extent of the necrotic myocardium of the left ventricle, which enhances gadolinium-DTPA contrast medium. The whole anterior wall of the left ventricle and parts of the inferior wall are infarcted. Healthy myocardium remains black.

ejection fraction of only 20%. Hence, he received a dual-chamber implantable cardioverter defibrillator for primary prophylaxis of sudden death according to the MADIT-II-trial criteria.

Discussion of case

Troponin and diagnostic confirmation of STEMI in patients with equivocal or confounding ECG

In 2000, a joint committee of the European Society of Cardiology and the American College of Cardiology (ESC/ACC) had recommended the use of troponins as the preferred cardiac marker and stated that an elevation of cardio-specific troponins above the 99th percentile of a healthy reference population in the

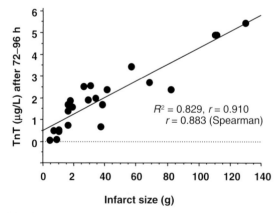

$R^2 = 0.829$, $r = 0.910$
$r = 0.883$ (Spearman)

Infarct size (g)

Figure 2.5 Correlation between cTnT after 72–96 hours and infarct size in grams determined by MRI in patients with STEMI. There is a significant correlation between infarct size and cTnT 72–96 hours after MI. In our patient cTnT after 72–96 hours was around 7 μg/L, which represents above 140-g infarct size.

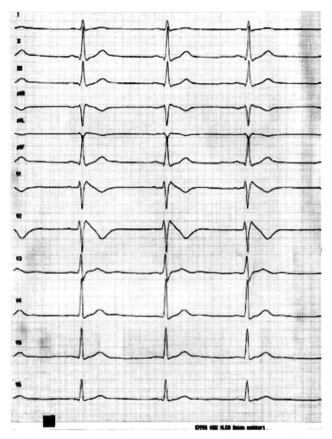

Figure 2.6 ECG of a patient with type 2 Brugada syndrome with the characteristic saddleback configuration, i.e., the high ST-segment elevation followed by a gradually descending ST segment and a positive or biphasic T wave. This pattern in Brugada syndrome is similar to the ECG pattern in our patient with RBBB and STEMI.

clinical setting of myocardial ischemia classifies for acute MI [1]. This decision was made because cTn are strictly intracellular and cardio-specific proteins, and consequently, their elevation in blood is the most convincing indicator of irreversible cardiomyocyte injury. Since not all patients with acute MI develop typical ST-segment elevations on the ECG, the new definition of MI distinguishes ST-segment elevation myocardial infarction (STEMI) and non-ST-segment elevation myocardial infarction (NSTEMI).

The allocation of a patient with clinical suspicion of MI to one of these diagnostic groups is of major importance for the therapeutic strategy.

In patients admitted with chest pain but without ST-segment elevation, the diagnosis of acute MI is made by an elevation of cTn. Hence, the diagnosis of NSTEMI relies on an elevated cTn level. It is known that in patients with NSTEMI, admission troponin levels are useful for risk stratification and allow identification of patients requiring administration of GP IIb/IIIa inhibitors and early invasive strategy [2].

In contrast, in patients with chest pain, typical ST-segment elevation in the ECG is highly specific for acute MI and cTn are neither required for the diagnosis of STEMI nor for the initiation of early therapy. The value of cTn in the setting of STEMI relies on the retrospective confirmation of the diagnosis and on risk prediction.

However, in a subset of patients, the interpretation of ECG may be difficult or even not possible despite retrospective confirmation of large acute MI. In the setting of a strictly posterior STEMI for example, ST-segment elevations are absent on standard 12-lead ECG but may be found on extended chest leads V7–V9. Frequently anterior ST-segment depressions are misinterpreted as reversible myocardial ischemia, and consequently, the diagnosis of a strict posterior acute MI due to an occluded left circumflex artery is missed or is made too late.

In other cases, the electrocardiographic diagnosis of STEMI is masked by preexistent or newly developed ECG changes like BBB or pacemaker rhythms. In the above-mentioned settings, the determination of cTn helps to diagnose or to exclude an acute MI.

The prevalence of BBB on arrival in patients with acute MI varies between 1.6 and 10.9% without marked difference between RBBB and LBBB [3, 4]. Although an RBBB does mask neither the repolarization phase nor the preexisting Q wave, minor ST-segment elevations in the anterior leads (i.e., V1–V4) can be missed due to pseudonormalization of the negative T waves. Wong *et al.* reported from data of the HERO-2 trial that the presence of an RBBB in the setting of an anterior STEMI is associated with a higher risk of death after 30 days (33% versus 12%) [5]. Our patient had a complete RBBB in the ECG on admission, which can mask the ECG diagnosis of anterior STEMI. In our patient, cTnT level on admission was 0.26 µg/L, which is well above the reference limit and thereby confirmed the diagnosis of acute MI.

Rarely, patients may falsely be labeled as having STEMI due to ST-segment elevations and may be exposed to the risk of thrombolytic therapy or coronary angiography without need. These pseudoinfarct patterns encompass the so-called *early repolarization pattern*. The early repolarization pattern is characterized by ST-segment elevations up to 0.5 mV in the midprecordial leads and is more common at slow than at rapid heart rates and more frequent in men than in women [6]. Another rare confounder showing ST-segment elevations in the right precordial leads is the *Brugada* syndrome (Fig. 2.6).

Troponin T or I and success of reperfusion therapy in STEMI

Primary goal in patients with STEMI is the early and complete restoration of the epicardial blood flow. But normal epicardial blood flow (TIMI flow grade 3) does not automatically mean normal tissue reperfusion since microvascular obstruction may persist [7]. Risk factors for microvascular obstruction include diabetes, advanced age, late reperfusion therapy, and male gender. An elevation of cTnT on admission may be associated with abnormal tissue perfusion due to microvascular obstruction [8] and helps to identify patients who may benefit from an adjunctive peri-interventional administration of GP IIb/IIIa inhibitors [9].

Troponin T and guidance of adjunctive medical therapy in STEMI

Adjunctive therapy with GP IIb/IIIa inhibitors in patients with STEMI and elevated cTnT on admission has been demonstrated to improve epicardial and myocardial perfusion as well as left ventricular function. However, no randomized study has ever demonstrated a significant reduction of short- or long-term mortality [9, 10]. Recently, an observational study gave first preliminary evidence that patients with a cTnT level being already elevated on admission showed less rapid cardiac marker washout 60 minutes after recanalization [9]. Administration of the GP IIb/IIIa inhibitor abciximab was found to accelerate marker washout in patients with positive admission cTnT levels suggesting improved tissue level reperfusion [9]. Forthcoming trials are needed to confirm whether patients with elevated cTn on admission will benefit from GP IIb/IIIa inhibitors.

Troponin T or I on admission and prognosis in STEMI

Besides the retrospective confirmation of acute MI in patients with STEMI, elevated cTn levels on admission imply an increased inhospital and long-term mortality [11, 12]. Patients with elevated troponin levels on admission more often develop congestive heart failure (23% versus 9%) or shock (30% versus 9%) during hospitalization [12]. Patients with elevated admission troponin values in conjunction with incomplete ST-segment resolution 60 minutes after fibrinolytic reperfusion therapy have a sixfold higher 1-year mortality compared to patients without cTnT elevation and with complete ST-segment resolution (18.2% versus 2.8%) [13]. Also when these patients are treated with primary PCI, elevated admission troponin levels predict a three to four times higher short- and long-term mortality [12, 14]. In these patients, primary PCI and thrombolytic therapy were shown to be less successful with respect to rates of complete reperfusion and sustained patency of the coronary vessel (TIMI flow grade 3), which is regarded as one of the possible reasons for the prognostic hazard of admission troponin. It has been speculated that more fibrin-resistant thrombi and microvascular no-reflow may play an important role [7, 15]. Possible reasons for the microvascular dysfunction include occlusion of capillaries at the center of the infracted zone either due to (1) preexisting microembolization of fragmented thrombus from unstable plaques [14, 16], (2) aggregation of blood cells, or (3) endothelial cell swelling as a consequence of ischemic edema [17].

Troponin T and infarct size in STEMI

Due to the short half-life of troponin T in blood of only about 90 minutes [18], the troponin T blood levels on Day 3 or 4 reflect degradation of the contractile machinery, which is a hallmark of irreversible cell injury. Thus, a troponin T elevation on Day 3 or 4 after symptom onset may be taken as definite proof of irreversible myocardial injury. Animal studies tried to establish a significant correlation between cTnT and infarct size. In an experimental study on 16 beagle dogs, in whom the LAD was ligated, the pathoanatomically measured infarct size correlated significantly with a single troponin measurement after 96 hours ($p = 0.0010$) [19]. In a similar study on 38 wild-type mice, the authors found a significant correlation between cTnT blood levels 24 hours after LAD ligation and the histological infarct size [20]. To show perfusion defect size in patients 72 hours after MI, Panteghini et al. [21] used single-photon emission computed tomography (SPECT) and found a significant correlation between cTnT at 72 hours and both the peak creatine kinase-MB (CK-MB) concentrations ($r = 0.76$; $p < 0.001$) and the perfusion defect size ($r = 0.62$; $p < 0.001$) [21]. For this time point, Licka et al. also found a significant correlation with scintigraphic infarct size [22]. We recently conducted a study on 44 patients with STEMI. Measurement of cTnT and infarct size using MRI was performed 72–96 hours after the index event. We found a highly significant correlation between cTnT and infarct size ($r_{Spearman} = 0.883$; $p < 0.0001$) (Fig. 2.3).

How many troponin measurements do we need in patients with STEMI?

While sampling protocols are straightforward in acute coronary syndrome without ST-segment elevations, no approved protocols are available in STEMI. Although not necessary for initiation of reperfusion therapy, a measurement of cTn on admission appears useful for short- and long-term risk stratification.

For retrospective confirmation of an acute STEMI, additional measurements are necessary in order to demonstrate a cTn concentration above the acute MI decision limit showing a typical rise and fall.

The cTn values at 12–24 hours reflect best washout of the cytosolic cTn pool, which is an indicator of success of reperfusion.

For estimation of infarct size, robust data are available for cTnT. For cTnT, measurement 72–96 hours after the onset of symptoms allows reliable estimation of infarct size. Recently published data from our group show that there is an excellent correlation ($r = 0.883$; $p < 0.0001$) between cTnT on Day 4 after the onset of symptoms and infarct size as assessed with contrast-enhanced MRI [23].

In patients with recurrent chest pain, additional cTn measurements may be required for identification of reinfarction [24].

In brief, we recommend at least three measurements of troponins in patients with STEMI. The first time point of measurement, also not necessarily needed to guide therapy, is on admission. Elevated admission troponins are useful for retrospective confirmation of MI especially in equivocal cases (e.g., atypical chest pain, uninterpretable ECG) and for estimation of prognosis including inhospital and long-term mortality. In addition, troponin elevations on admission are negatively correlated with reperfusion success, i.e., the TIMI flow following coronary intervention.

Only in patients with onset of symptoms 4–6 hours before admission and in whom admission troponin is still negative, another blood sample should be obtained 6–9 hours later.

In patients receiving thrombolytic therapy an additional troponin measurement 60–90 minutes after start of treatment may complement other noninvasive tools for noninvasive estimation of reperfusion success.

Finally, the last measurement between 72 and 96 hours after the index event allows estimation of infarct size.

References

1 Alpert JS, Thygesen K, Antman E, Bassand JP. Myocardial infarction redefined—a consensus document of the Joint European Society of Cardiology/American College of Cardiology Committee for the redefinition of myocardial infarction. *J Am Coll Cardiol* 2000;**36**: 959–969.
2 Sabatine MS, Morrow DA, Giugliano RP *et al.* Implications of upstream glycoprotein IIb/IIIa inhibition and coronary artery stenting in the invasive management of unstable angina/non-ST-elevation myocardial infarction: a comparison of the Thrombolysis In Myocardial Infarction (TIMI) IIIB trial and the Treat angina with Aggrastat and determine Cost of Therapy with Invasive or Conservative Strategy (TACTICS)-TIMI 18 trial. *Circulation* 2004;**109**:874–880.
3 Go AS, Barron HV, Rundle AC, Ornato JP, Avins AL, for the National Registry of Myocardial Infarction 2 Investigators. Bundle-branch block and in-hospital mortality in acute myocardial infarction. *Ann Intern Med* 1998;**129**:690–697.
4 Sgarbossa EB, Pinski SL, Gates KB, Wagner GS, for the Global Utilization of Streptokinase and t-PA for Occluded Coronary Arteries (GUSTO-I) Investigators. Predictors of in-hospital bundle branch block reversion after presenting with acute myocardial infarction and bundle branch block. *Am J Cardiol* 1998;**82**:373–374.
5 Wong CK, Stewart RA, Gao W, French JK, Raffel C, White HD. Prognostic differences between different types of bundle branch block during the early phase of acute myocardial infarction: insights from the Hirulog and Early Reperfusion or Occlusion (HERO)-2 trial. *Eur Heart J* 2006;**27**:21–28.
6 Mehta M, Jain AC, Mehta A. Early repolarization. *Clin Cardiol* 1999;**22**:59–65.
7 Ito H, Tomooka T, Sakai N *et al.* Lack of myocardial perfusion immediately after successful thrombolysis: a predictor of poor recovery of left ventricular function in anterior myocardial infarction. *Circulation* 1992;**85**:1699–1705.
8 Wong GC, Morrow DA, Murphy S *et al.* Elevations in troponin T and I are associated with abnormal tissue level perfusion: a Treat Angina with Aggrastat and Determine Cost of Therapy with an Invasive or Conservative Strategy-Thrombolysis in Myocardial Infarction (TACTICS-TIMI) 18 substudy. *Circulation* 2002;**106**:202–207.
9 Lehrke S, Giannitsis E, Katus HA. Admission troponin T, advanced age and male gender identify patients with improved myocardial tissue perfusion after abciximab administration for ST-segment elevation myocardial infarction. *Thromb Haemost* 2004;**92**:1214–1220.

10 Steen H, Lehrke S, Wiegand UK *et al.* Very early cardiac magnetic resonance imaging for quantification of myocardial tissue perfusion in patients receiving tirofiban before percutaneous coronary intervention for ST-elevation myocardial infarction. *Am Heart J* 2005;149:564.

11 Stubbs P, Collinson P, Moseley D, Greenwood T, Noble M. Prognostic significance of admission troponin T concentrations in patients with myocardial infarction. *Circulation* 1996;94:1291–1297.

12 Matetzky S, Sharir T, Domingo M *et al.* Elevated troponin I level on admission is associated with adverse outcome of primary angioplasty in acute myocardial infarction. *Circulation* 2000;102:1611–1616.

13 Bjorklund E, Lindahl B, Johanson P *et al.* Admission troponin T and measurement of ST-segment resolution at 60 min improve early risk stratification in ST-elevation myocardial infarction. *Eur Heart J* 2004;25:113–120.

14 Kim RJ, Chen EL, Lima JA, Judd RM. Myocardial Gd-DTPA kinetics determine MRI contrast enhancement and reflect the extent and severity of myocardial injury after acute reperfused infarction. *Circulation* 1996;94:3318–3326.

15 Giannitsis E, Muller-Bardorff M, Lehrke S *et al.* Admission troponin T level predicts clinical outcomes, TIMI flow, and myocardial tissue perfusion after primary percutaneous intervention for acute ST-segment elevation myocardial infarction. *Circulation* 2001;104:630–635.

16 Falk E. Unstable angina with fatal outcome: dynamic coronary thrombosis leading to infarction and/or sudden death. Autopsy evidence of recurrent mural thrombosis with peripheral embolization culminating in total vascular occlusion. *Circulation* 1985;71:699–708.

17 Lehrke S, Giannitsis E, Steen H, Katus HA. Cardiac troponin T in ST-segment elevation acute myocardial infarction revisited. *Cardiovasc Toxicol* 2001;1:99–104.

18 Katus HA, Remppis A, Looser S, Hallermeier K, Scheffold T, Kubler W. Enzyme linked immunoassay of cardiac troponin T for the detection of acute myocardial infarction in patients. *J Mol Cell Cardiol* 1989;21:1349–1353.

19 Remppis A, Ehlermann P, Giannitsis E *et al.* Cardiac troponin T levels at 96 hours reflect myocardial infarct size: a pathoanatomical study. *Cardiology* 2000;93:249–253.

20 Metzler B, Hammerer-Lercher A, Jehle J *et al.* Plasma cardiac troponin T closely correlates with infarct size in a mouse model of acute myocardial infarction. *Clin Chim Acta* 2002;325:87–90.

21 Panteghini M, Cuccia C, Bonetti G, Giubbini R, Pagani F, Bonini E. Single-point cardiac troponin T at coronary care unit discharge after myocardial infarction correlates with infarct size and ejection fraction. *Clin Chem* 2002;48:1432–1436.

22 Licka M, Zimmermann R, Zehelein J, Dengler TJ, Katus HA, Kubler W. Troponin T concentrations 72 hours after myocardial infarction as a serological estimate of infarct size. *Heart* 2002;87:520–524.

23 Steen H, Giannitsis E, Futterer S *et al.* Cardiac troponin T at 96 hours after acute myocardial infarction correlates with infarct size and cardiac function. *J Am Coll Cardiol* 2006;48: 2192–2194.

24 Apple FS, Murakami MM. Cardiac troponin and creatine kinase MB monitoring during in-hospital myocardial reinfarction. *Clin Chem* 2005;51:460–463.

CHAPTER 3

Therapeutic implications of cardiac troponins in ST-segment elevation and non-ST-segment elevation myocardial infarction

Tracy Y. Wang, John M. Castor, L. Kristin Newby

Case 1

A 65-year-old, male, retired engineer with a history of hypertension and ongoing tobacco use presented to the emergency room with chest pain. He woke that morning with a pressure sensation in his mid-chest associated with diaphoresis and nausea. He got out of bed, but pain worsened with exertion, and was then associated with lightheadedness. An ambulance was called. After receiving an aspirin and two sublingual nitroglycerins, he became pain-free. He was transported to the local hospital for further evaluation.

In the emergency department, his heart rate was 90 and regular, blood pressure 162/88, and oxygen saturation 98% on 2 L of nasal cannula. Estimated jugular venous pressure was 7 cm and no thyromegaly was noted. Lungs were clear to auscultation bilaterally. Cardiac examination was notable for normal S1, physiologically split S2, and presence of an S4. No murmurs were heard. Abdomen was without hepatomegaly, and extremities were warm without edema. Distal pulses were 2+ bilaterally.

A 12-lead electrocardiogram (ECG) showed normal sinus rhythm with left ventricular hypertrophy and 1-mm ST-segment depression in leads V2–V4. Chest X-ray showed no cardiopulmonary abnormalities. Initial laboratories 4 hours after symptom onset yielded normal blood counts and chemistries except for a troponin T of 0.16 ng/mL (local laboratory upper limit of normal, 0.1 ng/mL) and a creatine kinase-MB fraction (CK-MB) of 14 ng/mL (local laboratory upper limit of normal, 9 ng/mL). The patient remained pain-free and was admitted to the cardiac intensive care unit for further management.

In the intensive care unit, the patient was treated with enoxaparin and eptifibatide in addition to aspirin, β-blocker, statin and angiotensin-converting enzyme (ACE) inhibitor. His cardiac markers peaked at a troponin T of 0.22 ng/mL and a CK-MB of 20 ng/mL at 12 hours after symptom onset. Both markers trended down thereafter. The patient underwent cardiac catheterization on hospital day 2, which revealed a 95% hazy obstruction of the mid left anterior descending (LAD) artery, suggestive of fresh thrombus. His other major epicardial vessels were widely patent without significant obstructive lesions. He was given clopidogrel 600 mg and then underwent percutaneous implantation of a drug-eluting stent to the LAD lesion with a final result of <25% luminal obstruction. He remained on an eptifibatide infusion for 18 hours postprocedure. The remainder of his hospitalization was unremarkable and the patient was discharged on hospital day 4 to cardiac rehabilitation.

Discussion of Case 1

Approximately 5.5 million patients per year present to the emergency department with a primary complaint of chest pain. Recently, cardiac biomarkers have played an increasing role, in addition to clinical history and ECG, in identifying patients with acute coronary syndrome (ACS). Cardiac troponins are sensitive markers of myocyte necrosis released in the setting of thrombotic coronary obstruction or distal vascular microembolization of platelet aggregates. Cardiac troponins were introduced into clinical practice in 1989 (troponin I in 1992), and multiple studies have proven the power of cardiac troponins in the diagnosis and risk stratification of ACS patients. Elevated troponin levels in patients with ACS identify a population with an increased mortality risk proportional to the degree of elevation [1]. Further, the Global Use of Strategies to Open Occluded Coronary Arteries in Acute Coronary Syndromes (GUSTO) IIa troponin substudy showed that baseline troponin T concentration provides more prognostic information than CK-MB [2]. This suggests that patients with elevated levels are at higher risk and may benefit from more aggressive therapies.

Traditional antithrombotic therapies targeting these pathophysiologic mechanisms consisted of oral aspirin and intravenous unfractionated heparin (UFH). Low molecular weight heparins have a more predictable anticoagulant effect by more specific targeting of factor Xa, leading to reductions in thrombin generation and activity. Higher bioavailability because of less binding to plasma proteins also makes for a more predictable dose–response relationship that does not require routine laboratory monitoring. The Fragmin in Unstable Coronary Artery Disease (FRISC) study found that dalteparin reduced event rates in unstable coronary artery disease (CAD) compared with placebo [3]. In an analysis of the relative benefit of dalteparin versus UFH, regardless of troponin status, all patients had decreased events in the short-term (6 days) on dalteparin compared with placebo. However, long-term benefits of dalteparin use were noted only in patients with a troponin T level >0.1 µg/L, with a reduction in death or myocardial infarction (MI) from 14.2 to 7.4% (RR 0.52, 95% CI 0.32–0.83, $p < 0.05$) in the troponin-positive group [4].

The Efficacy and Safety of Subcutaneous Enoxaparin in Non-Q Wave Coronary Events (ESSENCE) trial compared enoxaparin with UFH and found enoxaparin to be superior in reducing the 30-day risk of death, MI, or recurrent angina (19.8% enoxaparin versus 23.3% UFH, $p = 0.016$) without significantly increasing bleeding risk [5]. This was confirmed in the Thrombolysis in Myocardial Infarction (TIMI) 11B study, which showed a sustained risk

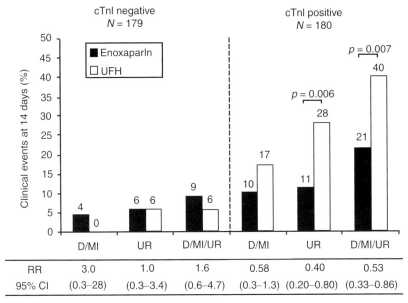

Figure 3.1 Clinical outcomes of troponin-positive vs. troponin-negative patients treated with enoxaparin compared with unfractionated heparin among CK-MB negative patients. Enoxaparin significantly reduced the rate of adverse events. (D, death; MI, myocardial infarction; UR, urgent revascularization, cTcl, cardiac troponin). (From Ref. [7].)

reduction with enoxaparin use (OR 0.85, 95% CI 0.72–1.00, $p = 0.048$) [6]. When these patients were risk stratified with troponin measurements, again a benefit was observed primarily in patients with positive admission troponin levels (Fig. 3.1). This demonstrates that measurement of troponin levels at presentation is useful in selecting patients, even those with normal CK-MB values, who are at higher risk of adverse outcomes and may benefit from more aggressive therapy with low-molecular-weight heparin.

If low-molecular-weight heparin is good, is a longer course of it better? Both FRISC II and TIMI 11B examined the efficacy of prolonged low-molecular-weight heparin therapy in preventing recurrent ischemia or need for revascularization. In FRISC II, a 3-month course of dalteparin improved the composite endpoint of death or MI at 1 month (3.1% versus 5.9%, OR 0.53, 95% CI 0.35–0.80, $p = 0.002$); this benefit was not sustained at 6 months [8]. TIMI 11B showed that outpatient enoxaparin for 43 days did not significantly add to the benefit of inpatient low-molecular-weight heparin use, but significantly increased major hemorrhage risk from 1.5 to 2.9% ($p = 0.021$) [7].

Glycoprotein IIb/IIIa inhibitors act at the platelet level to inhibit aggregation at the site of plaque rupture, which is a dominant feature in the pathophysiology of ACS. The C7E3 AntiPlatelet Therapy in Unstable Angina Refractory to Standard Treatment Trial (CAPTURE) was designed to determine whether use of abciximab in patients with refractory angina and significant coronary lesions awaiting revascularization improved clinical outcomes. Abciximab was given

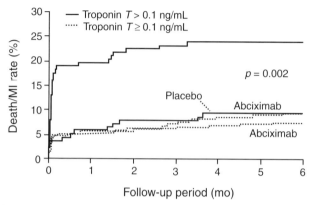

Figure 3.2 Cumulative incidence of death or MI among patients with non-ST-elevation ACS. Treatment of troponin-positive patients lowered risk to that similar to troponin-negative patients. (From Ref. [10].)

with intravenous UFH for 18–24 hours before coronary angioplasty and until 1 hour post-angioplasty. The study was stopped early because of a 29% lowering of the primary endpoint of death, MI, or urgent intervention at 30 days ($p = 0.012$) [9]. When stratified by troponin levels, troponin T-positive patients treated with abciximab had a similar risk of cardiac events to troponin T-negative patients, as shown in Fig. 3.2. Abciximab use reduced 6-month cardiac risk from 23.9 to 9.5% in troponin-positive patients as compared with 7.5 and 9.4% in troponin-negative patients treated with placebo and abciximab, respectively. Patients with refractory unstable angina and elevated troponin treated with abciximab had a relative risk of death or MI of 0.32 (95% CI 0.14–0.62) compared with troponin-negative patients. In contrast, CK-MB elevation did not predict treatment benefit with abxicimab [10].

The Platelet Receptor Inhibition in Ischemic Syndrome Management (PRISM) study randomized a population of ACS patients who were predominantly not revascularized, to treatment with tirofiban versus UFH [11]. Tirofiban lowered the risk of cardiac events during its 48-hour infusion, but no significant benefit was sustained at 30 days. However, in the troponin-positive population of this study, tirofiban lowered risk of death (OR 0.25, 95% CI 0.09–0.68, $p = 0.004$) and MI (OR 0.37, 95% CI 0.16–0.84, $p = 0.004$) in both medically managed patients as well as those undergoing revascularization. No treatment benefit was seen for troponin-negative patients [12]. The Platelet Receptor Inhibition in Ischemic Syndrome Management in Patients Limited by Unstable Signs and Symptoms (PRISM-PLUS) and Platelet Glycoprotein IIb/IIIa in Unstable Angina: Receptor Suppression Using Integrilin Therapy (PURSUIT) trials demonstrated incremental benefit when tirofiban or eptifibatide was added to UFH and aspirin; this benefit extends out to 6 months after randomization, supporting the hypothesis that early aggressive antiplatelet therapy leads to stabilization of coronary plaque [13, 14]. Patients

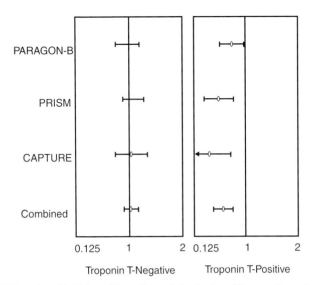

0.125   1   2 0.125   1   2

Troponin T-Negative   Troponin T-Positive

Figure 3.3 Odds ratios with 95% confidence intervals for death or MI among troponin-negative and -positive patients. Across trials, glycoprotein IIb/IIIa inhibitors consistently reduced risk in troponin-positive patients, OR 0.34; 95% CI 0.19-0.58. (From Ref. [15].)

who underwent percutaneous coronary revascularization derived the most benefit. The Platelet IIb/IIIa Antagonism for the Reduction of Acute coronary syndrome events in a Global Organization Network (PARAGON) B substudy prospectively showed that use of lamifiban with heparin neutralized the higher risk associated with a positive troponin in patients with non-ST-segment elevation ACS (see Fig. 3.3). This benefit was seen in both medically managed as well as revascularized patients [15].

Positive troponins in non-ST-segment elevation ACS correlate with severity of angiographic findings. Visible thrombus (14.6% versus 4.2%, $p = 0.004$), complex lesion characteristics (72% versus 53.9%, $p < 0.001$), and TIMI flow <2 (15.6% versus 5.1%, $p < 0.001$) were more frequent in troponin-positive patients on angiography [16]. The pathologic mechanism of ACS is disruption of the fibrous cap of an atherosclerotic plaque that initiates thrombosis. Angioscopy of troponin-positive patients shows a higher prevalence of yellow plaque, that is, vulnerable plaque with a large lipid core associated with a higher incidence of ACS [17]. While lesion morphology provides some prognostic information, particularly in regard to procedure-related risk, troponin is a more powerful predictor of cardiac risk than angiographic characteristics [16]. Abciximab improved TIMI flow and thrombus resolution significantly only in the troponin T-positive group. This supports the hypothesis that troponin release in patients with ACS suggests a more thrombogenic milieu with marked platelet activation which is more amenable to aggressive antiplatelet therapy.

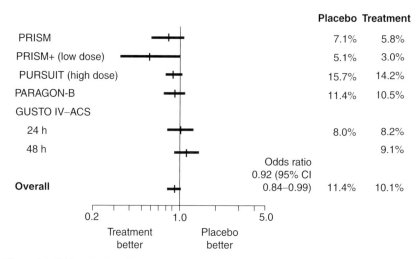

Figure 3.4 Odds ratio, 95% CI, and rates of death or MI across the major glycoprotein IIb/IIIa inhibitor trials showing its benefit in ACS patients. (From Ref. [19].)

A meta-analysis of CAPTURE, PRISM-PLUS, and PURSUIT determined that use of glycoprotein IIb/IIIa inhibitors before revascularization reduced risk of death or MI (2.9% versus 4.3%, $p = 0.001$), as well as risk of death or MI within 48 hours of percutaneous intervention (4.9% versus 8.0%, $p = 0.001$) [18]. This was challenged by the GUSTO IV-ACS trial, which randomized patients to 24- or 48-hour abciximab infusions versus placebo. Patients were excluded if early revascularization was planned. All patients received aspirin and either heparin or dalteparin. No improvement in outcome was noted; even troponin-positive and ST-segment depression groups did not receive any treatment benefit with abciximab [19]. This is in contrast to previous studies which showed benefit from glycoprotein IIb/IIIa use both with medical management or revascularization (Fig. 3.4). The explanation for the difference in results is unclear, but perhaps relates to infrequent use of early revascularization, suboptimal dosing regimens, or selection of patients at lower risk. The American College of Cardiology/American Heart Association (ACC/AHA) guidelines discourage abciximab use in patients with ACS not undergoing percutaneous intervention (class III) [20].

The hope was that intensive medical therapy with the above antithrombotic and antiplatelet regimens would improve coronary plaque stability and avoid invasive procedures. However, despite aggressive therapy, results are suboptimal. FRISC II randomized patients to a routine invasive versus an initial noninvasive treatment strategy and showed that the early invasive strategy reduced the composite risk of death or MI (OR 0.78, 95% CI 0.62–0.98, $p = 0.031$) [21]. Two-year follow-up of the FRISC II population showed the curves to continue to diverge with a sustained risk reduction of mortality (3.7% versus 5.4%,

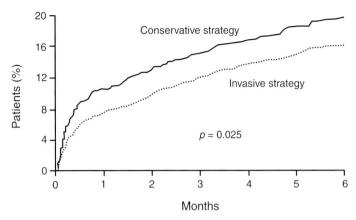

Figure 3.5 Cumulative incidence of death, MI or rehospitalization. The rate of adverse outcomes at 6 months was lower in the early invasive strategy group. (From Ref. [23].)

OR 0.68, 95% CI 0.47–0.98, $p = 0.038$) and MI (9.2% versus 12.7%, OR 0.72, 95% CI 0.57–0.91, $p = 0.005$) [22].

This was confirmed by the Treat Angina with Aggrastat and determine Cost of Therapy with an Invasive or Conservative Strategy (TACTICS)-TIMI 18 study, which showed a primary endpoint of death, nonfatal MI, or rehospitalization for ACS of 15.9% in the early invasive arm versus 19.4% in the conservative arm at 6 months (OR 0.78, 95% CI 0.62–0.97, $p = 0.025$) [23] (see Fig. 3.5). All patients were treated with aspirin, heparin, and tirofiban. In the troponin-positive group (54% of the study), there was a 39% relative risk reduction and a 10% absolute risk reduction with the use of the invasive strategy, whereas no difference was noted in the troponin-negative group ($p < 0.001$) [24]. Troponin was an independent and a more powerful predictor of benefit compared with other clinical indicators such as ST-segment depression, CK-MB, and TIMI risk score.

We may be getting to the point where medical therapies are advanced enough to stabilize plaque and avoid invasive procedures. A study by de Winter *et al.* randomized 1200 high-risk ACS patients with positive troponin levels to early invasive versus selective invasive management. Medical therapies for these patients included aspirin, early clopidogrel use, enoxaparin, periprocedural abciximab, and high-dose statin for lipid control. With this level of aggressive medical therapy, there was no significant difference between the early and selective invasive arms in terms of mortality and the composite endpoint of death, nonfatal MI, or rehospitalization [25]. Overall mortality was lower than previous studies (2.5%) despite selection of a high-risk population, suggesting that our therapies, both medical and invasive, are providing much better outcomes. Revascularization rates were higher in the selectively invasive groups (79% early and 54% selective versus 77% and 37% in FRISC II and 61% and 44% in TACTICS-TIMI 18). Much of the composite endpoint in the early invasive group was driven by a significantly higher incidence of periprocedural MI, which is of less certain prognostic significance.

In summary, elevated troponin levels identify patients with ACS who are at higher risk and who derive particular benefit from aggressive therapies such as use of low molecular weight heparin, glycoprotein IIb/IIIa inhibitors, and early invasive strategies. How are we doing? The Can Rapid Risk stratification of Unstable angina patients Suppress ADverse outcomes with Early implementation of the ACC/AHA guidelines (CRUSADE) initiative followed 23,298 patients with ACS. As before, troponin levels correlated with mortality risk. However, early therapies did not change based on the admission troponin level. Specifically, there was similar use of low molecular weight heparin (36.9% troponin-positive versus 37.5% troponin-negative) and glycoprotein IIb/IIIa inhibitor (34% versus 34%) in both troponin-positive and troponin-negative groups. Sixty-six percent of patients with a positive troponin did not receive any glycoprotein IIb/IIIa inhibitor. Despite evidence that patients presenting with baseline-positive troponins have a higher risk of mortality compared with patients with later-positive troponin results [26, 27], cardiac catheterization was, in fact, significantly underutilized in the patients with positive admission troponins compared with those with initial-negative then later-positive troponins [28]. When stratified by degree of troponin elevation, early aspirin, heparin, and glycoprotein IIb/IIIa inhibitor use was greater only in patients with major troponin elevations (greater than five times the upper limit of normal) (Table 3.1). Glycoprotein IIb/IIIa inhibitors were used in only 20–40% of patients across all levels of troponin elevation. Use of cardiac catheterization was higher in the troponin-negative cohort than in the cohort with troponin levels one to two times the upper limit of normal (Table 3.2) [29].

In conclusion, a positive troponin in non-ST-segment elevation ACS predicts higher risk and warrants aggressive therapy. Although ACC/AHA guidelines recommend using troponin levels to delineate treatment decisions [30], clinical adherence to these recommendations is poor. Substantial changes to clinical care algorithms need to be made to provide adequate evidence-based therapies.

Case 2

A 75-year-old man with chronic kidney disease on hemodialysis for the past 6 months and a history of hyperlipidemia, hypertension, and adult-onset diabetes mellitus presents to the emergency department with a chief complaint of increasing dyspnea in the last 24 hours.

On examination, he appears pale and diaphoretic. His heart rate is 101, blood pressure 90/55, respirations 21, and his oxygen saturation is 90% on 2-L nasal cannula. His cardiac examination reveals a regular rhythm with an S4. His lungs are clear to auscultation bilaterally.

A 12-lead ECG shows normal sinus rhythm with Q waves in leads II, II, and aVF consistent with an old inferior infarction. No acute ST-segment or T-wave abnormalities were noted. Laboratory testing revealed a troponin of

Table 3.1 Early therapies.*

Medication	Overall study cohort (n = 23,298)	Maximum troponin ratio			
		0–1 × ULN (n = 5291)	1–2 × ULN (n = 2499)	2–5 × ULN (n = 3825)	>5 × ULN (n = 11,683)
Aspirin, %	90.8	89.5	90.3	90.1	91.7
Heparin, %					
A	83.2	76.4	78.1	81.5	87.8
Unfractionated	53.6	47.8	48.0	50.2	58.4
Low molecular weight	36.4	34.2	35.7	37.2	37.3
Glycoprotein IIb/IIIa inhibitors, %	31.6	22.4	22.8	26.6	39.1
β-Blockers, %	76.9	73.0	75.3	76.8	79.0
Clopidogrel %	37.8	33.3	32.0	36.3	41.6

*Therapies delivered within 24 hours to eligible patients without listed contraindications.
†p < 0.001 for all medications comparing trends across the four categories of troponin elevation.
ULN, upper limit of normal.

Table 3.2 In-hospital cardiac procedures.*

Procedure	Overall study cohort (n = 23,298)	Maximum troponin ratio			
		0–1 × ULN (n = 5291)	1–2 × ULN (n = 2499)	2–5 × ULN (n = 3825)	>5 × ULN (n = 11,683)
Diagnostic cardiac catheterization, %	66.1	63.1	57.4	62.1	70.7
<24 h	29.8	26.1	22.9	25.8	34.2
<48 h	44.9	40.7	36.9	41.4	49.6
PCI, %	36.3	33.6	28.8	32.1	40.6
<24 h	17.3	14.2	11.8	14.3	20.8
<48 h	25.4	22.2	19.5	22.2	29.2
CABG, %	11.2	9.1	10.4	11.5	12.2

CABG, coronary artery bypass grafting; PCI, percutaneous coronary intervention; ULN, upper limit of normal.
*P < 0.001 for all procedures comparing trends across the four categories of troponin elevation.

0.23 ng/mL (upper limit of normal, 0.10 ng/mL) and CK-MB of 4 (upper limit of normal, 9 ng/mL). No prior cardiac markers were available for comparison. Investigation of noncardiac etiologies, including chest X-ray, basic chemistries, and a ventilation–perfusion scan, was negative. The patient was given aspirin, lopressor, and intravenous UFH, and was admitted for further evaluation.

On hospital day 2, an echocardiogram revealed an ejection fraction of 40% with inferior hypokinesis. His troponin peaked at 0.42 ng/mL 12 hours after admission, and then trended down. On hospital day 3, cardiac catheterization revealed a 75% distal right coronary artery lesion that was treated with a drug-eluting stent with good results. The patient was started on a statin, oral β-blocker, and clopidogrel. An ACE inhibitor was started as well but had to be discontinued due to hyperkalemia of 6.1 ng/mL two days after initiation. Patient was discharged on hospital day 5 without events.

Discussion of Case 2

In patients presenting with chest pain, data from the PARAGON B, GUSTO IIa, and CHest pain Evaluation by Creatine Kinase-MB, Myoglobin, and Troponin I (CHECKMATE) trials show that patients with both positive troponin and CK-MB levels had the highest 30-day risk of death or MI (OR 2.5, 95% CI 1.6–3.8) [31, 32]. However, an isolated positive troponin, even with a negative CK-MB level, carried an OR of 2.1 (95% CI 1.4–3.0) compared with an isolated positive CK-MB, OR 1.0 (95% CI 0.6–1.6) [33] (see Fig. 3.6).

The prevalence of CAD in patients with renal insufficiency is high and is a major cause of morbidity and mortality. In patients on dialysis, the prevalence of CAD is estimated at 40% [34] and cardiovascular disease accounts for almost 50% of deaths in patients with chronic renal insufficiency [35]. In a meta-analysis of acute MI mortality in patients over 65 years old, serum creatinine

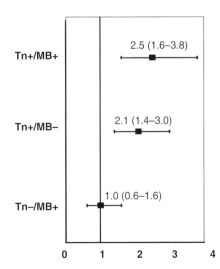

Figure 3.6 Adjusted OR and 95% CI for 30-day death or MI referenced to patients who are both MB- and troponin-negative. Patients who are troponin-positive have a higher risk of death or MI. (From Ref. [33].)

was the second most powerful predictor of 30-day mortality after presentation with cardiac arrest [36]. Patients with renal failure often have atypical presentations of ACS [37], so clinicians must rely on diagnostic modalities such as ECG and cardiac biomarkers for diagnosis.

Cardiac troponins are very specific markers of myocardial necrosis. With newer generation troponin assays, 50% of asymptomatic patients with renal failure, whether acute, chronic, or end stage, have elevated troponin levels. Troponin I is elevated in 7% of patients with advanced renal failure whereas troponin T is elevated between 17 and 53% of patients with renal failure [38, 39]. A higher proportion of troponin T (7% versus 3.5% troponin I) exists freely in the myocyte cytoplasm while the rest is bound within the sarcomere and therefore greater release of the unbound cytosolic troponin T may account for the higher specificity of troponin I in patients with renal failure. The cause of troponin elevation in end-stage renal disease (ESRD) has been debated. Uremia-induced skeletal muscle reexpression of cardiac troponin T, clinically silent micro-infarctions, left ventricular hypertrophy, and subclinical volume overload and heart failure have been postulated as potential sources of troponin elevation. Decreased renal clearance is unlikely to be the cause of elevated troponin; studies to date have not shown a relationship between degree of troponin elevation and creatinine clearance (CrCl) [40]. Improvement in renal function after renal transplantation does not alter the prevalence of troponin elevation [41]. Troponin I levels decrease up to 86% post-dialysis, while troponin T levels trend toward increasing post-dialysis [39]. Although dialysis membranes should clear only molecules smaller than intact troponin T or I, the thought is that troponin I may adsorb onto the membrane because of its hydrophobicity. Troponin T levels are thought to increase post-dialysis due to hemoconcentration.

In asymptomatic patients with renal dysfunction, troponin elevation has been shown to predict a two- to fivefold increase in all-cause mortality [42], suggesting a role for troponin in the clinical risk assessment of patients with renal disease. However, therapeutic consequences are unclear and the use of troponin as part of routine clinical risk stratification of renal patients is still being debated. However, the prognostic value of a positive troponin in the setting of suspected ACS and renal failure has been firmly established. An analysis from the GUSTO IV trial showed that patients presenting with chest pain and impaired CrCl who had troponin elevation still had significantly increased risk of 30-day risk of death and MI (OR 2.5, 95% CI 1.3–2.2, $p <$ 0.001) and should be treated aggressively [43].

The presence of ischemic symptoms, ECG changes, and an elevated troponin is generally sufficient evidence to diagnose ACS in renal patients. Confusion arises when renal patients present with atypical symptoms. ECG abnormalities such as left bundle branch block and left ventricular strain patterns are very common in end-stage renal patients, making the diagnosis more difficult [44]. In this setting, a rise in serum troponin is consistent with new myocardial damage, whereas an invariant serial troponin and CK-MB measurements, while still predictive of poor long-term prognosis, may indicate no new myocardial injury. Most trials evaluating therapies for ACS exclude patients with impaired CrCl. This has resulted in a general reluctance to use aggressive therapies such as glycoprotein IIb/IIIa inhibitors, fibrinolytic therapy, or percutaneous coronary intervention (PCI). Shlipak *et al.* showed that 1-year mortality post-MI in renal patients was an astounding 66% in comparison with 24% in patients with normal renal function [45]. Large clinical trials recruiting troponin-positive patients with renal dysfunction need to be performed to look at the efficacy and safety of therapies that are proven in patients with normal renal function.

Low molecular weight heparin, unlike UFH, is cleared primarily through the kidneys. Pharmacokinetic data for low molecular weight heparin have not been consistent. Cadroy *et al.* showed that in patients with ESRD, the half-life of enoxaparin was 1.7 times longer and clearance was twofold lower than in control patients [46]. However, another study by Brophy *et al.* showed that while use of enoxaparin in ESRD resulted in twofold prolongation of anti-factor Xa activity, clearance was not affected by the glomerular filtration rate and no dosage adjustments were needed [47].

TIMI 11A, while excluding patients with creatinine levels >2 mg/dL, showed that clearance of enoxaparin was reduced 22% in the group of patients with a CrCl levels <40 mL/min. Patients with this degree of renal impairment had increased peak and trough anti-Xa activity (mean trough was more than double that patients with normal CrCl) and were more likely to have major hemorrhagic events [48].

TIMI 11B and ESSENCE showed enoxaparin to significantly reduce the primary endpoint of death, MI, or urgent revascularization in patients with non-ST-segment elevation MI compared to UFH. In a subgroup analysis of these two studies, patients with renal impairment (CrCl levels <30 mL/min) had a higher rate of this primary endpoint regardless of treatment with either UFH or enoxaparin. Overall, patients with renal insufficiency had a higher bleeding risk compared to patients with normal renal function. There was no significant difference in benefit or bleeding risk between the UFH and enoxaparin group; however, this analysis was significantly underpowered (total of 143 patients) as most patients with renal insufficiency were excluded from the trial [49]. Collet *et al.* looked at enoxaparin dosing for ACS in patients with varying renal dysfunction. To achieve target anti-Xa levels between 0.5 and 1.0 IU/mL, patients with CrCl <30 mL/min required a final dosage of 0.64 mg/kg every 12 hours, whereas patients with CrCl between 30 and 59 mL/min required a dosage of 0.84 mg/kg every 12 hours [50]. In a small study of 72 patients with CrCl <40 mL/min, Choussat *et al.* demonstrated efficacy and safety of single-dose 0.5 mg/kg intravenous enoxaparin in patients undergoing elective PCI [51].

Bleeding complications with enoxaparin are significantly higher in patients with renal insufficiency. Gerlach *et al.* reported bleeding complications of 51% compared with 22% with normal renal function even in the setting of lower drug dose [52]. This has led to the recommendation that use of UFH, rather than low-molecular-weight heparin, is preferred in renal patients with a serum creatinine >2 mg/dL or CrCl <30 mL/min.

Glycoprotein IIb/IIIa inhibitors are highly underutilized in ACS; this is even more evident in patients with renal disease as most randomized studies excluded patients with renal dysfunction. In an observational study by Freeman *et al.*, 310 of 889 (34.9%) patients admitted for ACS had renal insufficiency. In-hospital mortality was significantly higher in patients with renal insufficiency (8.1% versus 2.6%, $p < 0.001$) even after adjustment for comorbidities. A glycoprotein IIb/IIIa inhibitor was used in 39.3% of patient with CrCl > 90 mL/min and 12.7% in CrCl < 30 mL/min ($p < 0.001$). When adjusted for level of renal dysfunction, glycoprotein IIb/IIIa inhibitor use was associated with a significant improvement in in-hospital mortality, but the adjusted OR for major bleeding in patients was 2.13 (95% CI 1.39–3.27, $p < 0.0001$) with renal insufficiency [53]. While PRISM-PLUS excluded patients with Cr >2.5 mg/dL, renal dysfunction predicted more high-risk angiographic features and worse outcome. Tirofiban reduced risk in all strata of renal function. Bleeding increased with addition of tirofiban to UFH; however, this risk was not amplified in patients with renal insufficiency, suggesting that tirofiban can be used in ACS patients with mild to moderate renal impairment [54].

The concern for increased bleeding risk is mostly based on the fact that glycoprotein IIb/IIIa inhibitors are primarily renally excreted. Tirofiban is 36–69% renally cleared, and half dose is recommended in patients with renal failure. Eptifibatide is contraindicated in dialysis patients and a reduction in infusion rate to 1 μcg/(kg min) is recommended for CrCl <50 mL/min. To date, no dose adjustment is recommended for abciximab as platelet-bound abciximab is cleared by the reticuloendothelial system. However, free circulating Fab fragments are still cleared by the kidneys.

The Enhanced Suppression of the Platelet IIb/IIIa Receptor with Integrilin Therapy (ESPRIT) trial looked at eptifibatide use in conjunction with PCI and excluded patients with a creatinine >4 mg/dL. In a subanalysis, patients with CrCl <60 mL/min had higher rates of adverse outcomes after PCI. Patients with lower CrCl received greater benefit from eptifibatide treatment (OR 0.53, 95% CI 0.34–0.83) compared to patients with higher CrCl (OR 0.68, 95% CI 0.49–0.94) without an increase in bleeding risk [55] (see Fig. 3.7). Currently, use of glycoprotein IIb/IIIa inhibitors is recommended for patients with mild to moderate renal insufficiency who present with ACS, with appropriate adjustment of infusion rates based on degree of renal impairment.

In general, patients with renal dysfunction are less likely to be prescribed proven therapies for ACS such as aspirin, β-blockers, heparin, or statins. Despite the fact that these patients tend to have more severe angiographic lesions, they are less likely to undergo invasive therapies such as PCI or coronary artery bypass grafting (CABG) [55]. An observational study of 4500 patients undergoing cardiac catheterization showed that in spite of the association of more severe angiographic lesions and higher mortality with renal insufficiency, a greater proportion of patients with renal insufficiency were managed medically after catheterization; 47.6% of patients with normal function underwent PCI

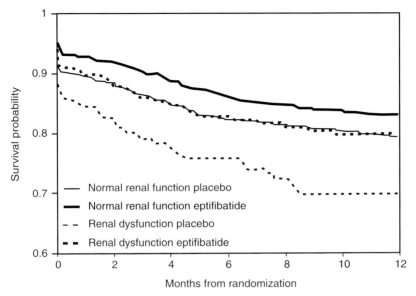

Figure 3.7 Kaplan Meier survival curves for patients stratified by renal function and eptifibatide use. Patients with renal dysfunction benefited from use of eptifibatide. (From Ref. [55].)

compared with 35.7% of patients with CrCl 60–90 mL/min and 15.9% with CrCl <30 mL/min [56]. While PCI was associated with improved survival over medical therapy in patients with normal renal function or mild renal insufficiency, this survival benefit was not noted in patients with severe renal dysfunction. In contrast, CABG was associated with improved survival over medical therapy at all levels of renal insufficiency, and CABG was better than PCI in patients with moderate to severe renal dysfunction. It is important to note that these observations were made in the non-drug eluting stent era.

To summarize, a positive troponin in the setting of typical symptoms in a patient with renal insufficiency predicts higher mortality and warrants aggressive therapy. However, current data are limited in that most studies exclude patients with renal dysfunction. UFH is recommended over low-molecular-weight heparins in this population. Glycoprotein IIb/IIIa inhibitors and PCI could be utilized more frequently in patients with mild to moderate renal insufficiency. Until studies that include patients with renal dysfunction are performed, we do not have any formal data to delineate appropriate therapies for ACS patients with renal insufficiency.

Case 3

A 54-year-old diabetic man noted vague epigastric discomfort and nausea after lunch. Four hours later, having no symptom relief from over-the-counter antacids, he drove himself to the local emergency department for further evaluation. On arrival in triage, he was noted to be pale and diaphoretic.

Heart rate was 106 and blood pressure 92/50. He was given an aspirin and three sublingual nitroglycerins without substantial relief of his discomfort. A 12-lead ECG showed 3-mm ST-segment elevation in V2–V5. Urgent cardiology consultation was obtained and the patient was transferred to a local tertiary facility for cardiac catheterization. En route, blood samples were drawn and patient was initiated on intravenous UFH and abciximab infusions.

Coronary angiography revealed a total occlusion of a large left anterior descending artery, which was treated with a drug-eluting stent with resolution of symptoms and ST-segment elevations. He received a clopidogrel load of 600 mg and remained on abciximab for another 12 hours post-procedure. Testing of his pre-catheterization blood samples revealed a troponin T of 2.3 ng/mL (upper limit of normal, 0.10 ng/mL) and a CK-MB of 24 ng/mL (upper limit of normal, 9 ng/mL). These cardiac enzymes peaked at 6 hours post-revascularization and then trended down. The patient had no recurrent symptoms. An echocardiogram showed moderate anteroapical hypokinesis with an estimated ejection fraction of 40%. The patient was started on daily aspirin, statin, β-blocker, and ACE inhibitor. He was discharged a few days later to cardiac rehabilitation.

Discussion of Case 3

The pathophysiologic substrate of ST-segment elevation MI (STEMI) is thrombotic occlusion of an epicardial coronary artery. Expedient restoration of flow to the obstructed artery is the key determinant of short- and long-term outcomes in these patients. When a STEMI patient presents to a hospital without interventional catheterization facilities, the decision to use fibrinolysis versus primary PCI depends on the time delay to PCI. A PCI strategy may not reduce mortality compared to immediate thrombolytic administration when a delay greater than 90 minutes is anticipated.

Cardiac biomarkers are used to evaluate and risk stratify patients with STEMI but not to determine the need for rapid reperfusion therapy. In the GUSTO trials, elevated baseline serum troponin T concentration was associated with increased cardiac mortality. In a troponin T substudy of GUSTO III, STEMI patients with positive admission troponin levels had a 30-day mortality of 15.7% compared with 6.2% ($p = 0.001$) in the troponin-negative group. When patients with STEMI undergo successful reperfusion, biomarkers are often detected earlier and rise more quickly to a peak level and then rapidly decline. The time to peak serum troponin T concentration also predicts clinical outcome (see Fig. 3.8). In one study, time to peak troponin >11 hours was associated with a lower cardiac event-free survival rate and with increased risk of reinfarction and target lesion re-intervention [57].

An elevated troponin level is hypothesized to reflect more tissue damage possibly due to longer periods of ischemia, lower success rates of reperfusion via either thrombolysis or primary angioplasty, and microvascular dysfunction due to distal microembolization and endothelial cell damage. Stubbs *et al.* found less effective reperfusion (50% versus 72%, $p = 0.006$) with streptokinase in patients with troponin T levels >0.2 ng/mL. Mortality rates were higher not

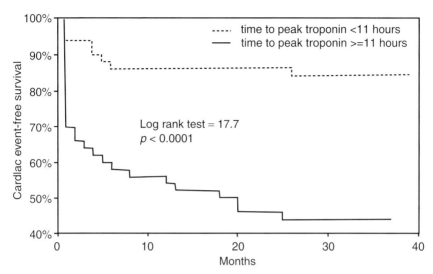

Figure 3.8 Kaplan-Meier event-free survival curve showing greater survival in patients whose time to peak troponin was < 11 hours compared to those whose time to peak troponin was > =11 hours. (From Ref. [57].)

only during the initial hospitalization, but were consistently higher as far out as 3 years (28% versus 7.5%, $p = 0.001$) [58]. In the TIMI 10B study, admission troponin levels were significantly lower in patients that achieved TIMI 3 flow after thrombolysis [59]. Lower rates of successful reperfusion with percutaneous intervention have also been reported in troponin-positive patients [60–62]. Giannitsis et al. looked at 140 patients with STEMI who presented within 12 hours of symptom onset and underwent primary PCI [62]. A positive admission troponin level predicted a 3.2-fold risk for incomplete epicardial reperfusion (TIMI flow <3) and was the strongest predictor of reperfusion success. Despite re-establishment of normal epicardial flow, troponin-positive patients had more impaired myocardial perfusion evidenced by lower 60-minute ratios of cardiac biomarkers. This correlated to clinical outcomes; troponin-positive patients had a higher all-cause and cardiac mortality at 9 months (18.8% versus 3.9%, $p = 0.05$ and 14% versus 3.9%, $p = 0.03$, respectively) [62].

While elevated baseline troponin levels have consistently predicted clinical outcome, the relationship between troponin levels and infarct size and post-infarct left ventricular function is still debated. Kurowski et al. showed that positive troponin levels are more often correlated with a depressed ejection fraction and the left anterior descending artery as the infarct-related artery [63]. In non-anterior MIs, a positive troponin discriminated high- and low-risk subgroups with a 30-day cardiac mortality of 9.6% versus 1.4% ($p = 0.04$) and 12-month cardiac mortality of 11.5% versus 1.3% ($p = 0.17$). In fact, cardiac mortality of a troponin-positive non-anterior STEMI was similar to that of a troponin-negative anterior STEMI. However, Ohlmann et al. did not find admission troponin levels to predict large enzymatic infarct size or ejection fraction. In contrast, later troponin levels measured up to 72 hours following PCI were shown to be correlated to infarct size and left ventricular function [64].

While patients with high-troponin levels on admission typically present later after symptom onset, even after adjustment for this, troponin elevation was an independent predictor of risk, suggesting that it is not only time to reperfusion that is important for survival. Factors other than myocardial salvage may be important for survival benefit, including microvascular flow reduction, microemboli, and higher thrombotic burden. Per ACC/AHA guidelines, reducing time to vessel patency remains the primary objective, and reperfusion therapy should not be contingent on biomarker testing [65]. However, the proven prognostic value of troponins in the setting of acute STEMI suggests more aggressive therapies for these patients.

Platelet glycoprotein inhibition in the setting of thrombolysis has been studied in several trials. TIMI 14 found that adding abciximab to tissue plasminogen activator improved TIMI 3 flow at 60 minutes (72% versus 43%, $p = 0.0009$) [66]. GUSTO V randomized patients to receive reteplase alone versus combination of half-dose reteplase plus full-dose abciximab. No mortality difference was noted at 30 days or 1 year, but combination therapy did reduce frequency of reinfarction (3.5% versus 2.3%, $p < 0.0001$). Significantly higher rates of bleeding were noted with severe bleeding occurring in 0.5% with thrombolysis alone versus 1.1% with combination therapy ($p < 0.0001$), especially intracranial bleeding in patients older than 75 years of age [67]. Therefore, addition of glycoprotein IIb/IIIa inhibitors to fibrinolytic therapy, in the absence of proven mortality benefit, is not recommended.

With percutaneous interventions, there is more of a role for glycoprotein IIb/IIIa inhibitor use. The Abciximab before Direct Angioplasty and Stenting in MI Regarding Acute and Long Term Follow-up (ADMIRAL) trial found that abciximab use with primary PCI significantly reduced the composite outcome of death, recurrent MI, and urgent target revascularization at both 30 days (6% versus 14.6%, $p = 0.01$) and 6 months (7.4% versus 15.9%, $p = 0.02$) [68] (see Fig. 3.9). Furthermore, earlier administration of glycoprotein IIb/IIIa inhibitors before PCI improved coronary patency [69].

Clopidogrel, a less potent antiplatelet agent than glycoprotein IIb/IIIa inhibitors, may provide incremental inhibition of platelet activation and aggregation which improves outcomes in STEMI patients without the higher bleeding risk. Sabatine *et al.* reported that the addition of clopidogrel to fibrinolytics and UFH improved the composite endpoint of occluded infarct-related artery on angiography, death, or recurrent MI from 32.7 to 15% (36% odd reduction, 95% CI 24–47, $p < 0.001$). No significant difference was noted in the incidence of bleeding complications [70]. This was confirmed in a large trial of almost 46,000 STEMI patients, half of which underwent thrombolysis, who were randomized to clopidogrel versus placebo on top of standard therapy (including aspirin). At 28 days, clopidogrel reduced the relative risk of death by 7% (7.5% versus 8.1% mortality, $p = 0.03$) and reduced the composite endpoint of recurrent MI,

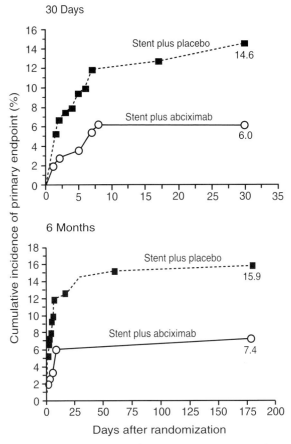

Figure 3.9 Cumulative incidence of death, reinfarction or urgent target vessel revascularization at 30 days and 6 months are both significantly reduced with the addition of abciximab therapy. (From Ref. [68].)

stroke, or death by 9% (event rate 9.3% versus 10.1%, $p = 0.002$) without any increase in bleeding risk [71]. In a substudy of the CLARITY trial, pretreatment with clopidogrel, given with thrombolytics at the time of presentation, significantly reduced 30-day risk of cardiovascular death, MI, or stroke (7.5% versus 12.0%, adjusted OR 0.59, 95% CI 0.43–0.81, $p = 0.001$; number needed to treat = 23) [72].

Low molecular weight heparin has emerged as an attractive alternative to UFH in STEMI patients. The Assessment of the Safety and Efficacy of a New Thrombolytic (ASSENT) III study randomized patients to UFH versus enoxaparin and found that patients who received UFH had a significantly higher composite outcome of death, reinfarction, and refractory ischemia (15.4% versus 11.4%, $p = 0.0001$) [73]. The efficacy and safety of enoxaparin use is currently being tested in a large clinical trial [74].

While none of these trials stratified patients according to their troponin levels, the worse prognosis associated with elevated troponins suggests use of these more aggressive measures to improve vessel patient and microvascular perfusion in an effort to reduce mortality and recurrent events. As with all MI patients, standard post-MI management, including aggressive β-blockade, renin–angiotensin system blockade, lipid control, and smoking cessation counseling, should be emphasized.

Financial disclosures

Dr. Newby has received consulting honoraria from Ischemia Technologies, Biosite, and Ortho-Clinical Diagnostics, and research grant support from Roche Diagnostics Corporation.

References

1 Antman EM, Tanasijevic MJ, Thompson B *et al.* Cardiac-specific troponin I levels to predict the risk of mortality in patients with acute coronary syndromes. *N Engl J Med* 1996;**335**:1342.

2 Ohman EM, Armstrong PW, Christenson RH *et al.* Risk stratification with admission cardiac troponin T levels in acute myocardial ischemia. *N Engl J Med* 1996;**335**:1333.

3 FRISC Study Group. Low molecular weight heparin (Fragmin) during instability in coronary artery disease (FRISC). *Lancet* 1996;**347**:561.

4 Lindahl B, Venge P, Wallentin L *et al.* Troponin T identifies patients with unstable coronary artery disease who will benefit from long term antithrombotic protection. *J Am Coll Cardiol* 1997;**29**:43.

5 Cohen M, Demers C, Gurfinkel EP *et al.* A comparison of low molecular weight heparin with unfractionated heparin for unstable coronary artery disease. *N Engl J Med* 1997;**337**:447.

6 Antman EM, McCabe CH, Gurfinkel EP *et al.* Enoxaparin prevents death and cardiac ischemic events in unstable angina/non Q wave MI. *Circulation* 1999;**100**:1593.

7 Morrow DA, Antman EM, Tanasijevic M *et al.* Cardiac troponin I for stratification of early outcomes and the efficacy of enoxaparin in unstable angina: a TIMI-11B substudy. *J Am Coll Cardiol* 2000;**36**:1812.

8 FRISC II Investigators. Long-term low molecular mass heparin in unstable coronary-artery disease: FRISC II prospective randomized multicentre study. *Lancet* 1999;**354**:701.

9 CAPTURE Investigators. Randomised placebo-controlled trial of abciximab before and during coronary intervention in refractory unstable angina: the CAPTURE study. *Lancet* 1997;**349**:1429.

10 Hamm CW, Heeschen C, Goldmann B *et al.* Benefit of abciximab in patients with refractory unstable angina in relation to serum troponin T levels. *N Engl J Med* 1999;**340**:1623.

11 PRISM Study Investigators. A comparison of aspirin plus tirofiban with aspiring plus heparin for unstable angina. *N Engl J Med* 1998;**338**:1498.

12 Heeschen C, Hamm CW, Holdmann B *et al.* Troponin concentrations for stratification of patients with acute coronary syndromes in relation to therapeutic efficacy of tirofiban. *Lancet* 1999;**354**:1757.

13 PRISM-PLUS Study Investigators. Inhibition of the platelet glycoprotein IIb/IIIa receptor with tirofiban in unstable angina and non Q wave myocardial infarction. *N Engl J Med* 1998;**338**:1488.

14 PURSUIT Study Investigators. Inhibition of platelet glycoprotein IIb/IIIa with eptifibatide in patients with acute coronary syndromes. *N Engl J Med* 1998;**339**:436.

15 Newby LK, Ohman EM, Christenson RH *et al.* Benefit of glycoprotein IIb/IIIa inhibition in patients with acute coronary syndromes and troponin T-positive status. *Circulation* 2001;**103**:2891.

16 Heeschen C, van den Brand MJ, Hamm CW *et al.* Angiographic findings in patients with refractory unstable angina according to troponin T status. *Circulation* 1999;**104**:1509.

17 Ohtani T, Ueda Y, Shimizu M *et al.* Association between cardiac troponin T elevation and angioscopic morphology of culprit lesion in patients with non-ST-segment elevation acute coronary syndrome. *Am Heart J* 2005;**150**:227.

18 Boersma E, Akkerhuis M, Theroux P *et al.* Platelet glycoprotein IIb/IIIa receptor inhibition in non-ST-elevation acute coronary syndromes: early benefit during medical treatment only, with additional protection during coronary intervention. *Circulation* 1999;**100**:2045.

19 GUSTO IV-ACS Study Investigators. Effect of glycoprotein IIb/IIIa receptor blocker abciximab on outcome in patients with acute coronary syndromes without early coronary revascularization: the GUSTO IV-ACS randomized trial. *Lancet* 2001;**357**:1915.

20 Braunwauld E, Antman EM, Beasley JW *et al.* ACC/AHA 2002 guideline update for management of patients with unstable angina and non-ST-segment elevation myocardial infarction. *Circulation* 2002;**106**:1893.

21 FRISC Investigators. Invasive compared with non-invasive treatment in unstable coronary artery disease: FRISC II prospective randomized multicentre study. *Lancet* 1999;**354**:708.

22 Lagerqvist B, Husted S, Kontny F *et al.* A long-term perspective on the protective effects of an early invasive strategy in unstable coronary artery disease. *J Am Coll Cardiol* 2002;**40**:1902.

23 Cannon CP, Weintraub WS, Demopoulos LA *et al.* Comparison of early invasive and conservative strategies in patients with unstable coronary syndromes treated with the glycoprotein IIb/IIIa inhibitor tirofiban. *N Engl J Med* 2001;**344**:1879.

24 Morrow DA, Cannon CP, Rifai N *et al.* Ability of minor elevations of troponin I and T to predict benefit from an early invasive strategy in patients with unstable angina and non-ST elevation myocardial infarction. *JAMA* 2001;**286**:2405.

25 de Winter RJ, Windhausen F, Cornel JH *et al.* Early invasive versus selectively invasive management for acute coronary syndromes. *N Engl J Med* 2005;**353**:1095.

26 Newby LK, Christenson RH, Ohman EM *et al.* Value of serial troponin T measures for early and late risk stratification in patients with acute coronary syndromes. *Circulation* 198;**98**:1853.

27 Antman EM, Sacks DB, Rifai N *et al.* Time to positivity of a rapid bedside assay for cardiac-specific troponin T predicts prognosis in acute coronary syndromes: a TIMI-11a substudy. *J Am Coll Cardiol* 1998;**31**:326.

28 Roe MT, Peterson ED, Pollack CV *et al.* Influence of timing of troponin elevation on clinical outcomes and use of evidence-based therapies for patients with non-ST-segment elevation acute coronary syndromes. *Ann Emerg Med* 2005;**45**:355.

29 Roe MT, Peterson ED, Li Y *et al.* Relationship between risk stratification by cardiac troponin level and adherence to guidelines for non-ST-segment elevation acute coronary syndromes. *Arch Intern Med* 2005;**165**:1870.

30 Braunwald E, Antman EM, Beasley JW *et al.* ACC/AHA guidelines for the management of patients with unstable angina and non-ST-segment elevation myocardial

infarction: executive summary and recommendations. A report of the American College of Cardiology/American Heart Association Task Force on Practice Guidelines (Committee on Management of Patients with Unstable Angina). *J Am Coll Cardiol* 2002;**40**:1366.

31 Petersen E, Pollack CV, Roe MT *et al.* Early use of glycoprotein IIb/IIIa inhibitors in non-ST-elevation acute myocardial infarction: observations from the National Registry of Myocardial Infarction 4. *J Am Coll Cardiol* 2003;**42**:45.

32 Ohman EM, Armstrong PW, White HD *et al.* Risk stratification with a point-of-care troponin T test in acute myocardial infarction. *Am J Cardiol* 1999;**84**:1281.

33 Rao SV, Ohman EM, Granger CB *et al.* Prognostic value of isolated troponin elevation across the spectrum of chest pain syndromes. *Am J Cardiol* 2003;**91**:936.

34 Foley RN, Parfrey PS, Sarnak MJ *et al.* Clinical epidemiology of cardiovascular disease in chronic renal disease. *Am J Kidney Dis* 1998;**32**(suppl 3):112.

35 Wolfe RA, Port FK, Webb RL *et al.* Annual data report of the United States renal data system VI: causes of death. *Am J Kidney Dis* 1998;**32**(Suppl):S81.

36 Krumholz HM, Chen J, Wang Y *et al.* Comparing AMI mortality among hospitals in patients 65 years of age and older. *Circulation* 1999;**99**:2986.

37 Aronow WS, Ahn C, Mercando AD *et al.* Prevalence of coronary artery disease complex ventricular arrhythmias and silent myocardial ischemia and incidence of new coronary artery events in older persons with chronic renal insufficiency and with normal renal function. *Am J Cardiol* 2000;**86**:1142.

38 McLaurin MD, Apple FS, Voss EM *et al.* Cardiac troponin I, cardiac troponin T, and creatine kinase MB in dialysis patients without ischemic heart disease: evidence of cardiac troponin T expression in skeletal muscle. *Clin Chem* 1997;**43**:976.

39 Wayand D, Baum H, Schatzle G *et al.* Cardiac troponin T and I in end-stage renal failure. *Clin Chem* 2000;**46**:1345.

40 Freda BJ, Wilson Tang WH, van Lente F *et al.* Cardiac troponins in renal insufficiency. *J Am Coll Cardiol* 2002;**40**:2065.

41 Fredericks S, Chang R, Gregson H *et al.* Circulating cardiac troponin T in patients before and after renal transplantation. *Clin Chim Acta* 2001;**310**:199.

42 Apple FS, Murakami MM, Pearce LA *et al.* Predictive value of cardiac troponin I and T for subsequent death in end stage renal disease. *Circulation* 2002;**106**:2941.

43 Aviles RJ, Askari AT, Lindahl B *et al.* Troponin T levels in patients with acute coronary syndromes, with or without renal dysfunction. *N Engl J Med* 2002;**346**:2047.

44 de Lemos JA, Hillis LD. Diagnosis and management of coronary artery disease in patients with end stage renal disease on haemodialysis. *J Am Soc Nephrol* 1996;**7**:2044.

45 Shlipak MG, Heidenreich PA, Noguchi H *et al.* Association of renal insufficiency with treatment and outcomes after myocardial infarction in elderly patients. *Ann Intern Med* 2002;**137**:555.

46 Cadroy Y, Pourrat K, Baladre MF *et al.* Delayed elimination of enoxaparin in patients with chronic renal insufficiency. *Thromb Res* 1991;**63**:385.

47 Brophy DF, Wazny LD, Gehr TW *et al.* Pharmacokinetics of subcutaneous enoxaparin in end-stage renal disease. *Pharmacotherapy* 2001;**21**:169.

48 Becker RC, Spencer FA, Gibson M *et al.* Influence of patient characteristics and renal function on factor Xa inhibition pharmacokinetics and pharmacodynamics after enoxaparin administration in non-ST-segment elevation acute coronary syndromes. *Am Heart J* 2002;**143**:753.

49 Spinler SA, Inverso SM, Cohen M *et al.* Safety and efficacy of unfractionated heparin versus enoxaparin in patients who are obese and patients with severe renal impairment: analysis from ESSENCE and TIMI 11B studies. *Am Heart J* 2003;**146**:33.

50 Collet JP, Montalescot G, Choussat R *et al.* Enoxaparin in unstable angina patients with renal failure. *Int J Cardiol* 2001;**80**:81.

51 Choussat R, Montalescot G, Collet JP *et al.* A unique, low dose of intravenous enoxaparin in elective percutaneous coronary intervention. *J Am Coll Cardiol* 2002;**40**:1943.

52 Gerlach AT, Pickworth KK, Seth SK *et al.* Enoxaparin and bleeding complications: a review in patients with and without renal insufficiency. *Pharmacotherapy* 2000;**20**:771.

53 Freeman RV, Mehta RH, Al Badr W *et al.* Influence of concurrent renal dysfunction on outcomes of patients with acute coronary syndromes and implications of the use of glycoprotein IIb/IIIa inhibitors. *J Am Coll Cardiol* 2003;**41**:718.

54 Januzzi JL, Snapinn SM, DiBattiste PM *et al.* Benefits and safety of tirofiban among acute coronary syndrome patients with mild to moderate renal insufficiency, results from the PRISM-PLUS trial. *Circulation* 2002;**105**:2361.

55 Reddan DN, Szczech LA, Tuttle RH *et al.* Chronic kidney disease, mortality and treatment strategies among patients with clinically significant coronary artery disease. *J Am Soc Nephrol* 2003;**14**:2373.

56 Reddan DN, Szczech LA, Bhapkar MV *et al.* Renal function, concomitant medication use and outcomes following acute coronary syndromes. *Nephrol Dial Transplant* 2005;**20**: 2105.

57 Karavidas AJ, Vrachatis AD, Alpert MA *et al.* Relation of troponin T release kinetics to long-term clinical outcome in patients with acute ST segment elevation myocardial infarction treated with a percutaneous intervention. *Catheter Cardiovasc Interv* 2002;**56**:312.

58 Stubbs P, Collinson P, Moseley D *et al.* Prognostic significance of admission troponin T concentrations in patients with myocardial infarction. *Circulation* 1996;**94**:1291.

59 Tanasijevic MJ, Cannon CP, Antman EM *et al.* Myoglobin, creatine kinase-MB and cardiac troponin I 60 minute ratios predict infarct-related artery patency after thrombolysis for acute myocardial infarction: results from the thrombolysis in myocardial infarction study (TIMI) 10B. *J Am Coll Cardiol* 1999;**34**:739.

60 Matetzky S, Sharir T, Domingo M *et al.* Elevated troponin I level on admission is associated with adverse outcome of primary angioplasty in acute myocardial infarction. *Circulation* 2000;**102**:1611.

61 Newby LK, Christenson RH, Ohman EM *et al.*, for the The GUSTO IIa Investigators. Value of serial troponin T measures for early and late risk stratification in patients with acute coronary syndromes. *Circulation* 1998;**98**:1853.

62 Giannitsis E, Muller-Bardordd M, Lahrke S *et al.* Admission troponin T level predicts clinical outcomes, TIMI flow and myocardial tissue perfusion after primary percutaneous intervention for acute ST-segment elevation myocardial infarction. *Circulation* 2001;**104**:630.

63 Kurowski V, Hartmann F, Killermann DP. Prognostic significance of admission cardiac troponin T in patients treated successfully with direct percutaneous interventions for acute ST-segment elevation myocardial infarction. *Crit Care Med* 2002;**30**:2229.

64 Ohlmann P, Monassier J, Michotey MO *et al.* Troponin I concentrations following primary percutaneous coronary intervention preduct large infarct size and left ventrial dysfunction in patients with ST-segment elevation acute myocardial infarction. *Atherosclerosis* 200;**168**:181.

65 Antman EM, Anbe DT, Armstrong PW *et al.* ACC/AHA guidelines for the management of patients with ST-elevation myocardial infarction: executive summary. A report of the American College of Cardiology/American Heart Association Task Force on practice guidelines. *J Am Coll Cardiol* 2004;**44**:671.

66 Antman EM, Giugliano RP, Gibson CM *et al.* Abciximab facilitates the rate and extent of thrombolysis: results of the TIMI 14 trial. *Circulation* 1999;**99**:2720.

67 Topol EJ, Califf RM, van de Werf F *et al.* Reperfusion therapy for AMI with fibrinolytic therapy or combination reduced fibrinolytic therapy with platelet GP IIb/IIIa inhibition: results of the GUSTO V trial. *Lancet* 2001;**357**:1905.

68 Montalescot G, Varragan P, Wittenberg O *et al.* Platelet GP IIb/IIIa inhibition with coronary stenting following AMI: results of the ADMIRAL trial. *N Engl J Med* 2001;**344**:1895.

69 Montalescot G, Borentain M, Payot L *et al.* Early vs. late administration of glycoprotein IIb/IIIa inhibitors in primary percutaneous coronary intervention of acute ST-segment elevation myocardial infarction. *JAMA* 2004;**292**:362.

70 Sabatine MS, Cannon CP, Gibson CM *et al.* Addition of clopidogrel to aspirin and fibrinolytic therapy for myocardial infarction with ST-segment elevation: the CLARITY-TIMI 28 study. *N Engl J Med* 2005;**352**:1179.

71 COMMIT collaborative group. Addition of clopidogrel to aspirin in 45 852 patients with acute myocardial infarction: randomised placebo-controlled trial. *Lancet* 2005;**366**:1607.

72 Sabatine MS, Cannon CP, Gibson CM *et al.* Effect of clopidogrel pretreatment before percutaneous intervention in patients with ST-elevation myocardial infarction treated with fibrinolytics: the PCI-CLARITY study. *JAMA* 2005;**294**:1224.

73 ASSENT-3 Investigators. Efficacy and safety of tenecteplast in combination with enoxaparin, abciximab, or unfractionated heparin: the ASSENT-3 randomized trial in acute myocardial infarction. *Lancet* 2001;**358**:605.

74 Antman EM, Morrow DA, McCabe CH *et al.* Enoxaparin versus unfractionated heparin as antithrombin therapy in patients receiving fibrinolysis for ST elevation MIL design and rationale for the enoxaparin and thrombolysis reperfusion for acute myocardial infarction treatment (ExTRACT-TIMI 25) study. *Am Heart J* 2005;**149**:217.

CHAPTER 4

Ischemic heart disease in the absence of overt coronary artery disease

Allan S. Jaffe

Introduction

The use of new, sensitive, and specific cardiac markers, i.e., the troponins, has caused the need to reassess our ideas concerning ischemic heart disease. It is becoming increasingly clear that what we consider ischemia, which by definition is "the inability of myocardial oxygen supply to keep track with myocardial oxygen demand," can occur even in the absence of overt epicardial coronary artery disease. Sometimes this is due to a coronary abnormality and sometimes due to increased myocardial demand that even normal coronary responses cannot overcome. Often some degree of necrosis is associated with such syndromes. Thus, in the patient who appears to have acute ischemic heart disease, consideration of other mechanisms other than solely epicardial disease is appropriate. In addition, it is now clear that the coronary angiogram itself is far from a perfect tool [1]. What sorts of abnormalities should we consider?
1 The epicardial coronary artery disease could be missed or underestimated.
2 There could be alterations in coronary vasomotion that changes the severity of a given epicardial coronary lesion.
3 There could be endothelial dysfunction without any detectable epicardial coronary abnormalities.
4 There could be small vessel involvement.
5 There could be normal coronary arteries in a circumstance where myocardial oxygen demand is extraordinarily high.
All of these mechanisms have been suggested and now complicate the management of patients with presumed ischemic heart disease. Some of these are likely why in TACTICS-TIMI 18 (Fig. 4.1), patients who presented with an elevated troponin and chest pain suggestive of acute coronary syndromes but normal or near-normal epicardial coronary arteries had an adverse prognosis compared to individuals who had normal troponins in the absence of epicardial coronary disease. Obviously, all the elevations may not have been due to coronary disease but having an elevated troponin absent evidence of epicardial coronary disease was as adverse prognostically as the mere presence of coronary artery disease itself. We will discuss as we look at cases how such abnormalities might occur but they become important today in interpreting biomarkers in the context of a presumed ischemic presentation.

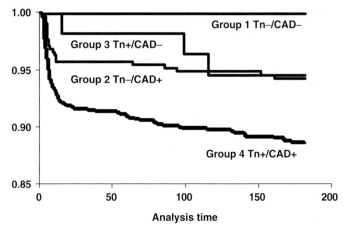

Figure 4.1 Events in patients with elevated troponin with and without coronary artery disease and those with normal troponins with and without coronary artery disease who present with acute coronary syndromes. Note increased number of events in patients with elevated troponins even with apparently normal coronary arteries. (Reproduced with permission from Ref. [2].)

Case 1

A 51-year-old woman who had a history of mild hypertension and mild hyperlipidemia was admitted with chest discomfort. She had been treated for hyperlipidemia which had been well controlled, but had been resistant to taking medications for hypertension. She was an exerciser who had a high-exercise tolerance. She denied any cardiopulmonary symptoms until the day of admission when she had substernal chest discomfort that lasted 2 hours. It radiated to her neck and transiently was associated with sweating. Her physical examination was unremarkable without hypertension on admission. Her electrocardiogram (ECG) revealed minor (<1 mm) lateral ST–T wave changes. Her troponin on admission was mildly elevated at 0.04 ng/mL and progressively rose to 0.8 ng/mL despite treatment with aspirin, IIB/IIIA antagonists, β-blockers, and nitroglycerin. She had a transthoracic echocardiogram that was read as totally unremarkable. Subsequently, she underwent cardiac catheterization and was shown to have "normal" coronary arteries. The question was what then was the etiology of her elevated troponins and chest pain. Despite the fact that she was not short of breath nor hypoxic, she underwent computed tomographic (CT) imaging to rule out pulmonary embolism, which was totally normal. Because the lateral ST–T wave changes the elevated troponin, a diagnosis of myocarditis was considered since involvement of the lateral wall is characteristic [2]. For this reason and because the suspicion of coronary ischemia was high clinically, she underwent magnetic resonance imaging (MRI). MRI with gadolinium demonstrated a small subendocardial area of delayed hyperenhancement in the inferior lateral wall indicative of a small area of focal injury (Fig. 4.2). She subsequently developed ventricular tachycardia but was

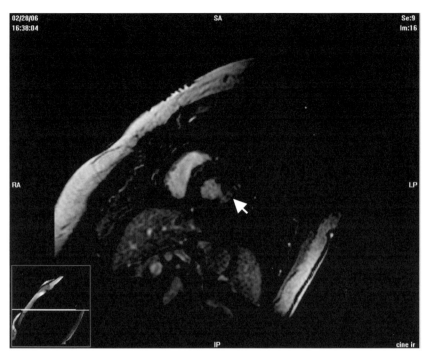

Figure 4.2 MRI in patient described in the text. Note area of hyperenhancement.

otherwise pain-free. She was treated with β-blocker and was discharged home on a statin and β-blocker. Subsequently, she has done well without recurrent chest discomfort. During follow-up, she has been able to continue to exercise for 30–45 minutes, although she is unhappy with the treatment with β-blocker, which keeps her from getting her heart rate higher and truncates her exercise tolerance. Nonetheless, she has continued to do well without recurrent chest discomfort.

Discussion of Case 1

The issue here is a complicated one. It is unclear what caused the minor amount of cardiac damage this woman suffered, but she is one of several such cases this investigator has observed just like this. She presented with chest pain, classic for angina, minor ECG changes, and elevated biomarkers, which met criteria for the diagnosis of myocardial infarction. We cannot exclude myocarditis in this woman, but there was very little else in her history or her subsequent course to confirm that, and classically, the changes on MRI seen with myocarditis involve the epicardium. Another, perhaps more attractive, possibility is that there were other mechanisms within her coronary vasculature to explain the focal cardiac damage that occurred. These could involve several different potential etiologies.

The first could be that since she was treated overnight with heparin and IIB/IIIA antagonists, by the time of angiography 12–18 hours later, evidence of thrombotic coronary artery occlusion, which may have been present acutely, may have resolved. This is certainly a possibility that cannot be totally excluded and would fit with early studies documenting patients with acute infarction and normal coronary arteries [3]. However, there was no overt lesion that was discernible. This, of course, does not mean that such a lesion was not present, but it certainly makes it somewhat less likely. However, coronary angiography clearly can miss areas of acute plaque rupture [1].

A second possibility is that the cause of the focal damage was related to alterations in coronary vasomotion. Coronary abnormalities and particularly those that are asymmetric can manifest substantial vasomotion [4]. Since the cross-sectional area of a pipe like the coronary artery is related to the square of the radius, it takes very little vasoconstriction to make a modest lesion, hemodynamically significant [5]. For example, it requires only a 10% change in the radius to change the cross-sectional area of a lesion from 47 to 76% if the entire lesion can respond with vasoconstriction. If only a percentage of a given lesion circumference can respond, then it may require a 60% lesion to constrict to make it clinically significant (i.e., 76%). In one small series of patients presenting with chest pain, those with elevated troponins manifested substantially more marked vasoconstriction in response to vasoconstrictors than those without elevations [6]. Thus in addition to missing a lesion angiographically, the lesion could be vasoactive, making a given lesion significant at one point in time but not at others.

Other possibilities include the possibility that focal necrosis could occur due to endothelial dysfunction alone whether in the epicardial coronary arteries or in the smaller vessels, which cannot be seen on the angiogram. In this particular individual endothelial function, studies were not done. However, the concept that endothelial function can be an abnormal absence of overt coronary artery disease and that patients can manifest vasoconstriction to substances that normally cause vasodilation is well established [7, 8]. It can lead to elevations in troponin and is associated with an adverse prognosis [8]. We do not totally understand the pathophysiology of these syndromes but there are starting to become ways to screen for it without doing invasive coronary studies. These approaches included forearm vascular reactivity studies [9] and tonometry of the upper extremity [10] with the presumption that abnormalities in those areas are frequently associated with abnormalities in the coronary vessels. This is at present a work in progress where additional research is necessary.

We do not know the exact etiology of this syndrome in this woman but her presentation was typical, her ECG suggestive, her markers classic, and her MR diagnostic. Several such patients have been observed lately. We cannot exclude the possibility that what was detected by MRI was an old insult and that this woman really had some other reason for her troponin elevations or that she has myocarditis that is atypical. Nonetheless, the clinical suspicion was high because of her classic presentation, and therefore, she was treated as if infarction was indeed present. It is suggested that when patients are so classic that one may not be able to rely solely on angiography for diagnosis.

Case 2

A 59-year-old woman presented with a 2- to 3-week history of chest pressure without associated symptoms and without relation to exertion. During the 24 hours prior to admission, the pain had became much more severe and radiated to her shoulders and across her chest, and she came to the emergency room. She had been a smoker, had taken estrogen replacement, and had mild hyperlipidemia and a history of fibromyalgia. Her physical examination revealed a normal blood pressure, normal pulse, and a normal physical examination. Her ECG is shown in Fig. 4.3 and showed only mild QT prolongation and T-wave inversion. Her cardiac troponin T (cTnT) on admission was 0.13 ng/mL, and she had mild hyperlipidemia and mild glucose intolerance. She was treated with aspirin, oxygen, IV nitroglycerin, metoprolol, heparin, morphine, Integrilin, and underwent urgent coronary angiography. Her coronary arteries were totally unremarkable; but after ventriculography was requested, subsequently, she was found to have a large akinetic apex suggestive of "apical ballooning." She was treated conservatively with β-blockers, antiischemics, and vasodilators. The antithrombotic therapy was stopped, and she gradually recovered without recrudescence.

Discussion of Case 2

This is becoming a more common circumstance. We now appreciate that women and particularly women who are older and most often postmenopausal can present after a traumatic, emotional, or physiological experience with chest pain, ST-segment elevation in the anterior leads, often with QT prolongation, modest elevations of biomarkers, and have a dyskinetic apex [11]. These individuals recover with supportive care. Right ventricular involvement can occur in a substantial number, and the dyskinetic area of the apex can be sufficiently extensive that patients end up with outflow tract obstruction. These patients respond extremely well to β-blockers. The etiology of this syndrome is unclear, but is associated with elevated troponins. There have been reports suggesting the syndrome is caused by increases in catecholamines, and it is argued that the cardiac apex may contain more β-receptors than other parts of the heart. Several studies have also shown that there is reduced blood flow to those areas despite normal coronary arteries. This has been confirmed with reduced thrombolysis in myocardial infarction (TIMI) flow grades as well as with echo and nuclear studies showing reduced perfusion in the areas that are hypocontractile. One must be careful since hypercontractile areas would be more perfused, and when one looks at perfusion in most circumstances, one is

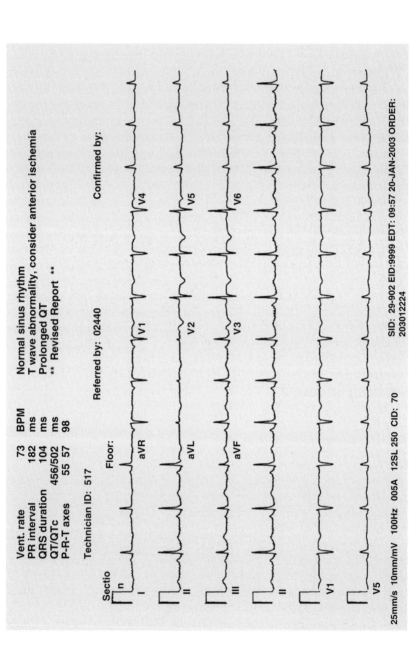

Vent. rate	73	BPM
PR interval	182	ms
QRS duration	104	ms
QT/QTc	456/502	ms
P-R-T axes	55 57	98

Normal sinus rhythm
T wave abnormality, consider anterior ischemia
Prolonged QT
** Revised Report **

Technician ID: 517

Referred by: 02440

Confirmed by:

Sectio

Floor:

n

I

II

III

II

V1

V5

aVR

aVL

aVF

V1

V2

V3

V4

V5

V6

25mm/s 10mm/mV 100Hz 005A 12SL 250 CID: 70

SID: 29-902 EID:9999 EDT: 09:57 20-JAN-2003 ORDER:
203012224

Figure 4.3

looking at relative perfusion; so increases in the hypercontractile areas and perhaps some downregulation in the hypocontractile areas could lead to apparent maldistribution of blood flow of a noncoronary etiology. Nonetheless, these findings have led to the suggestion that some patients may have small vessel disease as the potential etiology of their clinical syndrome of apical ballooning. This is a syndrome which again is associated with elevated troponins and needs to be kept in mind when patients present with apparent acute ischemia and normal coronary arteries.

Case 3

An 85-year-old woman with a long history of aortic stenosis, who had been followed for many years, presented with chest discomfort. She had not previously had syncope, congestive heart failure, nor angina, although in the past year, her degree of aortic stenosis had increased to significant range with a calculated valve area of 0.85 cm/m^2. She presented on the day of admission with chest discomfort typical of ischemic heart disease, mild hypotension, and shortness of breath. By the time she got to the emergency department, her chest pain syndrome had resolved and her ECG simply showed only left ventricular hypertrophy with ST–T wave changes. Her initial cTnT was less than 0.01 ng/mL but over the next 12 hours rose to as high as 0.68 ng/mL. Her physical examination was relatively unremarkable with a normal blood pressure, with a slightly slowed carotid with a transmitted murmur to the neck that was typical of the murmur of aortic stenosis in the elderly. Subsequently, cardiac catheterization revealed severe aortic stenosis with a gradient of 74 and a valve area of 0.77 cm/m^2 and normal coronary arteries.

Discussion of Case 3

This is a common situation where troponin can be elevated. Patients who have left ventricular hypertrophy are at risk for "supply–demand" ischemia even in the absence of overt coronary disease due to what some have called a "vulnerable subendocardium." Very often, coronary disease complicates aortic stenosis since they have common predictive features and can exacerbate this imbalance; but independent of that, the supply–demand relationships of the subendocardium can lead to ischemia. This is in large part because perfusion from the vessels in the subendocardium is dependent on intracavitary wall stress, which is increased in patients with decompensated aortic stenosis. In addition, there are fewer vessels per gram of myocardium in hypertrophied myocardium. Landmark work years ago by Buckberg and associates [12] has shown that increases in myocardial work as measured by the systolic time pressure index go up markedly and the diastolic time pressure index, a relative measure of perfusion, goes down, leading to ratios between these measures of supply and demand that can be associated with increased lactate production and ischemia. Aortic stenosis provides the model for this situation but the pathophysiology may be much more wide spread. This mechanism is likely the etiology of ischemia/injury and elevated troponins not only with aortic stenosis but with subaortic stenosis, hypertrophic cardiomyopathy, and perhaps in patients with severe hypertension with or without complicating arrhythmias. It is often difficult to tell why a particular patient may have an elevated troponin, say with hypotension, hypertension, or with arrhythmias, but one possibility could involve this mechanism of subendocardial ischemia. The importance of it clinically is that one needs to at least consider that as a possibility and then investigate the underlying etiology. If it is hypertrophic cardiomyopathy, treatment may require β-blockers. If it is aortic stenosis, it may well be surgical disease, and if it is hypo- or hypertension, it may relate to the better control of blood pressure and obviation of abnormalities in diastolic function. Nonetheless, this mechanism may undergird a substantial percentage of elevations of troponin due to ischemia in the absence of overt coronary artery disease.

References

1 Topol EJ, Nissen SE. Our preoccupation with coronary luminology. The dissociation between clinical and angiographic findings in ischemic heart disease. *Circulation* 1995;**92**: 2333–2342.

2 Abdel-Aty H, Boye P, Zagrosek A *et al*. Diagnostic performance of cardiovascular magnetic resonance in patients with suspected acute myocarditis: comparison of different approaches. *J Am Coll Cardiol* 2005;**45**:1815–1822.

3 Ammann P, Marschall S, Kraus M *et al*. Characteristics and prognosis of myocardial infarction in patients with normal coronary arteries. *Chest* 2000;**117**(2):333–338.

4 Yamagishi M, Nissen SE, Booth DC *et al*. Coronary reactivity to nitroglycerin: intravascular ultrasound evidence for the importance of plaque distribution. *J Am Coll Cardiol* 1995;**25**:224–230.

5 Brown BG, Bolson EL, Dodge HT. Dynamic mechanisms in human coronary stenosis. *Circulation* 1984;**70**:917–922.

6 Wang CH, Kuo LT, Hung MJ, Cherng WJ. Coronary vasospasm as a possible cause of elevated cardiac troponin I in patients with acute coronary syndrome and insignificant coronary artery disease. *Am Heart J* 2002;**44**:275–281.

7 Behrendt D, Ganz P. Endothelial function. From vascular biology to clinical applications. *Am J Cardiol* 2002;**90**(10C):40L–48L.

8 Lerman A, Zeiher AM. Endothelial function: cardiac events. *Circulation* 2005;**111**(3):363–368.

9 Anderson TJ, Gerhard MD, Meredith IT *et al*. Systemic nature of endothelial dysfunction in atherosclerosis. *Am J Cardiol* 1995;**75**:71B–74B.

10 Nigam A, Mitchell GF, Lambert J, Tardif JC. Relation between conduit vessel stiffness (assessed by tonometry) and endothelial function (assessed by flow-mediated dilatation) in patients with and without coronary heart disease. *Am J Cardiol* 2003;**92**:395–399.

11 Bybee KA, Prasad A, Barsness GW *et al*. Clinical characteristics and thrombolysis in myocardial infarction frame counts in women with transient left ventricular apical ballooning syndrome. *Am J Cardiol* 2004;**94**(3):343–346.

12 Hoffman JI, Buckberg GD. Pathophysiology of subendocardial ischaemia. *BMJ* 1975;**1**:76–79.

CHAPTER 5

So you think you have a "false-positive" troponin?

Jesse E. Adams

Introduction

Since the original observation in 1954 by Karmen *et al.* [1] of elevations of serum glutamic oxaloacetic transaminase in the circulation of patients who have suffered a myocardial infarction, markers of cardiac injury have become pivotal in guiding the evaluation and treatment of patients with diverse medical conditions. Over the last decade, utilization of measurement of serial levels of cardiac troponins (cTn) has supplanted measurement of levels of the MB fraction of creatine kinase (MB-CK) as the blood-based test of choice for diagnosis of myocardial infarction, due to both superior sensitivity and specificity for cardiac cellular necrosis. This evolution to a troponin standard as the preferred biomarker for the detection of myocardial necrosis was codified by a joint statement from the European Society of Cardiology and the American College of Cardiology in October of 2001 [2, 3].

A not so uncommon concern raised by clinicians regarding use of troponin proteins is the uncertainty if a particular patient has an elevation that is felt to be falsely positive. We should state at the outset that "false-positive" troponin values are quite rare, and it must be understood that usually the elevation of troponin protein is correctly indicating myocardial necrosis. In situations in which a potential false-positive troponin result is being considered, it usually is due to either greater sensitivity of the troponin testing when compared to the sensitivity of the alternative diagnostic test, occurs when a patient has a disease process that results in cardiac injury that does not require coronary artery disease, or can occur due to analytic issues that result in a false determination of the presence of troponin protein (Table 5.1).

Often the explanation of the apparent discrepancy between the results of troponin levels and other diagnostic testing lies in the relative superior sensitivity of cTn testing for small degrees of cardiac injury when compared to echocardiography, stress testing, or cardiac catheterization. Additionally, it must be appreciated that there are diverse disease processes that have been found to result in myocardial cell death that do not involve underlying coronary disease; a partial list is provided in Table 5.2, and many of these specific entities are discussed in greater detail in the following chapters [4, 5].

1 Troponin assay is more sensitive than the other diagnostic test
2 Myocardial cell death has occurred but not due to coronary artery disease
3 An analytic false-positive troponin result has occurred

A brief review of myocardial ischemia and necrosis pertinent to clinical practice

The spectrum of myocardial ischemia and necrosis as it applies to the clinical presentation of patients with coronary atherosclerotic disease has often been presented and will only be briefly reviewed here. Clinically, patients with atherosclerotic coronary artery disease are usually classified as having stable angina, unstable angina, non-Q-wave myocardial infarction, or Q-wave myocardial infarction. Two biologic transition points are of critical importance: first, an episode of plaque rupture, which leads to the transition from stable to unstable angina; and secondly, the onset of irreversible myocardial cellular necrosis, which signals the transition from unstable angina to myocardial infarction. It does not appear that plaque rupture will inevitably lead to the development of the clinical presentation of acute coronary syndrome; many patients have repeated episodes of plaque rupture before they transition to unstable angina from stable angina pectoris [6]. It has been found that patients who present for elective catheter-based interventions have areas of plaque rupture and ulceration independent from the anticipated site of intervention [7]. Also, intravascular ultrasound studies have shown that patients who present to the emergency department with acute coronary syndrome (ACS) will often have multiple sites of plaque rupture distant from the "infarct-related vessel" [8, 9]. Additionally, there is evidence to suggest that many patients that we classify as having unstable angina may have small amounts of myocardial cellular necrosis below the current detectability of our assays. Conceptually,

Table 5.2 Potential etiologies of myocardial injury and troponin elevations.

- Thrombotic occlusion of coronary arteries
- Cardiac contusion
- Anthracycline cardiac toxicity
- Pulmonary embolism
- Electrical shock
- Synchronized cardioversion
- Ablation therapy
- Cardiac surgery
- Ethenol septal ablation
- Thyrotoxicosis
- Pheochromocytoma
- Congestive heart failure
- Cocaine

the transition from "unstable angina" to "non-ST-segment elevation myocardial infarction" should occur when irreversible injury occurs to one cell. Our current troponin assays do not have this degree of sensitivity. However, progressive improvement in the available troponin assays has led to an increasing prevalence of those diagnosed with cardiac injury among those patients who present with ACS, just as occurred during the transition from a less sensitive marker (MB-CK) to troponin, increasing the clinician's ability to detect finer degrees of cardiac injury, which still have powerful prognostic significance [10, 11].

Once irreversible injury to cardiac cells occurs, levels of cTn predictably increase in the circulation with a typical delay of 6 hours. There is no evidence that levels of cTn become detectable in the absence of myocardial cell death. The cTnT molecule is usually released by itself, while the cTnI and cTnC molecules are most often released as a dimer, but both provide analogous clinical information in the majority of patients. Substantial modification of the troponin complex occurs prior to release from the cardiac cell, which at this time is not clinically useful but may allow for the development of future analytic assays that would further improve their diagnostic performance.

Case 1

A 56-year-old male comes to the emergency room with a complaint of indigestion that occurred shortly returning home after judging a chili cook-off. The epigastric pain occurred approximately 3 hours prior to presentation and lasted about 15–20 minutes. He has no history of heart disease, but he does have a brother who had a myocardial infarction 2 years prior. He is overweight with a body mass index of 28, has hypertension, and "borderline" diabetes mellitus. He does not know his cholesterol.

On arrival in the emergency room he is in no distress. He related the pain had been in his epigastrium, with no radiation, no associated nausea or diaphoresis, no acid taste in his mouth, and went away shortly after he sat down and had a glass of water. He has a history of gastroesophogeal reflux disease, and states that he did not want to come to the emergency room but that his wife insisted. His initial electrocardiogram (ECG) shows mild T-wave flattening in the lateral leads along with voltage criteria for left ventricular hypertrophy. Laboratory data were unremarkable except for a level of cTnT of 0.14 ng/mL (10% CV cutpoint < 0.1 ng/mL). A repeat level of cTnT 4 hours later was 0.19 ng/mL, while the next morning it was 0.12 ng/mL. His ECG the next morning was unchanged from that obtained on admission.

It was decided to take the patient to the cardiac catheterization laboratory due to his having "ruled in" for myocardial infarction by serial levels of troponin. However, at cardiac catheterization only "mild disease" was found in the circumflex and left anterior descending coronary arteries, and there was concern on the part of the invasive cardiologist as to whether the troponin levels were correct.

Discussion of Case 1

This is one of the most common situations that result in diagnostic insecurity on the part of clinicians—a patient whose story is not diagnostic with modest elevations of troponin protein but no corroboratory evidence on ECG, stress test, and/or cardiac catheterization. Currently, patients who present to the emergency department with complaints of chest discomfort are evaluated with a series of other diagnostic tests, often with a protocol-driven approach. After the initial diagnostic paradigm is utilized (preferably utilizing serial measurements of cardiac biomarkers and ECGs, with a concurrent assessment of the patients' pretest likelihood of disease) many patients will subsequently undergo either stress testing and/or coronary angiography. Discordant results between troponin testing and further diagnostic testing, especially with troponin elevations not corroborated by "significant" abnormalities on stress testing, echocardiography, and/or cardiac catheterization, have frequently resulted in challenges to the veracity of the diagnostic information provided by troponin testing. To address this requires in part a cogent understanding of the limitations of both stress testing and cardiac catheterization as well as issues particular to troponin assays.

A full review of stress testing is beyond the scope of this chapter or text, but suffice it to say that stress testing can be successfully performed via many different protocols. All patients who undergo stress testing will have electrocardiographic monitoring during the procedure. Attention will be paid to the presence or absence of ST-segment changes, which can indicate inducible cardiac ischemia. Unfortunately, the sensitivity and specificity of a stress ECG is incompletely robust for the detection of coronary artery disease. The sensitivity of a stress ECG is in the neighborhood of 60–65%, with a specificity for the detection of a 50% stenosis or greater on concurrent cardiac catheterization of 60–65%. Imaging modalities such as nuclear imaging or echocardiographic visualization are routinely utilized, which improve the sensitivity and specificity for the detection of cardiac disease. Conjoint imaging with echocardiographic visualization can be performed with both exercise stress and pharmacologic studies. The addition of nuclear imaging or echocardiographic imaging to a stress ECG evaluation improves both the sensitivity and specificity for the detection of coronary artery disease and subsequent cardiovascular risk. However, even with the addition of nuclear imaging or echocardiographic visualization the diagnostic performance of published studies have documented sensitivities and specificities of 80–85% for the detection of coronary artery disease, usually defined as stenosis of one or more coronary arteries greater than 50% [12, 13]. Thus, with sensitivities of this range, it must be *expected* that at times there will be patients who have had myocardial infarctions that will not be detected by stress testing. Most clinicians are aware and accept these limitations of stress testing and are not concerned when there is discordance between the results of the stress test and troponin values.

However, discordance between the results of cardiac catheterization and troponin testing is another issue. Clinicians at time have been quite concerned when there is discordance between troponin testing and cardiac catheterization, with troponin elevations but a lack of high-grade disease documented on the angiogram. This is both due to the fact that cardiac catheterization is frequently performed (rather than stress testing) when troponin elevations are found and cardiac catheterization is often viewed as the "gold standard" for the detection of atherosclerotic disease. A cardiac catheterization is performed via the introduction of radiopaque contrast into each of the epicardial coronary arteries, producing a "lumenogram" that can demonstrate obstruction or atherosclerotic impingement on the coronary lumen. While cardiac catheterization is often viewed as the gold standard, it has several important limitations, especially when applied to a population of patients who present with ACS. First and foremost, Topol and Nissen have described in great detail the limitations of a diagnostic cardiac catheterization for the detection of plaque rupture, intra-plaque hemorrhage, or plaque erosion [14]. It is rare in studies involving cardiac catheterization for these lesions to be detected. Yet intravascular ultrasound studies have consistently found that ruptured plaque is frequently present in patients who present with ACS [9, 15]. Plaque disruption is present not only in the "infarct-related" vessel, but in other locations within the epicardial coronary tree as well. Additionally, we know that patients who present with chest discomfort due to ACS frequently have thrombus formation at the site of plaque disruption. Thrombus can be missed by cardiac catheterization due to several reasons. First, the thrombus can be laminar and not visualized by the angiogram. Second, the thrombus can be within the plaque due to intra-plaque hemorrhage and not intralumenal, again not amenable to visualization by the angiogram. Third, our usual standard of care for patients with ACS includes rapid use of anticoagulant and antiplatelet strategies; any delay in performance of the cardiac angiogram will decrease the sensitivity for detection of the thrombus. All of these influences will decrease the sensitivity of cardiac catheterization to detect lesions in patients with ACS. A current appreciation of the complexity of the pathobiology of atherothrombosis and ACS requires an understanding (and ultimately detection) of the vessel wall pathology, and in this aspect both stress testing and cardiac catheterization are lacking. It should thus be anticipated by clinicians that patients with acute coronary syndromes would at times have cardiac catheterizations that would show a lack of high-grade stenosis.

This patient presented with a combination of risk factors for coronary artery disease and developed a rising and falling pattern of cTnT in the setting of chest discomfort. Thus, he meets the criteria set out in the 2001 definition for myocardial infarction; he should be viewed as having had a non-ST-segment myocardial infarction [2]. The lack of a "significant" abnormality demonstrated on cardiac catheterization is understandable in light of the above discussion; it is likely that had intravascular ultrasound been performed on this patient, an acute plaque rupture would have been demonstrated. Appropriate medical therapy should be instituted and aggressive risk factor modification is indicated.

Case 2

A 62-year-old female with a history of "mild" coronary arterial disease treated with medical therapy was an unrestrained driver in a two-car collision and was brought to the emergency room. She was conscious and had a blood pressure 136/68 mm Hg, heart rate 96 beats/min, and a respiratory rate 18 breaths/min. She complained of pain in her chest and left wrist. Radiography found a left wrist fracture as well as a fracture of the sternum. No other injuries were present. An ECG showed normal sinus rhythm with a left anterior fascicular block and T-wave flattening in the lateral leads. Laboratory data on arrival were entirely normal; the troponin I value was <0.03 ng/mL (normal <0.03 ng/mL). The patient was admitted for treatment of her injuries and observation. A troponin level obtained 6 hours later was elevated at 1.78 ng/mL and the next morning had risen to 2.2 ng/mL. An echocardiogram was performed and showed a mildly enlarged right ventricle with free wall hypokinesis, trace tricuspid regurgitation with a calculated pulmonary arterial pressure of 22 mm Hg, normal left ventricular size and function with an ejection fraction of 65%, and normal valvular structure and function. The patient continued to complain of chest pain. Because of her history of coronary arterial disease, the positive troponin values, and the uncertainty as to whether her chest pain was due to angina or the sternal fracture, the patient was taken to the cardiac catheterization laboratory where no change in her mild coronary artery disease was found.

Discussion of Case 2

This is a classic case of a patient with a cardiac contusion and represents one of the many situations where myocardial cell death is understood to occur but in which no evidence of a culprit lesion in the coronary anatomy is expected to be found. A fundamental issue that can at times obfuscate the clinical interpretation of troponin elevations is the fact that levels of cTn will increase after myocardial cellular injury regardless of the cause. Many disease states not associated with myocardial infarction have been found to have small degrees of cardiac injury and can be associated with elevations of troponin proteins (see Table 5.1). Troponin elevations can be seen in these illnesses for several reasons, which can occur concomitantly. First, the disease process can directly cause damage to the cardiac myocytes as is the case here. Secondly, some illnesses can cause a sufficiently prolonged supply–demand mismatch to result in irreversible cardiac injury. Finally, if a patient has underlying atherosclerotic disease, there is less cardiac circulatory reserve and a myocardial infarction can occur in the setting of increased myocardial oxygenation demand during acute systemic illness. Thus, troponin elevations in situations such as sepsis, pulmonary embolism, cardiac contusion, and the like can cause diagnostic difficulties if the clinician does not understand the mechanism of troponin release and the contemporary understanding of these situations.

Cardiac contusion occurs due to blunt trauma that produces concussive injury to the myocardium. Generally, this is due to blunt trauma to the anterior chest wall and results in injury to the right ventricle (due to compressive deceleration injury against the sternum). In cardiac contusion, it has been appreciated for many years that damage to the myocardium can occur and that cardiac contusion can complicate the immediate care of these patients. Previous work with MB-CK demonstrated that accurate detection with this analyte was compromised by the interference with skeletal muscle injury [16, 17]. Animal models have shown that damage to the heart by direct blunt trauma in experimental models results in cardiac cell death and subsequent release of cTn into the circulation [18]. Interestingly, small amounts of cardiac injury have been shown to result in transient elevations of cTn, while more significant injury results in prolonged elevations of cTn as seen in patients with acute myocardial infarction [19]. In addition, animal models have demonstrated that the degree of elevation of cTnI and cTnT found after graded cardiac contusion correlates with the delivered force and the amount of injury documented on histologic examination [20]. Levels of cTnI have been measured in patients who present with blunt chest wall trauma; elevations of cTn have been found to correlate with those patients more likely to have deleterious clinical events, while those patients without troponin elevations by 6 hours are unlikely to have clinically significant cardiac contusion or future cardiac events [21]. Indeed, investigators have stressed the usefulness of troponin testing in conjunction with electrocardiography for the exclusion of cardiac contusion, obviating the need for further testing (specifically avoiding the need for subsequent echocardiography) [22]. Additionally, levels of cTn appear to be more sensitive for the detection of cardiac injury than biplane transesophageal echocardiography; all patients with wall motion abnormalities detected by biplane transesophageal echocardiography have been found to have elevations of troponin, while lower degrees of troponin positivity are not found to correlate with detectable abnormalities on echocardiography [23]. It must be remembered, however, that echocardiographic visualization of the heart yields diagnostic information on injuries that may not be associated with troponin elevations.

Thus, this patient had elevations of cTn that correctly indicated damage to myocardium. However, this was not due to underlying atherosclerosis. Studies of patients with cardiac contusion find that the right ventricle is the most often affected ventricle (due to its location behind the sternum and deceleration injury to the right ventricle against the inside of the sternum). Additional pathologic studies on patients who have died of cardiac contusion have found pathologic evidence of direct injury as well as contraction band necrosis in the right ventricle with normal coronary anatomy and no atherosclerosis in the right coronary artery. Thus, clinicians should not be concerned with a disparity of troponin elevations and the presence of coronary artery disease, and should understand that elevations of troponin only indicate cardiac cell death without indicating a pathologic cause. The presence of elevations in troponin protein is indicative of increased short-term risk and the patient should be managed accordingly.

Case 3

A 29-year-old farmer presented to the emergency department with a complaint of chest pain. Upon questioning by the emergency department physician, the patient related that the pain was constant, had started over the weekend, and was worse when he lifted objects or raised his arms over his head. Additionally, the patient related that his wife had given him a new gym membership and he had lifted weights for the first time since he had graduated from college, yet had followed the same weight program that he had used when he played college football.

His physical examination was remarkable only for diffuse chest pain in the left pectoralis muscle. Pressure at this point or pushing with his left arm against resistance reproduced his pain. The patient had no cardiac history and no cardiac risk factors. The emergency room physician diagnosed the patient as having a muscle strain involving his left pectoralis muscle and prepared to discharge the patient with an appropriate therapy, but the nurse then reported that his level of cTnI (drawn on arrival per protocol in this patient with "chest pain") was elevated with a value of 1.4 ng/mL (10% CV cutpoint <0.03 ng/mL). An ECG was obtained and was normal, but because of the troponin elevation he was admitted for observation. His chest pain was relieved by local heat and Naprosyn. Subsequent ECGs remained normal; serial troponin I measurements obtained every 4 hours were 1.40 ng/mL, 1.38 ng/mL, 1.44 ng/mL, and 1.40 ng/mL. A repeat troponin performed 5 days later returned a value of 1.42 ng/mL. A measurement of cTnT was sent on the fourth sample and was undetectable.

Discussion of Case 3

In the first two cases, we discussed patients that had elevations of troponin in which the troponin measurements correctly indicated damage to myocardium, the first with acute coronary syndrome and the second with cardiac contusion. In this case, the patient has no symptoms that would indicate cardiac injury. Based on the clinical history provided, the patient's pretest likelihood of having coronary artery disease is low. When the patient presented to the emergency department with chest pain, he was felt to have chest wall pain. When the initial level of troponin returned with an elevated level, the patient was admitted overnight for monitoring and serial measurements of troponin. Once the levels of troponin returned with essentially identical results, the concern of the patient's clinicians for acute coronary syndrome decreased and the patient was discharged home. The patient had a later follow-up sample sent as well as the measurement for cTnT (since the hospital utilizes cTnI as the standard measurement) to confirm the presence of a false-positive troponin result.

Cardiac troponin assays are two-site "sandwich" assays with a "capture" antibody that captures the troponin molecule and fixes it to the analytic surface, and a separate "tag" antibody that serves as the detector [24]. Human antianimal antibodies can arise in a variety of situations and are seen in clinical practice as IgM, IgG, IgA, and occasionally IgE [25]. Often the term "heterophile antibodies" is used in this situation as the specific initial antibody challenge is usually not defined. False-positive troponin levels due to heterophile antibodies have been reported for every troponin assay; oftentimes a specific antibody will affect more than one analytic assay. Elevations of cTn due to heterophile antibodies should be considered when a patient presents with a troponin elevation that manifests a nonevolving pattern (there is a lack of the typical "rising and falling" pattern seen in patients who present with myocardial infarction). Obviously, consideration of a heterophile antibody causing a false measurement of cTn will only occur if serial measurements of troponin are routinely performed. The strategy, employed by some laboratories, of stopping collections of troponins in patients as soon as the first sample turns positive must be discouraged.

Once a false-positive troponin elevation is suspected, serial measurements beyond the usual 8–16 hours time frame should be obtained. Communication by the clinician with the laboratory is critical; the laboratorian can then employ several techniques to define if a heterophile antibody is present, often both by analyzing the sample with alternative troponin assays as well as by adding various human antianimal antibody blocking agents to the sample and then reanalyzing for the level of troponin present.

In this patient, the presence of a heterophile antibody was confirmed in the initial sample by the use of blocking agents; subsequent analysis showed the presence of a human antimouse antibody. The patient's occupation as a farmer may well have facilitated this antibody development. The patient was counseled as to the presence of this antibody and the effect that it would have on troponin testing for an undefined future period (as heterophile antibodies can persist for months or years). The patient was also given a card to carry in his wallet with this information, with the recommendation of initial laboratorian involvement if future troponin measurements were clinically necessary.

Conclusion

Clinicians are at times concerned that an elevated level of troponin in a particular patient is not correct. The most common occasions in which this occurs is in situations where the sensitivity of troponin proteins is greater than the other diagnostic test (including cardiolite stress tests, echocardiography, and diagnostic catheterization), other illness that results in myocardial cell death without requiring decreased myocardial blood supply, and analytic false positives (see Table 5.1). Usually a careful attention to the patient's history and pertinent pathophysiology, the pattern of the troponin elevations (rising and falling patterns that would be consistent with myocardial cell death versus persistent elevations or a single isolated marked elevation with otherwise normal values), and a determination of the patient's pretest likelihood of disease will usually resolve any questions. It must be remembered that in the majority of the time the results of troponin testing are providing robust prognostic information regarding the patient's status. It should be rare that with a consideration of the above issues that a clinician cannot comfortably resolve any questions regarding troponin results.

References

1 Karmen A, Wroblewski F, Ladue JS. Transaminase activity in human blood. *J Clin Invest* 1954;**34**:126–133.

2 Alpert JS, Thygesen K, Antman E, Bassand JP. Myocardial infarction redefined—a consensus document of the Joint European Society of Cardiology/American College of Cardiology Committee for the Redefinition of Myocardial Infarction. *J Am Coll Cardiol* 2000;**36**: 959–969.

3 Apple FS, Wu AH, Jaffe AS. European Society of Cardiology and American College of Cardiology guidelines for redefinition of myocardial infarction: how to use existing assays clinically and for clinical trials. *Am Heart J* December 2002;**144**(6):981–986.

4 Morrow DA. Cardiac-specific troponins beyond ischemic heart disease. In: AHB Wu, ed. *Cardiac Markers*, 2nd edn. Humana Press, Totowa, NJ, 2003:149–170.

5 Apple FS, Morrow DA. Cardiac troponins in conditions other than acute coronary syndromes. In: Morrow DA, ed. *Cardiovascular Biomarkers: Pathophysiology and Disease Management*. Humana Press, Totowa, NJ, 2006:139–159.

6 Van Belle E, Lablanche J-M, Bauters C, Renaud N, McFadden EP, Beertrand ME. Coronary angioscopic findings in the infarct-related artery within 1 month of acute myocardial infarction. Natural history and the affect of thrombolysis. *Circulation* 1998;**97**:26–33.

7 Schoenhagen P, Stone GW, Nissen SE *et al.* Coronary plaque morphology and frequency of ulceration distant from culprit lesions in patients with unstable and stable presentation. *Arterioscler Thromb Vasc Biol* October 1, 2003;**23**(10):1895–1900.

8 Kerensky RA, Wade M, Deedwania P *et al.*, for the Veterans Affairs Non-Q-Wave Infarction Strategies in Hospital (VANQWISH) Trial Investigators. Revisiting the culprit lesion in non-Q-wave myocardial infarction: results from the VANQWISH trial angiographic core laboratory. *J Am Coll Cardiol* 2002;**39**:1456–1463.

9 Goldstein JA, Demetriou D, Grines CL *et al.* Multiple complex coronary plaques in patients with acute myocardial infarction. *N Engl J Med* 2000;**343**:915–922.

10 Jaffe AS, Ravkilde J, Roberts R *et al.* It's time for a change to a troponin standard. *Circulation* 2000;**102**:1216–1220.

11 Morrow DA, Cannon CP, Rifai N *et al.* Ability of minor elevations of troponin I and T to predict benefit from an early invasive strategy in patients with unstable angina and non-ST elevation myocardial infarction. *JAMA* 2001;**286**:2405–2412.

12 Klocke FJ, Baird MG, Lorell BH *et al.*, for the ACC; AHA; ASE. ACC/AHA/ASNC guidelines for the clinical use of cardiac radionuclide imaging—executive summary: a report of the American College of Cardiology/American Heart Association Task Force on Practice

Guidelines (ACC/AHA/ASNC Committee to Revise the 1995 Guidelines for the Clinical Use of Cardiac Radionuclide Imaging). *J Am Coll Cardiol* October 1, 2003;**42**(7):1318–1333.

13 Cheitlin MD, Armstrong WF, Aurigemma GP *et al.*, for the ACC; AHA; ASE. ACC/AHA/ASE 2003 guideline update for the clinical application of echocardiography: summary article. A report of the American College of Cardiology/American Heart Association Task Force on Practice Guidelines (ACC/AHA/ASE Committee to Update the 1997 Guidelines for the Clinical Application of Echocardiography). *J Am Soc Echocardiogr* October 2003;**16**(10):1091–1110.

14 Topol EJ, Nissen SE. Our preoccupation with coronary lumenology; the dissociation between clinical and angiographic findings in ischemic heart disease. *Circulation* 1995;**92**: 2333–2342.

15 Asakura M, Ueda Y, Yamaguchi O *et al.* Extensive development of vulnerable plaques as a pan-coronary process in patients with myocardial infarction: an angioscopic study. *J Am Coll Cardiol* 2001;**37**:1284–1288.

16 Adams JE, Davila-Roman VG, Besey PQ, Blake DP, Ladenson JH, Jaffe AS. Improved detection of cardiac contusion with cardiac troponin I. *Am Heart J* 1996;**131**:308–312.

17 Swaanenburg JC, Klaase JM, DeJongste MJ *et al.* CKMB-activity and CKMB-mass as markers for the detection of myocardial contusion in patients who experienced blunt trauma. *Clin Chim Acta* 1998;**272**:171–181.

18 Meier R, van Griensven M, Pape HC, Krettek C, Chawda M, Seekamp A. Effects of cardiac contusion in isolated perfused hearts. *Shock* 2003;**19**:123–126.

19 Okubo N, Hombrouck C, Fornes P *et al.* Cardiac troponin I and myocardial contusion in the rabbit. *Anesthesiology* 2000;**93**:811–817.

20 Berttichant JP, Robert E, Polge A *et al.* Release kinetics of cardiac troponin I and cardiac troponin T in effluents from isolated perfused rabbit hearts after graded experimental myocardial contusion. *J Trauma* 1999;**47**:474–480.

21 Collins JN, Cole FJ, Weireter LJ, Biblet JL, Britt LD. The usefulness of serum troponin levels in evaluating cardiac injury. *Am Surg* 2001;**67**:821–825.

22 Velmahos GC, Karaiskakis M, Salim A *et al.* Normal electrocardiography and serum troponin I levels preclude the presence of clinically significant blunt cardiac injury. *J Trauma* 2003;**54**:45–50.

23 Mori F, Zuppiroli A, Ognibene A *et al.* Cardiac contusion in blunt chest wall trauma: a combined study of transesophogeal echocardiography and cardiac troponin I determination. *Ital Heart J* 2001;**2**:222–227.

24 Wu AHB. Analytic issues for the clinical use of cardiac troponin. In: Morrow DA, ed. *Cardiovascular Biomarkers: Pathophysiology and Disease Management*. Humana Press, Totowa, NJ, 2006:27–40.

25 Yeo K-TJ, Hoefner DM. Interferences in immunoassays for cardiac troponin. In: AHB Wu, ed. *Cardiac Markers*, 2nd ed. Humana Press, Totowa, NJ, 2003:187–197.

CHAPTER 6

Use of cardiac troponin in patients in non-ischemic pathologies and exposure to environmental toxins

Fred S. Apple

Case 1

A 16-year-old male with no previous history of coronary artery disease was found unconscious in a closed-door garage with the car engine running. The maximum time the patient could have been exposed to the exhaust fumes was 3 hours. When emergency personnel arrived, no gross trauma was identified. The patient was unresponsive to verbal stimuli, pupils were pinpoint and unreactive bilaterally, heart rate was tachycardic, decerebrate posturing was present, and Babinski signs were upgoing bilaterally. The patient was placed on 100% oxygen, transferred to the emergency department, sedated, and intubated. Carbon monoxide (hemoglobin) concentration at this time was 31% and the patient was metabolically acidotic. Chest X-ray showed no infiltrates or pneumothorax. The ECG showed nonspecific anterolateral ST–T abnormalities in leads I, a VL, and VW-V6. The patient was transferred to the hyperbaric chamber for two sessions of 90 minutes at 2.4 atm. Clinical neurologic assessment demonstrated diffuse anoxic metabolic encephalopathy, and a CT scan revealed diffuse decreased attenuation in white matter and globus pallidus consistent with CO poisoning. At presentation (see table), cTnI was within normal limits (<0.3 µg/L) but increased to 2.2 µg/L over time.

Post exposure (h)	Total CK (URL 300 U/L)	cTnI (URL < 0.3 µg/L)
3.5	3178	0.03
10.5	4013	1.7
16.5	4629	2.2
24.5	4332	1.9

Case 2

The patient, a 44-year-old male, is admitted to the hospital with a 2 week history of recurrent upper chest pain. The patient had been in excellent health, and is both a nonsmoker and a coffee drinker. He has a known history for 5 years of elevated total cholesterol, ranging from 230 to 260 mg/dL. He has been a jogger (20–30 miles per week) for 2–3 years, and has been training for his first marathon (26.2 miles). On the day prior to admission, he was running the Twin Cities Marathon, when at 22 miles he developed chest pain which forced him to stop and walk for 3–5 minutes during which time the pain resolved. He completed the run in 4 hours and 20 minutes, 45 minutes slower than anticipated. After the race he went home. On the day following the race, he was being seen in his doctor's office for his yearly routine scheduled physical, prior to leaving on a vacation. However, his ECG was normal, but he was admitted for a rule out MI (myocardial infarction) workup based on his symptoms of chest and elbow pain. During his 20 hours in the hospital, and although he was ruled out for an MI based on his ECG and normal echocardiogram, his cTnT values, increased above the 99th percentile (<0.01 ng/mL), were as follows: 0 hour at presentation 0.02 ng/mL, 6 hours 0.02 ng/mL, 12 hours 0.01 ng/mL. During this time his total CK values were 3520 U/L, 2220 U/L, and 1065 U/L, respectively. He was given the diagnosis of exertional strain of the heart post-extreme exercise (marathon race) and scheduled for a return visit for 6 months.

Case 3

A 43-year-old female with no past medical history of any pathology or drug or alcohol use is admitted 1.5 hours after acute chest pain at 2350 hours. Her presenting ECG shows an ST elevation with sinus tachycardia, with at rate at 165. While giving a history, she admits to snorting cocaine 2 hours prior to presentation, during which her acute onset of chest pain occurred almost immediately. She was emergently taken to the catherization laboratory, during which time her ECG normalized prior to angiography. At angiography none of her coronaries showed evidence of occlusion. The final diagnosis was MI secondary to cocaine induce vasospasm. The laboratory findings for her cardiac biomarkers were as follows.

Time (h)	Total CK (U/L)	cTnT (ng/mL)	CKMB (ng/mL)
Presentation	450	0.09	14.0
5.3	874	0.89	76.0
15.5	2516	4.89	221

Discussion of Cases 1, 2, and 3

We have learned a great deal over the past 6–10 years pertaining to the valuable role that cTnI and cTnT play in defining evidence of myocardial necrosis when increased above the 99th percentile reference limit [1–4]. Determining the pathologic etiologies responsible for cardiac troponin (cTnI or cTnT) increases can be frustrating for many clinicians in their attempt to properly interpret their clinical value. We now know that an acute MI is predicated on an increased cardiac troponin above the 99th percentile reference limit in the clinical setting of ischemia; with either a rising or fall pattern on serial samples obtained over a 6–12 hour time period after the index clinical event. Further, as the analytical quality of cardiac troponin assays have improved (i.e., second-, third-, and fourth-generation assays now measure values at <20 pg/mL), assays are detecting smaller and smaller amounts of myocardial cell necrosis; including patients with etiologies that are not ischemia and not acute coronary syndrome based. Table 6.1 is representative of a list of pathologies responsible for cardiac cell death resulting in increases of cTn that are not ACS. In addition, the newer generation assays demonstrate a clinical specificity of approximately 75–85% in patients presenting to rule out ACS and MI. This shows that 15–25 patients out of 100 who have an increased cTn above the 99th percentile reference limit do not have an MI, but need to be worked up for another clinical etiology. Further, as shown in Table 6.1, it is also well documented that in the large majority of non-ischemic causes for increased cardiac troponin, values are associated with adverse clinical outcomes. Therefore, the important clinical question regarding an increased cardiac troponin in a non-ischemic setting, where an MI

Table 6.1 Diagnostic pathologies associated with increased cardiac troponin concentrations without an ischemic presentation and in the absence of acute coronary syndromes.

1	Congestive heart failure*
2	Trauma, cardiac contusion
3	Cardioversion, electrical defibrillation
4	Pulmonary embolism, edema*
5	Sepsis, septic shock*
6	Myocarditis
7	Exercise, vital exhaustion
8	Stroke*
9	Non-cardiac, vascular surgery
10	End-stage renal disease*
11	Hypertension
12	Hypotension
13	Critically ill intensive care patients*
14	Aneurysmal subarachnoid hemorrhage
15	Drugs of abuse toxicity, including ethanol
16	Chemotherapy
17	Heart surgery, transplantation
18	Polymyositis, dermatomyositis
19	Cardiomyopathy
20	Rhabdomyolysis, trauma (non-chest)
21	Hematologic malignancies
22	Acute pericarditis
23	Amyloid cardiomyopathy
24	Idiopathic dilated cardiomyopathy
25	Neonates
26	Lung disease

*Literature evidence for role of cardiac troponin for risk stratification for short- and or long-term adverse outcomes.

is not in the differential, is when to decide to "chase" these values to provide appropriate clinical care for the patient.

The earliest report that identified hospitalized patients without acute MI that had increased cTnT concentrations was in 79 patients randomly sampled within 12 hours of admission from medical and surgical units [5]. cTnT increases ranged from 0.13 μg/L to as high as 7.8 μg/L (normal ≤ 0.1μg/L) in a varied group of pathologies, including lung cancer, drug overdoses, small bowel obstruction, stroke, end-stage renal disease, pneumonia, and scleroderma. Over the past 20 years since this report, numerous case reports and clinical studies have carefully demonstrated that cTnT and cTnI are the preferred specific biomarkers to detect myocardial injury [6] in the clinical setting of non-myocardial ischemic presentations. This chapter briefly reviews the literature for studies and case presentations of non-ischemic presentations that have documented increased cardiac troponins. Clinicians need to recognize that an increased cardiac troponin does not necessarily equate to acute MI and does not indicate a false positive finding. The challenge for a differential diagnosis rests in the understanding that cardiac troponin increases mean "think heart."

Miscellaneous pathologies

Cases of cTnI and/or cTnT increases have been reported in a wide variety of miscellaneous pathologies indicating myocardial injury secondary to the primary diagnosis. These include aneurysmal subarachnoid hemorrhage [7], polymyositis/dermatomyocytis [8], rhabdomyolysis/skeletal muscle injury not involving the chest [9], hematologic malignancies [10], acute pericarditis [11], and lobar lung disease [12]. In one of the most interesting observations reported, cTnI was preserved through time, with immunoreactivity found in mummified abdominal tissue from Horemkenesi, a craftsman excavating and decorating the tombs of the Pharaohs (c. 1050 BC), who died of a heart attack [13].

Drug-induced myocardial damage

Observations regarding cTn increases in (a) patients treated with certain types of antineoplastic agents, (b) patients presenting to hospitals following alcohol and drug abuse, and (c) therapeutic drug-induced cardiac toxicity have been reported [14]. Both acute (within hours) and chronic (days to weeks) myocardial toxicity effects (including ischemia, arrhythmias, myocarditis, pericarditis, cardiomyopathy, and MI) following dosing of the anthracyclines 5-fluorouracil, doxorubicin, and daunorubicin have resulted in both minimal and large cTnI increases. Reports have documented both a medication dose-dependent type of myocyte injury being responsible for troponin increases, even without electrocardiographic or echocardiographic findings. Numerous drugs of abuse have also been associated with increases of cTn, without evidence of ischemia. These include heavy alcohol consumption, cocaine and amphetamines, CO exposure, theophylline overdose, propofol, snake bites, and during treatment with fluvastatin [15–17].

Heart failure

Increased concentrations of cTnI and cTnT have been found in patients with congestive heart failure (CHF). CHF is a dynamic process with spontaneous, progressive severity, and is structurally characterized by cellular degeneration and multiple foci of myocardial cell death. The specific underlying mechanisms remain unclear. In the majority of HF patients studied, cardiac troponins were detected in patients with advanced CHF predominantly involving New York Heart Association (NYHA) III and IV classifications [18].

Trauma

Both cTnI and cTnT have been shown to be increased in trauma patients, especially following cardiac contusion. In the large majority of cardiac trauma patients studied, small to moderate increases in cTn are found, implying that the extent of injury is small in the majority of patients. Monitoring cTn was able to differentiate the majority of patients who demonstrated isolated increased CKMB values which were indicative of skeletal muscle damage. In one representative study of 44 blunt chest trauma patients, 37 of these trauma patients without cardiac contusion had CKMB increases without cTnI increases [19]. In the six patients with evidence of cardiac injury by echocardiography, all six had increased cTnI values, based on serial sampling over 24 hours following presentation.

Electrical cardioversion therapy

Minor increases of both cTnT and cTnI following direct-current cardioversion in patients presenting with atrial or ventricular fibrillation occur in less than 50% of patients [20]. It appears that the percentages of patients reported with increases are dependent upon what cardiac troponin concentration was used as a reference cutoff. Overall, the data suggest occult, asymptomatic myocardial injury can occur following electrical cardioversion, and does not appear related to the number of shocks or to the amount of energy delivered.

Pulmonary emboli

Both cTnT and cTnI have been shown to be increased in more than one third to one half of patients clinically diagnosed with pulmonary embolism, although the number of patients studied are small ($N < 200$) [21]. cTnI helped to identify patients with right ventricular dysfunction who had a greater amount of lung defects and was associated with poor long-term survival and provided an independent prediction of mortality in patients with acute cardiogenic pulmonary edema.

Sepsis

Numerous reports have established that both cTnI and cTnT are biomarkers of myocardial injury in sepsis and septic shock. Septic patients presenting to both tertiary care, urgent care, and intensive care settings, without known documented heart disease demonstrate, in 50% of cases, increased cTn findings.

The mechanism responsible for the microbiological role for causing minor myocardial damage is not completely understood. Patients presenting with worse left ventricular function showed greater increases of cTn, and were often older compared to those with normal cTn values [22].

Myocarditis

Several studies have established that cTnI and cTnT detect myocyte injury in myocarditis [23]. cTn monitoring provided sensitive evidence of clinically suspected myocarditis in the first month after the onset of heart failure symptoms. However, it has been shown that negative results do not exclude the presence of the disease.

Stroke

The relationship between cTnT concentrations at hospital admission and mortality in patients admitted with an acute ischemic stroke has been established [24]. In one study of 181 patients admitted over 9 months, cTnT concentrations monitored over 72 hours after admission demonstrated that a peak cTnT level >0.1 µg/L had a 40% risk of mortality versus 13% for patients with a normal value, with a relative risk of death of 3.2.

Non-cardiac surgery

Numerous studies have now confirmed the successful role of monitoring either cTnI or cTnT during or post non-cardiac surgery to detect a perioperative MI. In one study of 96 patients undergoing vascular surgery, serial cTnI monitoring confirmed eight patients who had new cardiac abnormalities detected during echocardiography [25]. cTnI monitoring differentiated the high incidence (19%) of false positive CKMB increases associated with skeletal muscle release of CKMB. Routine postoperative monitoring of cTnI and cTnT has also identified patients following vascular surgery who had an increased risk for short-term mortality.

Critically ill

cTnI has long been recognized as an independent biomarker of mortality among critically ill patients. The initial observational study examining 209 admissions to a medical and respiratory intensive care unit, showed that 32 (15%) had an increased cTnI [26]. However, only 12 of these 32 patients (37%) were recognized by the medical staff; with 20 patients (63%) unrecognized without the assistance of cTnI. Mortality in patients with increased cTnI was 40% compared to 15% in patients with normal troponin values. These findings were confirmed in a study that associated increased short-term mortality in non-cardiac ill emergency department patients [27].

Exercise

Several studies have observed cTnI and cTnT increases in highly trained young and older athletes during training and following athletic competition. The majority of reports have addressed marathon runners and triathletes [28, 29]. The early literature confounded the presence of increased CKMB in athletes with myocardial injury; dispelled with the evidence that CKMB enriched skeletal muscle, injured during intense exercise, was responsible for the increased serum CKMB values. Substantial cTn increases have been reported as follows: ultracyclists (cTnI increase in 34% of 38 participants); 6 of 23 Ironman triathletes, along with abnormalities in their echocardiogram; cTnT and cTnI increases in over 10% of marathon runners evaluated in at least five different studies within 6–24 hours post race; increases in cTnT in arduous training military recruits. Extreme exercise using 3–5 hours of forced swimming in a rat model showed substantial increases in cTnT that corresponded with histological evidence of localized myocyte damage [30]. However, in human subjects, studies have demonstrated normal post-race quantitative antimyosin myocardial imaging in asymptomatic marathon runners (excluding silent myocardial cell necrosis by imaging), even in presence of increased cardiac troponin evidence of myocardial cell death. Long-term risk stratification or outcome studies in these apparently health endurance athletes have not been examined, as it is difficult to catch up to these individuals, and keep them in one place long enough to evaluate.

Newborn infants/pediatrics
cTnT and cTnI concentrations have been described in cord blood and for reference determinations in newborns and pediatric patients. In one study, 12 of 209 neonates showed increased cTnT levels at the time of delivery. Increases were associated with exposure to magnesium sulfate therapy to the mother prior to birth [31]. It has been suggested that infants with respiratory distress at birth had increased cTnT levels. In a study of 18 infants, it was shown that gestational age and birth weight influenced cTnI levels, with preterm infants having higher cTnI values. In older pediatric patients, up to 29 months, cTnI values are generally not increased.

End-stage renal disease
Cardiac disease is the major cause of death in patients with end-stage renal disease (ESRD), accounting for approximately 45% of all deaths. In dialysis patients, about 20% of cardiac deaths are attributed to acute MI. One challenge confronting the nephrology community is to explore more aggressive treatment modalities for cardiovascular disease in these patients. Recent evidence demonstrates that serum or plasma cTnT and cTnI are important predictors of long-term, all-cause mortality, and cardiovascular mortality in patients with ESRD [32]. Cardiac troponin increases are not a spurious finding, as the biomarker is indeed elevated. Troponin elevations detected in outpatient dialysis patients are a powerful predictor of all-cause mortality for cTnT and cTnI. Elevated versus normal cTnT defined by the 99th percentile cutoff was associated with a two- to fourfold increased risk of death over 2–3 years. Several studies substantiate the cTnT, cTnI difference observed in rates of increases,

and demonstrate differences between different cTnI assays [33]. Using 99th percentile cutoff, 85% (*n* = 339) of cTnT versus only 5–19% (*n* = 20–76; Dade cTnI versus Beckman cTnI assays) of cTnI concentrations were increased. Additional studies are needed to elucidate the mechanism responsible for the cTnI/cTnT differences found in ESRD patients. Regardless of the mechanisms of myocardial injury in ESRD patients, findings continue to substantiate and add to the growing literature demonstrating the prognostic power of cardiac troponin testing for predicting mortality in ESRD patients. One plausible, cost-effective scenario is the developing role of outpatient cardiac troponin testing. Incorporation of quarterly or semi-annual cardiac troponin monitoring in ESRD patients may assist in initiating more aggressive treatment of underlying CAD, detection of subclinical myocardial injury, and assist in treatment therapies before renal transplantation.

References

1 Jaffe AS, Ravkilde J, Roberts R *et al.* It's time for a change to a troponin standard. *Circulation* 2000;**102**:1216–1220.

2 Joint European Society of Cardiology/American College of Cardiology Committee. Myocardial infarction defined—a consensus document of the Joint European Society of Cardiology/American College of Cardiology Committee for the redefinition of myocardial infarction. *J Am Coll Cardiol* 2000;**36**:959–969.

3 Braunwald E, Antman EM, Beasley JW *et al.* ACC/AHA guidelines for the management of patients with unstable angina and non-ST-segment elevation myocardial infarction. *J Am Coll Cardiol* 2000;**36**:970–1062.

4 Apple FS, Wu AHB, Jaffe AS. European Society of Trial Cardiology and American College of Cardiology guidelines for redefinition of myocardial infarction: how to use existing assays clinically and for clinical trials. *Am Heart J* 2002;**144**:981–986.

5 Apple FS, Wu AHB, Valdes R, Jr. Serum cardiac troponin T concentrations in hospitalized patients without acute myocardial infarction. *Scand J Clin Lab Invest* 1996;**56**:63–68.

6 Apple FS. Tissue specificity of cardiac troponin I, cardiac troponin T, and creatine kinase MB. *Clin Chim Acta* 1999;**284**:151–159.

7 Parekh N, Venkatesh B, Cross D *et al.* Cardiac troponin I predicts myocardial dysfunction in aneurysmal subarachnoid hemorrhage. *J Am Coll Cardiol* 2000;**36**:1328–1335.

8 Kobayashi S, Tanaka M, Tamura N, Hashimoto H, Hirose S. Serum cardiac troponin T in polymyositis/dermatomyositis. *The Lancet* 1992;**340**:726.

9 Lavoinne A, Hue G. Serum cardiac troponins I and T in early post-traumatic rhabdomyolysis. *Clin Chem* 1998;**44**:667.

10 Missov E, Calzolari C, Davy J *et al.* Cardiac troponin I in patients with hematologic malignancies. *Cor Art Dis* 1997;**8**:537–541.

11 Bonnefoy E, Godon P, Kirkorian G *et al.* Serum cardiac troponin I and ST-segment elevation in patients with acute pericarditis. *Eur Heart J* 2000;**21**:832–836.

12 Brandt R, Filzmaier K, Hanrath P. Circulating cardiac troponin I in acute pericarditis. *Am J Cardiol* 2001;**87**:1326–1328.

13 Miller R, Callas DD, Kahn SE, Ricchiuti V, Apple FS. Evidence of myocardial damage in mummified human tissue. *JAMA* 2000;**284**:831–832.

14 Cardinale D, Sandri M, Martinoni A *et al.* Left ventricular dysfunction predicted by early troponin I release after high-dose chemotherapy. *J Am Coll Cardiol* 2000;**36**:517–522.

15 Herman Eugene, Ferrans VJ. The use of cardiac biomarkers for the detection of drug-induced myocardial damage. In: Wu AHB, ed. *Markers in Cardiology*. Human Press, Totowa, NJ, 2001:211–234.

16 McLaurin M, Apple FS, Henry TD, Sharkey SW. Cardiac troponin I and T levels in patients with cocaine associated chest pain. *Ann Clin Biochem* 1996;**33**:183–186.

17 Stelow R, Johari V, Smith S, Crosson J, Apple FS. Propofol-associated rhabdomyolysis with cardiac involvement in adults: chemical and anatomic findings. *Clin Chem* 2000;**46**:577–581.

18 Missov E, Mair J. A novel biochemical approach to congestive heart failure: cardiac troponin T. *Am Heart J* 1999;**138**:95–99.

19 Adams J, Davila-Roman V, Bessey P *et al.* Improved detection of cardiac contusion with cardiac troponin I. *Am Heart J* 1996;**131**:308–312.

20 Georges J, Spentchian M, Caubel C *et al.* Time course of troponin I, myoglobin, and cardiac enzyme release after electrical cardioversion. *Am J Cardiol* 1996;**78**:825–827.

21 Perna E, Macin S, Parras J *et al.* Cardiac troponin T levels are associated with poor short- and long-term prognosis in patients with acute cardiogenic pulmonary edema. *Am Heart J* 2002;**143**:814–820.

22 Wu A. Increased troponin in patients with sepsis and septic shock: myocardial necrosis or reversible myocardial depression? *Intensive Care Med* 2001;**27**:59–61.

23 Smith S, Ladenson J, Mason J, Jaffe A. Elevations of cardiac troponin I associated with myocarditis. *Circulation* 1997;**95**:163–168.

24 James P, Ellis C, Whitlock R *et al.* Relation between troponin T concentration and mortality in patients presenting with an acute stroke: observational study. *BMJ* 2000;**320**:1502–1504.

25 Adams J, Sicard Gr, Allen B *et al.* Diagnosis of perioperative myocardial infarction with measurement of cardiac troponin I. *N Engl J Med* 1994;**330**:670–674.

26 Guest T, Ramanathan A, Tuteur P *et al.* Myocardial injury in critically ill patients: a frequently unrecognized complication. *JAMA* 1995;**273**:1945–1949.

27 Wright R, Williams B, Cramner H *et al.* Elevations of cardiac troponin I are associated with increased short-term mortality in non-cardiac critically ill emergency department patients. *Am J Cardiol* 2002;**90**:634–636.

28 Rifai N, Douglas PS, O'Toole M, Rimm E, Ginsburg G. Cardiac troponin T and I electrocardiographic wall motion analyses, and ejection fractions in athletes participating in the Hawaii Ironman Triathlon. *Am J Cardiol* 1999;**83**:1085–1089.

29 Apple FS, Rogers MA, Sherman WM, Casal DC, Ivy JL. Creatine kinase MB isoenzyme adaptations in stressed human skeletal muscle. *J Appl Physiol* 1985;**59**:149–153.

30 Chen Y, Serfass RC, Mackey-Bojack S, Kelly KL, Titus JL, Apple FS. Cardiac troponin T alterations in myocardium and serum of rats following stressful, prolonged intense exercise. *J Appl Physiol* 2000;**88**:1749–1755.

31 Shivvers S, Wians F, Jr, Keffer J, Ramin S. Maternal cardiac troponin levels during normal labor and delivery. *Am J Obstet Gynecol* 1999;**180**:122–123.

32 Apple FS, Murakami MA, Pearce L, Herzog C. Predictive value of cardiac troponin I and T for subsequent death in end-stage renal disease. *Circulation* 2002;**106**:2941–2945.

33 Apple FS, Murakami MA, Pearce L, Herzog C. Multi-biomarker risk stratification on N-terminal pro-B-type natriuretic peptide, high-sensitivity C-reactive protein, and cardiac troponin T and I in end-stage renal disease for all-cause death. *Clin Chem* 2004;**50**:1–7.

CHAPTER 7

Cardiac troponins in patients with congestive heart failure

Jesse E. Adams

Introduction

Markers of cardiac injury have become pivotal in guiding the evaluation and treatment of patients with diverse medical conditions, and over the last decade, utilization of measurement of serial levels of cardiac troponins has supplanted measurement of levels of the MB fraction of creatine kinase (MB-CK) as the blood-based test of choice for diagnosis of myocardial infarction, due both to superior sensitivity and specificity for cardiac cellular necrosis [1]. This evolution to a troponin standard for the detection of myocardial necrosis was codified by a joint statement from the European Society of Cardiology and the American College of Cardiology in October 2001 [2].

However, increased utilization of cardiac troponins has generated contemporary controversies regarding unanticipated elevations of troponin proteins. Challenges and adjustments are a normal part of the evolutionary progression in the clinical application of cardiac biomarkers, and we have seen this in regards to troponin measurements when applied in diverse clinical situations beyond the central application of troponin testing in patients with chest discomfort. Many of these specific situations are explored in additional chapters of this book.

Congestive heart failure (CHF) is the most common cardiac admitting diagnosis in the United States, and the incidence of CHF is increasing worldwide. Many patients will present to their physicians or to emergency departments with a primary complaint of dyspnea, sometimes with an additional component of chest discomfort. In some of these patients the diagnosis of CHF is overt, while in other patients who present with dyspnea a much wider range of diagnostic possibilities must be entertained. In all of these patients blood-based markers are a key component of a contemporary diagnostic approach, and troponin measurements will often (and appropriately) be obtained in such patients. Elevations of troponin will occur routinely in patients who present with a diagnosis of CHF and at times result in diagnostic uncertainty.

Case 1

A 54-year-old Hispanic female presents to the emergency department with complaint of increasing dyspnea of 5 day duration. She has noted increasing lower extremity edema as well as orthopnea, but denies chest discomfort. She has a history of an ischemic cardiomyopathy with an ejection fraction of 25%. Six months ago she had a positive stress test; a cardiac catheterization showed three-vessel coronary arterial disease with four out of four patent bypass grafts. Her current medical therapy consists of enteric-coated aspirin 81 mg daily, lisinopril 20 mg daily, carvedolol 12.5 mg twice daily, digoxin 0.125 mg daily, lipitor 20 mg daily, and spironolactone 25 mg daily. She has also been treated with furosemide and potassium but recently stopped this diuretic because of frequent urination. Her exam is notable for a loud S3, an elevated jugular venous pressure, bibasilar rales, and moderate bilateral lower extremity edema. Her electrocardiogram shows mild T wave flattening unchanged from her prior study. Samples obtained on admission yield a level of BNP that is elevated at 982 pg/mL, but her cardiac troponin I is elevated at 0.26 ng/mL (99% cutpoint is 0.1 ng/mL). A repeat troponin level 4 and 8 hours later shows no change.

Discussion of Case 1

The central question in interpreting the results of the troponin results in this patient is whether the patient's presentation is primarily due to CHF or to acute coronary syndrome. The presence of elevations of troponin proteins is a critical component of a contemporary diagnosis of acute myocardial infarction. However, it must be understood that all troponin elevations do not equate to a diagnosis of a myocardial infarction. Ultimately, troponin elevations must be understood as indicative of myocardial cellular death, but the presence of a single elevation of troponin does not speak to the cause of the cardiac cellular necrosis.

Troponin elevations are well described in patients who present with CHF. Typically, they manifest a lower degree of elevation, and usually demonstrate a relatively "flat" curve. There is usually little change over the time of the "rule-out" serial measurements in contrast to the rising and falling pattern seen in patients who present with an acute myocardial infarction. Troponin elevations due to decompensated CHF are indicative of increased risk in the near term. Troponin elevations in patients with CHF do not require the presence of underlying coronary arterial disease; such elevations can occur in patients with non-ischemic cardiomyopathies as well. Indeed, various studies have found that elevations of cardiac troponins are found in 10–25% of patients who present with CHF. And while some have considered that elevations of troponin in patients who present with CHF could indicate underlying myocarditis, this has not been found to be the case. While there are some data in patients who present with myocarditis that indicate that brief troponin elevations do in fact occur, troponin is not a sensitive diagnostic technique in patients with myocarditis. It is believed that troponin elevations in patients with CHF is indicative of ventricular and myofibrillar remodeling. And while some have suggested that patients with CHF and elevations of troponin proteins may particularly benefit from implantation of a defibrillator, no data as yet are available to answer this supposition.

Detection of elevated levels of cardiac troponins in the circulation of patients who present with CHF corresponds both with a greater severity as well as worsened prognosis [3]. Patients with CHF who manifest elevations of cardiac troponins have a greater incidence of death, both in the short-term as well as the long-term; they also have a greater rate of readmission as well. The pattern of troponin elevation in this population is important as well; patients with persistent elevations have a much greater incidence of cardiovascular events when compared with those that demonstrate only transient elevations on arrival.

Thus, this patient's elevated levels of troponin protein were due to her decompensated CHF, likely due to her cessation of her prescribed diuretics complicated by dietary indiscretion. While she initially received anti-ischemic therapy, these were discontinued by her primary cardiologist the next morning after the serial troponin measurements were available and all treatment was focused on her volume overload and CHF. She diuresed 11 pounds prior to discharge with complete relief of her symptoms; medical and dietary compliance was stressed as a necessary component for longer term success.

Case 2

A 52-year-old African American male presented to the emergency department with a primary complaint of dyspnea. This patient had no prior cardiac history but had not seen a physician for 12 years when he had had a vasectomy. Patient had been feeling well until the day of presentation, when he developed severe dyspnea as well as with activity. He has worked as a deliveryman for United Parcel Service for 18 years, and has noted increasing fatigue lately. He denies any chest discomfort but has been having "lots of heartburn" lately, both at rest as well as during the day with activity, and he currently has this indigestion feeling at presentation. His physical exam is noteworthy for obvious distress and dyspnea, rales at the left base, jugular venous distention of 10 cm, and an absence of lower extremity edema. His electrocardiogram demonstrates a left bundle branch block; no prior electrocardiogram is available for review. Initial blood work is unremarkable except for an elevated level of BNP of 672 and an elevation of cardiac troponin I of 0.18 ng/mL (10% CV cutpoint of 0.03 ng/mL).

Discussion of Case 2

In this patient it is not yet clear as to what is responsible for the conjoint elevation of troponin and BNP. In the first case we discussed troponin elevations that can occur in patients who present with CHF as the primary pathophysiologic derangement. Conversely, levels of BNP can (and frequently do) occur in patients who present with acute coronary syndrome. Unfortunately, since BNP is sometimes viewed (erroneously) as simply a "test for heart failure" patients with elevations of BNP are sometime immediately diagnosed with CHF without a consideration of alternative diagnoses.

In this patient, the history would be quite unusual for decompensated (chronic) CHF, and we must ascertain the etiology of the troponin elevation. While a left bundle branch block can certainly occur in patients with left ventricular dysfunction, it also is indicative of increased risk in patients who present with acute coronary artery syndrome.

Because of the rapidity of the patient's onset, his symptoms, the left bundle branch block of unknown duration, and his cardiac risk factors, he was taken emergently to the cardiac catheterization laboratory where severe three-vessel coronary arterial disease including significant left main stenosis was found. Hemodynamic stabilization and anti-ischemic therapy, including intra-aortic balloon pulsation, were utilized and the patient underwent emergent coronary artery bypass grafting.

In conclusion, in any patient who presents with dyspnea and is found to have an elevated level of natriuretic peptide, the clinician must always consider if the patient could have a primary ischemic presentation due to underlying coronary artery disease.

Case 3

A 66-year-old male with a history of non-ischemic cardiomyopathy and an ejection fraction of 20% by echocardiography 6 months prior presented to his physician's office with a complaint of worsened dyspnea, orthopnea, increased lower extremity edema, and a gradual 15 pound weight gain. He had increased his furosemide on his own but had continued to get worse. At this point he gets short of breath when he walks across the room. Physical exam confirms the weight gain as well as bilateral rales and jugular venous distention to 12 cm. A point-of-care BNP was run in the physician's office and returned a value of 1252 ng/mL. He was sent to the hospital with a diagnosis of CHF, where the admission evaluation additionally demonstrated bilateral interstitial infiltrates on the chest radiograph and an electrocardiogram that was unchanged from one obtained 6 months earlier. The patient's initial laboratory data was largely unremarkable except for a troponin level that was elevated (cardiac troponin I of 0.82 ng/mL, 10% CV < 0.03 ng/mL). The patient was admitted and intravenous diuresis was instituted; his afterload reduction was advanced. Spironolactone was also initiated. After 4 days he had lost 12 pounds; repeat laboratory data that day showed no change in renal function or electrolytes; BNP was improved but still elevated at 472 ng/mL. A repeat troponin level was obtained and was increased at 0.74 ng/mL. A repeat echocardiogram showed no change from the prior echocardiogram of 6 months earlier; the patient's ejection fraction remained at 20–25%. The patient was discharged home and returned for follow-up to his physician's office 5 days later; a repeat BNP at that time was 220 ng/mL, with a troponin level (run at the hospital on the same assay and analyzer) of 0.38 ng/mL.

Discussion of Case 3

In this case we have a patient who presents with a fairly classic case of an acute exacerbation of CHF in a patient with a history of a non-ischemic cardiomyopathy. On arrival the patient demonstrated a significant elevation of natriuretic peptides as would be expected. However, despite his apparent improvement, he continued to manifest elevations of BNP and troponin.

Studies have demonstrated that the degree of elevation of both BNP and troponin on arrival are inversely related to cardiovascular morbidity and mortality [3–6]. As in the situation with patients who present with chest pain, serial measurements over an 8–12 hour period are recommended; studies that have evaluated the use of cardiac troponins in patients with CHF have generally utilized cutpoints similar to those in patient with chest pain, although there has been disparity between utilization of the manufacturer's recommended limit based on the original receiver–operator curve (ROC) and the more contemporary decision threshold predicated on a 10% CV threshold or 99th percentile cutpoint.

Additionally, there is evidence that ongoing measurement of troponins provides additional information regarding the prognostic status of the patient. One study that investigated this phenomenon was published in 2004 by Perna and colleagues [7]. They prospectively followed 115 outpatients with a history of CHF for 1 year. All patients had an ejection fraction less than 40%, and roughly two thirds had a history of coronary arterial disease. Blood samples were collected at baseline and 3, 6, and 12 months and assayed for levels of cardiac troponin T, with a value of greater than 0.02 ng/mL defined as abnormal. At 18 months, patients with no episodes of an elevation of cardiac troponin T had a CHF hospitalization-free survival rate of 63%, while those patients with a single elevated cardiac troponin T result had only a 43% CHF hospitalization-free survival rate. Those patients with consistently elevated measurements of cardiac troponin $T > 0.02$ ng/mL fared the worst, with only a 17% CHF hospitalization-free survival rate ($P = 0.0001$). Along with hospitalization in the last year and a functional CHF class of III or IV, detectable levels of cTnT were independently associated with prognosis. The authors suggested a role for monitoring of cTnT levels to identify high-risk patients. And again, as noted above some investigators have suggested that given that the primary etiology of death in this population is arrhythmic that patients with persistent or frequent elevations of cardiac troponins (and/or BNP) would potentially benefit the most from implantable defibrillators, but there are currently no studies that address this question.

Another variable in the assessment of risk in patients who present with CHF is the presence and degree of BNP elevations and their relationship with the absence or presence of cardiac troponins. This interaction is often not appreciated but is a very powerful indicator of risk in patients who present with CHF. There appears on anecdotal evidence that once a patient is admitted with CHF and there is no concern for acute coronary syndrome to dismiss any cardiac troponins elevations and to ascribe any such elevations as "simply due to the

CHF." However, this approach ignores the powerful information provided to the clinician by these biochemical markers. In addition to the independent prognostic information provided by the presence of either natriuretic peptides or cardiac troponin, the presence of elevations of both cardiac troponin and natriuretic peptides in the patient at presentation indicates a greatly increased risk of mortality. In one study involving 238 patients with advanced CHF, Horwich and colleagues determined that the joint presence of both of these markers was associated with a 12-fold increased risk of long-term mortality [8]; this finding has been corroborated by other investigators [6, 7].

This patient presented with an exacerbation of his chronic CHF. The presence of both BNP and troponin elevations was indicative of increased risk, which was magnified by the persistence of their elevations. Aggressive titration of medical therapy is warranted, close and frequent follow-up is needed, and if the patient meets the criteria then replacement of his defibrillator with a biventricular defibrillator would be reasonable.

Case 4

A 67-year-old female visiting from Santiago Chile with a history of prior admissions for "water on the lung" presents to the emergency department with increasing dyspnea and lower extremity edema. The patient does not speak English and the family members accompanying the patient state that she has been compliant with her medications but can offer no other historical information. The patient has 3+ lower extremity edema and bibasilar rales. The electrocardiogram shows evidence of left ventricular hypertrophy with left ventricular strain pattern; the chest radiograph demonstrates bibasilar infiltrates. The initial laboratory data are unremarkable except for a BNP level of 2740 ng/mL and an elevation of cardiac troponin I of 0.20 ng/mL (10% CV cutpoint of 0.03 ng/mL). Repeat troponin levels at 4 and 8 hours yield results of 0.18 and 0.22 ng/mL, respectively. Intravenous diuretics are started and the patient begins to promptly diurese with marked clinical improvement. An echocardiogram demonstrates marked concentric left ventricular hypertrophy with an ejection fraction of 70–75%, evidence of diastolic dysfunction, and normal valvular function. An adenosine cardiolyte is performed the next morning and shows an ejection fraction of 82% with no evidence of ischemia.

Discussion of Case 4

This patient presents with CHF due to a hypertrophied left ventricle and left ventricular diastolic dysfunction. Diastolic dysfunction is a common etiology of CHF, especially in women and in those of advancing age. While CHF due to diastolic dysfunction has been felt in the past to confer less risk, more recent studies have demonstrated that the risk is greater than previously appreciated. Indeed, more recent investigations have ascribed similar risk to those who present with CHF regardless of the underlying ejection fraction [9]. Thus, it becomes important to stratify patients who present with CHF on presentation to allow accurate and adequate treatment.

Elevations of cardiac troponin have been reported to be found routinely in patients who present with CHF and diastolic dysfunction or left ventricular hypertrophy and preserved systolic function [10, 11]. Elevations of cardiac troponins in these patients are associated with worse prognosis, just as is the case with in those patients who present with CHF and diminished left ventricular function. Perna and colleagues reported on a mixed group of 159 patients with decompensated CHF and no acute coronary event [12]. Elevations of cardiac troponins (in this study cardiac troponin T) were associated with greater end-systolic and end-diastolic diameters and well as greater left ventricular mass. Data indicated that the elevations of cardiac troponins (felt to be indicative of ongoing myofibrillar degradation as well as ventricular remodeling) were associated with a sixfold increase in death or refractory heart failure. And while the current case is in a patient who presented to the emergency department with CHF, similar conclusions apply to patients who are ambulatory and seen in outpatient settings. Troponin levels (along with New York Heart Association Class) have been found to be independent predictors of prognosis in stable ambulatory patients. A recent study investigated the presence of troponin positivity in a population of ambulatory outpatients with a history of CHF and preserved systolic function (defined as an ejection fraction greater than 40%) [13]. In this study, 39% of the patients manifested at least one episode of an elevated level of cardiac troponin T. Those patients who demonstrated an elevation of cardiac troponin did worse with a significant decline in their heart failure hospitalization-free survival as well as overall prognosis. The authors concluded that elevations of cardiac troponins in patients with a history of CHF were indicative of ongoing myocardial injury and portended progressive impairment. Accordingly, clinicians must consider troponin elevations in patients with CHF to be potent predictors of risk in patients with both systolic as well as diastolic heart failure.

References

1 Adams JE, Bodor G, Davila-Roman V *et al.* Cardiac troponin I: a marker with high specificity for cardiac injury. *Circulation* 1993;**88**:101–106.

2 Myocardial infarction redefined—a consensus document of the Joint European Society of Cardiology/American College of Cardiology Committee for the redefinition of myocardial infarction. *J Am Coll Cardiol* 2000;**36**:959–969.

3 Sugiura T, Takase H, Toriyama T *et al.* Circulating levels of myocardial proteins predict future deterioration of congestive heart failure. *J Card Fail* 2005;**11**:504–509.

4 Perna ER, Macin SM, Cimbaro Cannella JP *et al.* Minor myocardial damage detected by troponin T is a powerful predictor of long-term prognosis in patients with acute decompensated heart failure. *Int J Cardiol* 2005;**99**:253–261.

5 Missov E, Mair J. A novel biochemical approach to congestive heart failure: cardiac troponin T. *Am Heart J* 1999;**138**:95–99.

6 Ishii J, Nomura M, Nakamure Y *et al.* Risk stratification using a combination of cardiac troponin T and brain natriuretic peptide in patients hospitalized for worsening congestive heart failure. *Am J Cardiol* 2002;**89**:691–695.

7 Perna ER, Macin SM, Cimbaro Cannella JP *et al.* Ongoing myocardial injury in stable severe heart failure: value of cardiac troponin T monitoring for high-risk patient identification. *Circulation* 2004;**110**:2376–2382.

8 Horwich TB, Patel J, MacLellan WR *et al.* Cardiac troponin I is associated with impaired hemodynamic, progressive left ventricular dysfunction, and increased mortality rates in advanced heart failure. *Circulation* 2003;**108**:833–838.

9 Bursi F, Weston SA, Redfield MM *et al.* Systolic and diastolic heart failure in the community. *JAMA* 2006;**296**:2209–2216.

10 Angheliou GO, Dickerson RP, Ravakhah K. Etiology of troponin I elevation in patients with congestive heart failure and low clinical suspicion of myocardial infarction. *Resuscitation* 2004;**63**:195–201.

11 Setsuta K, Seino Y, Ogawa T *et al.* Use of cytosolic and myofibril markers in the detection of ongoing myocardial damage in patients with chronic heart failure. *Am J Med* 2002;**113**:717–722.

12 Perna ER, Macin SM, Cimbaro Canella JP *et al.* High levels of troponin T are associated with ventricular remodeling and adverse in-hospital outcome in heart failure. *Med Sci Monit* 2004;**10**:CR90–CR95.

13 Macin SM, Perna ER, Cimbaro Canella JP *et al.* Increased levels of cardiac troponin-T in outpatients with heart failure and preserved systolic dysfunction are related to adverse clinical findings and outcome. *Cor Art Dis* 2006;**17**:685–691.

CHAPTER 8

Troponins and the critically ill patient

Jose Antonio Perez, Luciano Babuin, Allan S. Jaffe

Introduction

Troponins are the biomarkers of choice for the detection of myocardial damage and the diagnosis of acute myocardial infarction [1, 2]. In patients with acute coronary syndromes (ACS) troponin elevations define a high-risk group [3] and provide guidance for therapeutic decision making [4]. Using the 99th percentile of a normal reference population as cutoff to define elevations, both the diagnostic and prognostic accuracy are maximized [1].

However, the increased sensitivity of contemporary troponin assays leads to identification of some degree of cardiac damage in a variety of noncoronary-related disease states as well including many associated with critical illness. Since 1995, when the initial article by Guest and colleagues was published [5], several studies have reported that a substantial number of critically ill patients have elevated troponins [5–9]. The percent of elevations varies from as low as 15% to as high as 71% (depending on the sensitivity of the assay used and the cutoff value chosen to define an elevation) [5–9]. Despite the different percent of elevations the mortality rate in patients with elevations is consistently 1.5- to 3-fold higher than those without elevations (depending on the subset of patients involved and the extent of the follow-up) [5–9]. A partial listing with putative mechanisms is included as Table 8.1.

The cause for these elevations in critically ill patients is no doubt multifactorial but they certainly reflect myocardial damage. The first consideration in regard to the etiology of this damage is that these patients may have occult coronary artery disease [10]. However, there are many other putative mechanisms one also could consider. These include vulnerability of the ventricular subendocardium to changes in wall stress and hypoperfusion, especially if left ventricular hypertrophy is present [11]. A similar mechanism can affect the RV in situations where acute pulmonary hypertension (e.g., due to pulmonary embolism) can increase wall stress and thus reduce subendocardial perfusion [12]. Similarly, vasoactive drugs increase myocardial work and thus can induce ischemia secondary to a discrepancy between demand and supply [13]. In one sense such changes could be considered ischemic but certainly not in the conventional sense. However, there are also several additional situations when direct cardiac injury can occur. These include cardiac contusion secondary to chest trauma, cardioversion or defibrillation (including ICD firings). In addition, agents such as catecholamines and chemotherapy agents,

Table 8.1 Elevated troponins without overt coronary heart disease.

Possible diminished O_2 supply

−Coronary spasm, perhaps including small vessel spasm in apical ballooning
−Myocardial bridging (secondary tachycardia)
−Coronary vasculitis
−Severe hypoxia

Possible increased O_2 demand

−Any cause of tachycardia (sustained)
−Vital exhaustion
−Sepsis
−Cutaneous burns > 30%

Possible diminished supply and increased demand

−Severe ventricular hypertrophy (i.e., hypertrophic obstructive cardiomyopathy)
−Non-cardiac surgery
−Severe aortic stenosis and hypertrophic cardiomyopathy
−Acute and chronic heart failure
−Increase cathecholamines (stroke, subarachnoid bleed, seizures, cocaine use, pheochromocytoma)
−Severe pulmonary hypertension (primary or secondary as pulmonary embolism)
−Aortic dissection
−Pulmonary embolism

Possible direct damage

−Inflamation (myocarditis, pericarditis)
−Chemotherapy drugs (adriamycin, 5-fluorouracil, herceptin)
−Catecholamines
−Heart trauma (pacing, contusion, ablation, cardioversion, defibrillation, cardiac surgery, endomyocardial biopsy)

Other potential causes

−Hypothyroidism
−Infiltrative diseases as amyloidosis, hemochromatosis, and sarcoidosis
−Rhabdomyolysis with cardiac injury
−Hemolytic uremic syndrome

and circulating toxins such as TNF alpha and heat shock protein can be directly myocardiotoxic [14].

These factors may be exacerbated by arrhythmias, metabolic or respiratory acidosis, changes in thoracic pressure induced by mechanical ventilation with high positive end-expiratory pressure, hypoxia, hypercarbia, anemia, heart failure, renal failure, and the recognized pro-thrombotic propensity of critically ill patients kept at bed rest. This can make determination of the mechanism of a given elevation difficult to discern. However, it is now clear that troponin elevations define a high-risk group but it is not clear at present what the appropriate treatment is. Of importance is the fact that these elevations occur with relatively common disease presentations.

The cases below are illustrative of the problems marked by such elevations in troponin.

Case 1: gastrointestinal bleeding

A 59-year man was transferred from another hospital after vomiting (approximately 550 mL) bright red blood. Emergency esophagogastroduodenoscopy (EGD) documented a large ulcer located at the lesser curve of the stomach with profuse bleeding and an old healed ulcer in the pyloric region. The ulcer was fulgurated and the patient was stabilized with blood and volume replacement.

At the time of admission, he was dizzy and fatigued but denied chest pain, palpitations and/or dyspnea. He denied alcohol use or abuse of aspirin or nonsteroidal anti-inflammatory pain agents. He was a nonsmoker and had no known additional risk factors for coronary artery disease; moreover, there were no symptoms suggestive for cardiovascular disease in his past medical history.

On physical examination, he was pale and appeared dehydrated and was vomiting blood. His temperature was normal, blood pressure 80/45 mm Hg, heart rate 125 beats/min, and respiration rate 30 times/min. He was passing maroon stool per rectum.

Laboratory results of note on admission were: hematocrit 17.1%; hemoglobin 5.7 g/dL; elevated white blood cell (WBC) count (14×10^9/L); platelet count and INR were normal. His BUN was mildly elevated (34 mg/dL) with a normal creatinine (1.1 mg/dL). At the time of admission his cardiac troponin T (cTnT) was 0.03 µg/L and later during the day it increased to 0.07 µg/L. Both those values are above the 99th percentile for cTnT (which is <0.01 µ/L) and the second one is above the concentration where the coefficient of variation for the cTnT assay is ≤10% (which is 0.035 µ/L). His electrocardiogram (ECG) showed right bundle branch block (RBBB); unchanged from a previous tracing. An arterial blood gas done on admission showed a mild acidosis with a PO_2 of 85 mm Hg and a PCO_2 of 30 mm Hg on room air. His chest radiogram demonstrated mild pulmonary congestion without cardiomegaly. An echocardiography showed a left ventricle of normal size and wall thickness, without regional wall motion abnormalities, but with a moderately reduced ejection fraction (EF = 39%); aortic sclerosis without stenosis, mild–moderate aortic regurgitation, and an estimated pulmonary artery systolic pressure of 45 mm Hg.

The patient received four packed red blood cells but did not require support with pressors or inotropes. He continued to deny chest pain. After 2 days, repeat EGD showed a nonbleeding ulcer and his hematocrit was 32%. By this time, his ejection fraction had returned to normal (>50%). He was discharged from the intensive care unit (ICU) on a proton pump inhibitor and antibiotics for newly diagnosed Helicobacter pylori.

Discussion of Case 1

This gentleman did not have a history of cardiovascular disease nor cardiovascular risk factors. He presented with sudden and severe gastrointestinal (GI) bleeding, and documented cardiac injury, marked by elevated troponins and ventricular dysfunction. His ECG did not suggest acute coronary disease and he did not have regional wall motion abnormalities by echocardiogram. He was easily stabilized and subsequently, his ejection fraction normalized. The etiology and significance of his elevated troponin is unclear and it may require long-term follow-up to establish its potential significance.

However, this patient is far from atypical. In some studies, the frequency of elevated troponins in patients with severe enough bleeding to warrant ICU monitoring and treatment is as high as 13–14%. Some of these elevations are no doubt due to exacerbation of underlying coronary disease. However, that did not appear to be the case in this patient. Given that fact, what then might explain his elevated troponin? First and most evident was his huge sudden blood loss that was estimated at about 550 mL. Reduced intravascular volume, resultant hypotension, and a marked reduction in oxygen carrying capacity were present. Tachycardia was due to appropriate sympathetic activation. This was additionally increased by the urgent EGD, a clinically critical procedure, which has been demonstrated in several studies to be safe even in patients with acute myocardial infarction. Why such minor elevations of troponin are associated with such marked reductions in ejection fraction is difficult to explain as well. There is evidence that severe physiological and emotional stresses can lead to myocardial injury and dysfunction similar to that seen with myocardial stunning. That is often the case with critically ill patients who manifest modest or minor elevations in troponin despite marked reductions in cardiac performance. Fortunately, cardiac function, as this case, usually improves as the patient stabilizes, in keeping with the troponin levels, which usually suggest only minor amounts of cardiac injury. Recent, as yet unpublished data indicate that those patients with elevations of troponin manifest an increased risk for cardiovascular events during follow-up. Thus, this gentleman will require cardiovascular surveillance during follow-up.

Case 2: acute respiratory failure

A 67-year-old lady, with a history of moderate chronic obstructive pulmonary disease (COPD) due to a >40 year pack history of smoking, was found unresponsive in the nursing home where she lived. She was brought to the local hospital and found to be in hypercapnic respiratory failure ($PCO_2 = 105$ mm Hg). At that time, she was intubated, ventilated, and transferred to Mayo Clinic for further evaluation. The patient's relatives said she had complained of shortness of breath for several days prior to the event and had been treated with oral antibiotic therapy. They denied other cardiovascular risk factors other than well-controlled type 2 diabetes and a past history of smoking but she had stopped 20 years before. To their knowledge, she had never had a cardiovascular event or symptoms of cardiovascular disease.

Upon arrival, the patient was disoriented with a respiratory rate of 33 and a heart rate of 98 beats/min. Blood pressure was 100/40 mm Hg, and temperature was 38.7°C. There were coarse breath sounds with bibasilar crackles over both lung fields. Her chest X-ray showed infiltrates in the left lower lung, atelectasis in the right lower lung and possible pulmonary congestion. An arterial blood gas showed pH $= 7.29$; $PO_2 = 125$ mm Hg, and $PCO_2 = 86$ mm Hg on synchronized intermittent mandatory ventilation (SIMV) with an FIO_2 of 50%. Other laboratory results were unremarkable except for a WBC count of 20×10^9/L with a left shift. Admission cTnT was 0.04 µ/L and subsequently rose to 0.09 µ/L but became undetectable 24 hours later. Her ECG had Q waves in the inferior leads of questionable significance. Echocardiography showed moderate pulmonary hypertension with a moderately dilated right ventricle, mild tricuspid regurgitation, and inferior hypokinesis with an ejection fraction of 42%.

The patient received an intensive respiratory pharmacological support including inhalators, corticoids, and antibiotics for presumed pneumonia. Low doses of dopamine plus diuretics were used as well. No other organ dysfunction was noted. She slowly improved and after 9 days in the ICU, the patient was weaned from the ventilator and transferred to the ward. She was discharged 8 days later on oxygen. Twenty-nine days after discharge, the patient suffered a cardiac arrest and died.

Discussion of Case 2

This patient had a history of moderate COPD and diabetes without known cardiovascular complications and had respiratory failure partially related to well-documented pulmonary infection. There were, however, mild signs of heart failure on the chest radiography on admission and her echocardiogram revealed reduced ejection fraction (EF) and regional wall motion abnormalities. Troponins were elevated but only transiently. There were no significant ECG changes. Given the frequency of coronary artery disease in diabetics, which often can be occult, one would have to consider the possibility of occult coronary artery disease as the etiology of the troponin elevations. Perhaps this woman had an infarction in the days or weeks prior to hospitalization. Infarction can be relatively silent or at least unappreciated in diabetics. She then could have developed heart failure and nosocomial pneumonia on the substrate of increased lung water. This would fit with her reduced LV function and the mild pulmonary congestion detected radiographically. It is also possible that what occurred prior to admission in response to the stress of her respiratory compensation was extension of infarction. In diabetics, coronary disease must always be a consideration since diabetes is considered a coronary artery risk equivalent. In addition, smoking is a risk factor for both COPD and coronary heart disease so individuals frequently have both. Indeed, as many as 25% of patients with acute respiratory failure (ARF) who die have been reported to have concurrent myocardial infarction.

Whether underlying coronary artery disease was or was not present, it is likely that the severe increase in myocardial oxygen demand hypoxemia, the increased work of breathing, acidemia, and severe hypercarbia also contributed to an imbalance between myocardial oxygen supply and demand. Furthermore, β_2 agonists and fever can produce tachycardia and the use of catecholamines not only increase myocardial work out of proportion to increases in coronary blood flow but also have direct myocardiotoxic effects.

However, this patient had a more abrupt rise and fall in troponin than is usually seen. This pattern has been associated with pulmonary embolism (PE) and sepsis and may have been a hint as to the underlying pathophysiology. It is thus worth, monitoring patients like this if there is suspicion of PE to see how rapidly the elevations resolve. Acute pulmonary hypertension which could have been associated with her COPD and backward heart failure could cause a similar pattern.

In almost every study or critically ill patients, elevations in troponin have prognostic significance, both short and long term. Thus, even if the short-term results appear favorable, continued surveillance is advised for patients whose troponins were elevated. As in this woman, they often harbor undetected abnormalities that led to the troponin elevation. In this case, an autopsy was performed and this woman had both pulmonary emboli as well as a recent extension of a prior inferior myocardial infarction.

Case 3: sepsis

A 71-year-old woman came to the emergency department with increasing difficulty breathing, fever, chills, and nausea over the past 12 hours. On arrival she was in severe respiratory distress and lacked even a palpable blood pressure. She was immediately intubated and a dopamine infusion was begun.

The patient's past medical history was remarkable for dyslipidemia, polyendocrinopathy with lymphocytic adrenalitis, Hashimoto thyroiditis, pernicious anemia, and splenectomy in 1998 for idiopathic thrombocytopoenia purpura (ITP). She had hip surgery in 2001. She was on levothyroxine, B12 vitamin, and atorvastatin.

Upon arrival to the ICU, her blood pressure was 70/35 mm Hg, heart rate was 120 beats/min, respiratory rate was 29 times/min, and temperature was 34.9°C. She was treated with mechanical ventilation, pressors, and antibiotics. Her physical examination revealed dullness and crackles at her left lung base. She had severe metabolic acidosis and respiratory failure. On an FIO_2 of 100%, she had a PO_2 of 88 mm Hg, a PCO_2 of 26 mm Hg, and a pH of 7.01. In addition, her INR was 10.5 and there appeared to be disseminated intravascular coagulopathy by blood smear. There was also mild renal dysfunction with a Cr of 1.7 mg/dL and a BUN of 68 mg/dL. Mild anemia (hematocrit = 30.4%) was present along with an elevated white count to 11,600 with a left shift. cTnT was 0.04 μ/L and rose to 0.16 μ/L thereafter. An ECG manifested mild T changes abnormalities and an echocardiography (TTE) on admission showed normal left ventricular size with an LVEF of 65%. The next day, however, her ejection fraction had fallen to 37%. No new regional wall motion abnormalities were present. Chest X-ray showed a left basal infiltrate, bilateral pleural effusions, and increased interstitial markings thought due to pulmonary venous congestion. Blood cultures were positive for Streptococcus pneumoniae.

The hemodynamic pattern derived from the placement of a Swan–Ganz catheter was compatible with septic shock with a high cardiac output and low peripheral vascular resistance. The patient was treated with vasopressin and phenylephrine to maintain her blood pressure. She was also given pharmacologic doses of hydrocortisone.

The patient was successfully resuscitated from two cardiac arrests. Thereafter, the family decided that the patient should become DNR (do not resuscitate) and she expired the next morning.

Discussion of Case 3

This patient clearly had septic shock, likely secondary to a respiratory infection. She had no known cardiovascular disease despite a history of hyperlipidemia. She was at high risk for Streptococcus septicemia given her prior splenectomy. She presented with septic shock secondary with multisystem organ failure with involvement of the kidneys, brain, liver, respiratory, hematologic, and cardiovascular systems at admission. In patients with septic shock, there is a relationship between the degree of troponin elevation and both the extent of LV dysfunction and the need for pressor support. Elevations are also a risk factor for subsequent mortality.

Elevated troponin levels, either troponin I (cTnI) or cTnT, have been reported in between 36 and 68% of critically patients with sepsis or septic shock. The differences between studies reflect issues likely relate to patient selection, the organisms involved and the assays and cutoff values used to define troponin elevations.

The cause of these troponin elevations in patients with sepsis is multifactorial. A variety of potentially toxic cytokines have been described in septic patients. Substances such as endotoxins, tumor necrosis factor (TNF)-α, cytokines such as interleukins (IL) 1β, IL 6, and reactive oxygen species all can produce myocardial depression.

This patient, as the other critically ill patients, was hypotensive, tachycardic, on pressors, and mechanically ventilated. All of these factors and the increased contractility needed to increase cardiac output likely resulted in supply–demand imbalance and can lead to the troponin elevations.

Concluding remarks

These patients are typical of the critically ill patients who have troponin elevations. Most have multisystem organ failure rather than one solitary diagnosis. Although elevations of troponin could represent the unmasking of coronary artery disease, they could also be due to a variety of other hemodynamic, toxic, or inflammatory comorbidities. Patients at risk, in addition to being critically ill, often have other characteristics that might put them at risk. Ventricular hypertrophy is a good example. Hypertrophy is associated with a reduction in the number of blood vessels per gram of myocardium in the subendocardium. In addition, the subendocardium is dependent on the intracavitary pressure for coronary perfusion from blood vessels that tend to be straight and thus sensitive to wall stress. Moreover, this area is profoundly involved in the increases in contractility required by catecholamines, endogenous or exogenous, which are increased in the critically ill patients. Thus, there is reduced blood flow and thus reduced oxygen delivery at a time when there are marked increases in myocardial oxygen requirements due to the increased work of the heart. In addition, myocardial stretch itself along with the multiple cytokines released during systemic septic stress can increase the degree of myocardial apoptosis. Such abnormalities can effect both the ventricle and the atria.

Regardless of the etiology, multiple studies have confirmed the adverse prognostic importance of troponin elevations both short and long term [5–9]. That likely reflects the fact that regardless of the mechanism of elevation, those patients with elevations harbor serious heart disease exacerbated by the stress of the illness. The implications for treatment are complex. Perhaps the best way to treat the patients is focusing on the underlying processes that led to the critical illness maximally without regard to the cardiac effects with the idea that compensation of the underlying critical illness will impact positively on the heart as well. However, to the extent that we can employ therapies that improve myocardial oxygen and reduce demand rather than those that negatively impact on that balance, that might from first principles be more efficacious. This is an area where much more research is required.

References

1 Alpert JS, Thygesen K, Antman E, Bassand JP. Myocardial infarction redefined—a consensus document of the Joint European Society of Cardiology / American College of Cardiology Committee for the redefinition of myocardial infarction. *J Am Coll Cardiol* 2000;**36**: 959–969.

2 Jaffe AS, Ravkilde J, Roberts R *et al.* It's time for a change to a troponin standard. *Circulation* 2000;**102**:1216–1220.

3 Antman EM, Tanasijevic MJ, Thompson B *et al.* Cardiac-specific troponin I levels to predict the risk of mortality in patients with acute coronary syndromes. *N Engl J Med* 1996;**335**:1342–1349.

4 Morrow DA, Cannon CP, Rifai N *et al.* Ability of minor elevations of troponins I and T to predict benefit from an early invasive strategy in patients with unstable angina and non-ST elevation myocardial infarction: results from a randomized trial. *JAMA* 2001;**286**:2405–2412.

5 Guest TM, Ramanathan AV, Tuteur PG, Schechtman KB, Ladenson JH, Jaffe AS. Myocardial injury in critically ill patients. A frequently unrecognized complication. *JAMA* 1995;**273**:1945–1949.

6 Wu TT, Yuan A, Chen CY *et al.* Cardiac troponin I levels are a risk factor for mortality and multiple organ failure in noncardiac critically ill patients and have an additive effect to the APACHE II score in outcome prediction. *Shock* 2004;**22**:95–101.

7 Landesberg G, Vesselov Y, Einav S, Goodman S, Sprung CL, Weissman C. Myocardial ischemia, cardiac troponin, and long-term survival of high-cardiac risk critically ill intensive care unit patients. *Crit Care Med* 2005;**33**:1281–1287.

8 King DA, Codish S, Novack V, Barski L, Almog Y. The role of cardiac troponin I as a prognosticator in critically ill medical patients: a prospective observational cohort study. *Crit Care* 2005;**9**:R390–R395.

9 Quenot JP, Le Teuff G, Quantin C *et al.* Myocardial injury in critically ill patients: relation to increased cardiac troponin I and hospital mortality. *Chest* 2005;**128**:2758–2764.

10 Gunnewiek JM, Van Der Hoeven JG. Cardiac troponin elevations among critically ill patients. *Curr Opin Crit Care* 2004;**10**:342–346.

11 Hamwi SM, Sharma AK, Weissman NJ *et al.* Troponin-I elevation in patients with increased left ventricular mass. *Am J Cardiol* 2003;**92**:88–90.

12 Giannitsis E, Muller-Bardorff M, Kurowski V *et al.* Independent prognostic value of cardiac troponin T in patients with confirmed pulmonary embolism. *Circulation* 2000;**102**:211–217.

13 Kim LJ, Martinez EA, Faraday N *et al.* Cardiac troponin I predicts short-term mortality in vascular surgery patients. *Circulation* 2002;**106**:2366–2371.

14 Wu AH. Increased troponin in patients with sepsis and septic shock: myocardial necrosis or reversible myocardial depression? *Intensive Care Med* 2001;**27**:959–961.

CHAPTER 9

Cardiac troponins and renal failure

Suresh Pothuru, Christopher deFilippi

Introduction

Cardiac troponins have redefined the diagnosis of myocardial infarction and revolutionized the management of acute coronary syndromes (ACS) [1, 2]. Current cardiac troponin assays are sensitive and can diagnose small episodes of myocardial necrosis [3]. Cardiac troponins have proved their utility not only as diagnostic markers of myocardial injury and important prognosticators, but as critical tests for directing therapy in ACS [2–6]. In patients with kidney disease, cardiac troponins remain reliable prognostic markers of short-term mortality in the setting of an ACS [7]. However, patients with end-stage renal disease (ESRD) represent a unique population where the presence of sporadic or persistent cardiac troponin elevations in the absence of symptoms is common [8–14].

The troponin complex regulates contraction of striated muscle cells. The complex consists of three subunits: troponin C—which binds to calcium ions, troponin I (cTnI)—which binds to actin and inhibits actin–myosin interactions, and troponin T (cTnT)—which binds to tropomyosin and attaches the troponin complex to the thin filament [15]. The troponin complex is present in both skeletal and cardiac muscle cells. However, skeletal and myocardial troponin T and I are encoded by different genes and the resultant protein molecules are immunologically distinct allowing for the development of assays for the cardiac-specific isoforms. The detection of cTnT in asymptomatic ESRD patients on dialysis challenged this concept. Initially, there was controversy regarding expression of cardiac troponin T in skeletal muscle in patients with ESRD [16, 17]. However, speculation that skeletal muscle in patients with uremia might re-express cTnT was not confirmed and ultimately neither cTnT mRNA or the cTnT protein were found in skeletal muscle of patients with ESRD [18, 19]. Though there was modest cross-reactivity with skeletal muscle troponin T based on the first generation of this commercial assay, this problem was resolved in later generations of the assay and detectable levels of cTnT remain common in ESRD patients [20].

Normally, cardiac troponin T (cTnT) and cardiac troponin I (cTnI) are not detectable in the peripheral blood of healthy persons and troponin elevations are almost always associated with some cardiac pathology [21]. The presence of elevated levels of cTnT and cTnI indicates cardiac myocyte damage, but is not always synonymous with an ACS. This could be the result of a variety of conditions including trauma, toxin exposure, and inflammation [22]. In the setting of a possible ACS the near absolute specificity of cardiac troponins for myocardial injury is widely accepted. The American College of Cardiology (ACC) and European Society of Cardiology (ESC) consensus document state, "there is no discernible threshold below which an elevated value of cardiac troponin would be deemed harmless" [1]. The ACC/ESC guidelines recommend that a single cutoff point be chosen such that a myocardial infarction will be diagnosed, as a result of myocardial ischemia, if cTnT or cTnI are detected at least once within 24 hours after the index clinical event at a level exceeding the 99th percentile of the values measured in a normal control population with an acceptable imprecision of 10% or less. The caveat is that the clinical context and the patient population in which troponin levels are elevated will determine the need for testing multiple levels and subsequent management.

Diagnosing heart disease with cardiac troponin assays in ESRD patients

The clinical context is very important in evaluating a patient with elevated cardiac troponins, including the patient presenting symptoms, ECG abnormalities and other clinical data. The typical rise and fall of cardiac troponins indicate the presence of an ACS. On the other hand, a chronic modest elevation of cardiac troponin in a patient with renal failure may not represent an acute myocardial infarction but nevertheless has important prognostic implications. This is best studied in patients with ESRD, but elevations of troponins can be found in ambulatory patients with chronic kidney disease (CKD) not requiring renal replacement therapy [19]. The prognostic significance of this finding is less certain.

Chronic cTnT level elevations in patients with ESRD were reported in the mid-1990s. With the first-generation cTnT assay that had a greater cross reactivity with skeletal muscle, the majority of dialysis patients showed increased values [17, 23]. However, even with the second and third generation more cardiac specific assays, increased cTnT values were found in about 35–65% of ESRD patients on hemodialysis with the percent of patients with elevated values in part dependent on the cutoff used [8–12]. The exact mechanism of clearance of cardiac troponins is unknown. The reticuloendothelial system is postulated as an agent for clearance given the relatively large size of the troponin molecule. The troponin molecules might also be fragmented into smaller molecules, though a recent biochemical study has found that most of the circulating cTnT in the dialysis population is in the free intact form and is identical in molecular weight and elution pattern to cTnT found in patients with ACS [24]. Cardiac TnT levels are increased after dialysis potentially because of concentration effects, while cTnI levels are decreased [9]. Cardiac TnI levels were uniformly reduced after dialysis irrespective of the dialysis membrane type. Absorption of the cTnI molecule onto the dialysis membrane is one possible mechanism postulated for this finding. Hence, it is recommended that troponin levels be checked pre-dialysis, if used in the evaluation of asymptomatic patients with ESRD. Multiple mechanisms have been postulated to explain cardiac troponin elevations in ambulatory asymptomatic ESRD patients. Elevated troponin levels may reflect damage to myocytes from epicardial atherosclerotic disease with distal embolization leading to small vessel occlusion and myocyte cell death or could be secondary to myocyte damage from non-atherosclerotic mechanisms. Asymptomatic ESRD patients on hemodialysis may have either sporadic or permanent elevations of cTnT or cTnI. In patients without symptoms, signs, or other corroborating evidence of an ACS, the significance of transient or chronic elevations is uncertain.

Cardiovascular causes account for a significant percentage of deaths in patients with ESRD [25]. Overall mortality among patients on hemodialysis is as high as 240 deaths per 1000 patient years. Cardiovascular causes account for up to 40–45% of all deaths in patients with ESRD [25] (Fig. 9.1). The incidence of myocardial infarction also is substantially greater in patients with ESRD compared to those without renal disease and even in those patients with CKD not requiring dialysis (Fig. 9.2). In the setting of ACS, even small degrees of troponin elevations have predicted increased risk of death and cardiac events [7]. Over 7000 patients being evaluated for suspected ACS enrolled

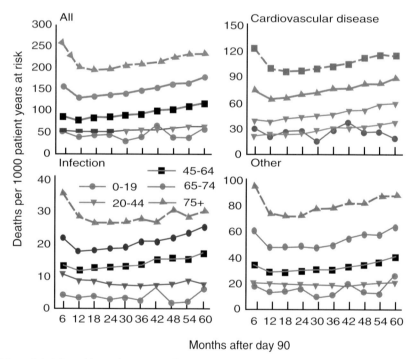

Figure 9.1 Adjusted interval cause-specific mortality, by age USRDS ADR 2005 data. (Available at www.usrds.org)

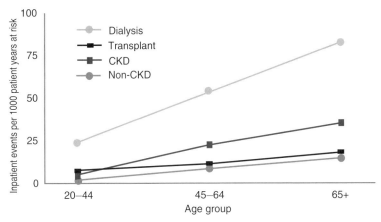

Figure 9.2 Adjusted rates of myocardial infarction, by age USRDS ADR 2005 data. (Available at www.usrds.org)

in the GUSTO IV trial were analyzed. The primary end point was a composite of death or myocardial infarction within 30 days. Cardiac TnT elevations were independently predictive of risk across the entire spectrum of renal dysfunction after adjusting for confounders, though the number of patients with severe renal disease ($n = 10$) was too small for definitive conclusions [7]. This study supports the value of troponin measurements in patients with renal impairment who present with symptoms suggestive of ACS. The implication is that a rise and fall of cardiac troponin levels in ESRD patients with signs and symptoms of an ACS can remain diagnostic. However, it is important to recognize the diagnostic accuracy of changing cardiac troponin levels during presentation for myocardial infarction has not been definitively studied in this population.

Prognosis of ESRD patients based on cardiac troponin levels

It is increasingly evident that elevated levels of cardiac troponins in patients with ESRD in settings other than that of suspected ACS also appear to be strongly associated with a higher incidence of major cardiac events and death [11–14]. This link is even stronger if troponin levels are used in conjunction with elevated C-reactive protein levels [11]. Measures to risk stratify and alter morbidity and mortality favorably are potentially important in the management of these high-risk patients. Cardiac disease is especially difficult to diagnose as atypical presentations and silent myocardial ischemic events are common in the ESRD population. Cardiac troponins have been studied as tools for risk stratification in ESRD patients. A significant body of clinical evidence now points to the increased risk of death and major cardiac events in patients with ESRD who have chronic asymptomatic elevations in cardiac troponins [14].

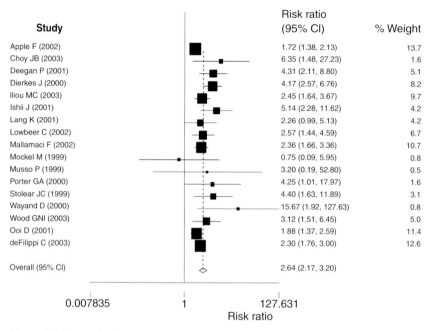

Figure 9.3 Forest plot of primary studies evaluating abnormally elevated cardiac troponin T and all-cause mortality in ESRD patients from 17 primary studies that reported all-cause mortality. (See Ref. [14])

A recent meta-analysis by Khan *et al.* [14] of 28 studies that included 3931 patients, the majority of whom were on hemodialysis, summarizes the literature on this topic. Patients were followed for an average of 23 months. Studies utilized the later generation cTnT assay and multiple cTnI assays. The majority of these studies evaluated cTnT levels for predicting all-cause mortality. There was a consistent association between elevated cTnT levels and increased risk of death with the pooled analysis revealing a relative risk of 2.64; 95% CI, 2.17–3.20 (Fig. 9.3). Eight studies in this meta-analysis evaluated cTnT levels and the outcome of cardiac death. The authors also concluded that elevated cTnT was strongly associated with a significant increase in long-term cardiac death (RR, 2.55; 95% CI, 1.93–3.37; $p < 0.001$) (Fig. 9.4). Of the 12 studies examining cTnI, elevated cTnI levels were associated with an increased total mortality (RR, 1.74; 95% CI, 1.27–2.38; $p = 0.001$). However, the risk of cardiac death was highly variable in the six studies that studied the outcome of cardiac death and troponin I (Figs. 9.5 and 9.6). Cardiac TnT levels were also found to be an independent predictor of mortality after adjusting for age, diabetes, and presence of known coronary disease in 15 of 16 studies that performed a multi-variate analysis. In contrast, of the eight troponin I studies that controlled for these confounding variables, only two

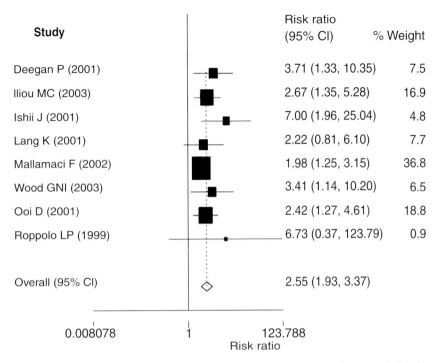

Figure 9.4 Forest plot of primary studies evaluating abnormally elevated cardiac troponin T and cardiac death in ESRD patients from eight primary studies that reported cardiac deaths. (See Ref. [14])

studies showed that troponin I was independently associated with mortality. In conclusion, asymptomatic elevation in ESRD patients of either cardiac troponin is a predictor of all-cause mortality, though the current data for cTnT for this application are more robust. Less information is available for predicting cardiovascular death, but cTnT level appears to be more predictive than cTnI for this prognostic application in ESRD patients.

Prognosis is important, but only part of the picture when using biomarkers to manage patients. An editorial by Michael Lauer in the journal *Circulation* succinctly summarized the state of current information regarding cardiac troponin levels in asymptomatic ESRD patients by stating that, "Even if we don't know what we are diagnosing when we find an elevated troponin level in a dialysis patient, we know that we have hit on an important prognostic measure that identifies an increased risk of death. We may want to know exactly what it is we are diagnosing so that this knowledge can help us develop the test to its next level, namely, as a guide to definitive therapy" [26]. The remainder of this chapter will explore evidence pointing toward or away from specific cardiac pathology responsible for troponin elevations in CKD. To illustrate these points, cases will be presented.

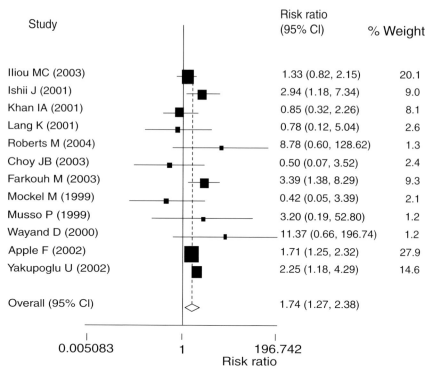

Figure 9.5 Forest plot of primary studies evaluating abnormally elevated cardiac troponin I and all-cause mortality in ESRD patients from 12 primary studies that reported all-cause mortality. (See Ref. [14])

Case presentations

Case 1

This case explores the association of elevated cTnT levels with coronary artery disease and myocardial infarction in asymptomatic ESRD patients. A 70-year-old African American male with diabetes who has been on hemodialysis for approximately a year is evaluated for renal transplantation. He ambulates distances greater than two blocks without symptoms of dyspnea or chest pain. He denies a history of prior cardiovascular events or known coronary disease. His echocardiogram shows no regional wall motion abnormalities or left ventricular hypertrophy (LVH). His left ventricular ejection fraction is estimated to be >55%. A cTnT level is measured at 0.104 ng/mL (normal is <0.03 ng/mL). A cardiac magnetic resonance imaging study with delayed late gadolinium enhancement is done as part of a research protocol to look for evidence of prior myocardial infarction (Fig. 9.7). A small region of gadolinium enhancement is seen in the apex of the left ventricle. Gadolinium enhancement detected by magnetic resonance imaging is known to identify regions of myocardial necrosis [27]. Coronary angiography is performed and shows multi-vessel coronary

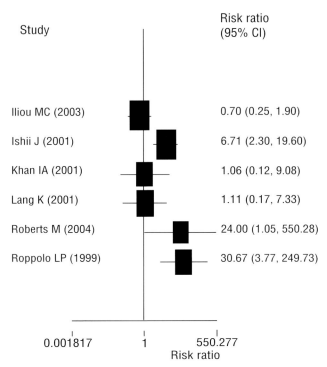

Study

Risk ratio
(95% CI)

Iliou MC (2003)	0.70 (0.25, 1.90)
Ishii J (2001)	6.71 (2.30, 19.60)
Khan IA (2001)	1.06 (0.12, 9.08)
Lang K (2001)	1.11 (0.17, 7.33)
Roberts M (2004)	24.00 (1.05, 550.28)
Roppolo LP (1999)	30.67 (3.77, 249.73)

0.001817   1   550.277
Risk ratio

Figure 9.6 Forest plot of primary studies evaluating abnormally elevated cardiac troponin I and cardiac death in ESRD patients from six primary studies that reported cardiac deaths. (See Ref. [14])

artery disease including a total occlusion of the left anterior descending artery (Fig. 9.8).

Discussion of Case 1

Several studies have found a correlation between elevated cardiac troponin levels in ESRD patients and the presence of epicardial coronary artery occlusive disease. Silent or subclinical myocardial infarctions have also been postulated to occur in ESRD patients with sporadic or chronic elevations of cardiac troponins even in the absence of epicardial coronary disease. A study by Ooi *et al.* [28] found areas of myocardial fibrosis, scarring, and recent myocardial infarctions at autopsy in ESRD patients even with modest troponin elevations. In a prospective study of ambulatory ESRD patients, our group found that the extent and severity of angiographically documented coronary disease increased with higher quartiles of cTnT elevation [11] (Fig. 9.9). Sharma *et al.* [29] demonstrated that, in ESRD patients, using a troponin T cutoff level of 0.04 ng/mL resulted in a detection of nearly twice as many patients with positive dobutamine stress echocardiogram evidence of ischemia as well as angiographic evidence of presence of coronary disease. However, not all data

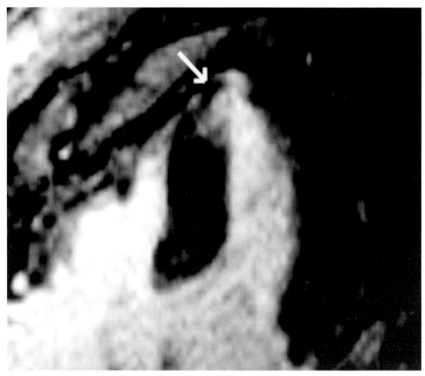

Figure 9.7 Case 1: cardiac magnetic resonance image shows gadolinium enhancement of the apex of left ventricle (arrow) thought to be consistent with myocardial infarction (age of infarct is unknown).

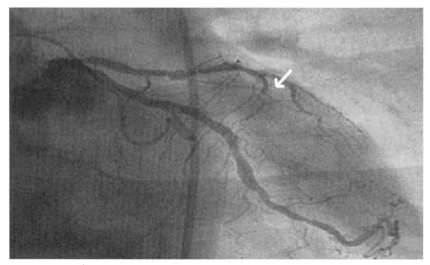

Figure 9.8 Case 1: coronary angiogram image shows the left coronary system with multi-vessel coronary disease and total occlusion of the left anterior descending artery (arrow).

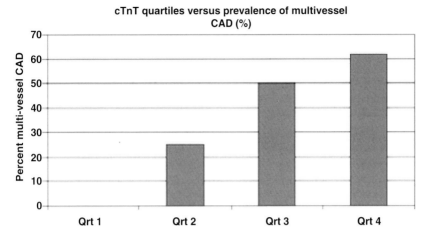

Figure 9.9 Prevalence of multi-vessel coronary disease based on quartiles of cardiac troponin T levels in asymptomatic ambulatory ESRD patients volunteering for coronary angiography ($n = 67$). cTnT, cardiac troponin T; Qrt, Quartiles; cTnT Qrt 1, < 0.029 ng/mL; cTnT Qrt 2, 0.029–0.064 ng/mL; cTnT Qrt 3, 0.065–0.116 ng/mL; cTnT Qrt 4, $\geq$0.116 ng/mL. (See Ref. [11])

have been consistent with these findings. Obialo *et al.*, in a study of ESRD patients with possible ACS, have questioned the strength of the relationship between cTnT and angiographic coronary disease [30]. In this retrospective study including 29 ESRD patients with presumed ACS with elevated cTnT levels, half the patients had normal coronary arteries. In a recently completed study by our group, we used cardiac magnetic resonance imaging to determine the prevalence of myocardial infarctions as detected by late gadolinium enhancement in ESRD patients without a history of myocardial infarction or depressed left ventricular function. We evaluated 13 patients with elevated cTnT levels (>0.07 ng/mL) and 13 patients with very low or undetectable cTnT levels (<0.03 ng/mL). We identified only three patients out of 13 in the elevated cTnT level group who had evidence by MRI of myocardial infarctions (versus 0 of 13 in the low cTnT group). It is therefore likely that clinically silent acute myocardial infarctions represent only one of several possible etiologies to explain troponin elevations in asymptomatic ESRD patients.

Case 2

This case examines the possible etiologies of cTnT elevations in asymptomatic ESRD patients without coronary disease. A 56-year-old African American male with ESRD on hemodialysis undergoes cardiac assessment as part of an evaluation for renal transplantation. He has hip pain that limits his walking beyond two blocks. He also has dyspnea on exertion on climbing more than 28 steps. He has no prior history of coronary disease and has no other cardiac symptoms. An adenosine thallium stress test shows "evidence for myocardial ischemia in the anterior wall of the left ventricle." There were no areas suggestive of prior

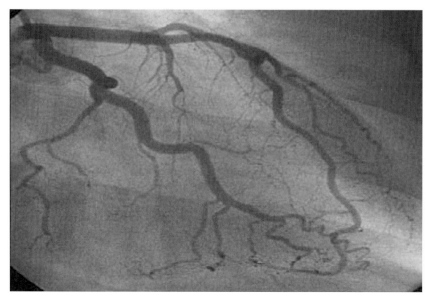

Figure 9.10 Case 2: coronary angiogram image shows the left coronary artery system in the right anterior oblique view. There is no evidence of epicardial coronary artery disease.

infarction. Resting left ventricular function was normal. Cardiac TnT levels were elevated at 0.156 ng/mL. He underwent echocardiography that showed LVH. He is referred for a cardiac catheterization that shows some mild luminal irregularities, but no obstructive coronary artery disease (Fig. 9.10). Subsequently the patient participated in a research study and underwent cardiac magnetic resonance imaging, which shows severe LVH with wall thickness approaching 2 cm, normal wall motion and no evidence of delayed gadolinium enhancement (Fig. 9.11).

Discussion of Case 2

As illustrated in this case, elevated troponin levels in ESRD patients are not always associated with the presence of epicardial coronary disease. Other mechanisms are probably responsible and several hypotheses have been advanced to explain this finding. LVH with resultant increased wall stress and ischemia due to impaired microvascular flow has been postulated as responsible for troponin elevations. Several studies have found an independent association between cardiac troponin levels and left ventricular mass [31–35]; however, this has not been a consistent finding [11, 29]. One explanation to explain these disparate findings is that echocardiography may not be accurate at estimating left ventricular mass in ESRD patients [36]. In a study by our group, magnetic resonance imaging was used to measure left ventricular mass in ESRD patients and no difference was found in the prevalence of LVH in relation to cTnT levels. There are possibly other mechanisms besides epicardial coronary

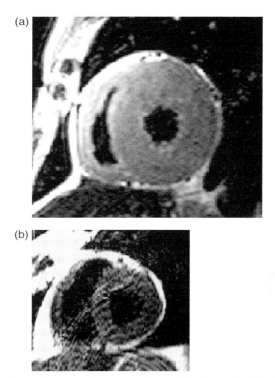

Figure 9.11 Case 2: cardiac magnetic resonance image of the short-axis of the left ventricle shows (a) severe LVH. (b) A short-axis image from a different patient without LVH is shown for reference.

disease and LVH accounting for the increased cardiac and all-cause mortality in these patients. A recent study by Mark *et al.* [37] found a pattern of diffuse late gadolinium enhancement within the myocardium on cardiac magnetic resonance imaging in 14% of their ESRD subjects indicating possibly another mechanism besides epicardial atherosclerosis (suggested by a pattern of isolated subendocardial gadolinium enhancement). The authors suggest that this pattern may represent myocardial fibrosis and be an alternative form of uremic cardiomyopathy. Interestingly, in a separate study, Aioki *et al.* [38] studied ESRD patients with dilated cardiomyopathy (DCM) and normal coronary angiograms and found that interstitial fibrosis was extensive in these patients and survival was inversely related to the extent of fibrosis on endomyocardial biopsy. The autopsy findings by Ooi *et al.* showing cTnT elevation in the presence of fibrosis and congestive heart failure support the concept that a variety of pathologies can lead to myocyte cell death and cardiac troponin release [28]. Uremia-induced changes in the ventricular myocardium including fibrosis might account for troponin elevations in ESRD patients who do not have epicardial coronary disease and helps explain the link between elevated troponin levels and increased mortality in ESRD patients.

Summary

Cardiac troponin elevations, particularly cTnT, are common in patients with ESRD and CKD. These troponin elevations are of cardiac origin. The mechanisms of cardiac injuries resulting in these elevations are diverse and likely result from epicardial coronary disease, LVH, microvascular disease, and potentially myocardial fibrosis causing cardiomyopathy among others. In the setting of an ACS, the utility of troponin measurement has been well validated in patients with CKD and provides valuable information to guide therapy and prognosticate. Troponin elevations in a non-ACS setting in ESRD patients are associated with decreased survival and an increase in both all-cause and cardiac mortality. Further work is still needed to better understand how the myocardium is injured in ESRD patients, which lead to troponin elevations. A better understanding of these issues could result in improved treatment options in this high-risk patient population.

References

1 Alpert JS, Thygesen K, Antman E, Bassand JP. Myocardial infarction redefined—a consensus document of the Joint European Society of Cardiology/American College of Cardiology Committee for the redefinition of myocardial infarction. *J Am Coll Cardiol* 2000;**36**:959–969.

2 Braunwald E, Antman EM, Beasley JW *et al.* ACC/AHA 2002 guideline update for the management of patients with unstable angina and non–ST-segment elevation myocardial infarction: a report of the American College of Cardiology/American Heart Association task force on practice guidelines (Committee on the management of patients with unstable angina). 2002. Available at http://www.acc.org/clinical/guidelines/unstable/unstable.pdf.

3 Jaffe AS, Ravkilde J, Roberts R *et al.* It's time for a change to a troponin standard. *Circulation* 2000;**102**:1216–1220.

4 Morrow DA, Cannon CP, Rifai N *et al.* Ability of minor elevations of troponins I and T to predict benefit from an early invasive strategy in patients with unstable angina and non-ST elevation myocardial infarction: results from a randomized trial. *JAMA* 2001;**286**:2405–2412.

5 Hamm CW, Heeschen C, Goldmann B *et al.*, for the c7E3 Fab Antiplatelet Therapy in Unstable Refractory Angina (CAPTURE) Study Investigators. Benefit of abciximab in patients with refractory unstable angina in relation to serum troponin T levels. *N Engl J Med* 1999;**340**:1623–1629.

6 Heeschen C, Hamm CW, Goldmann B, Deu A, Langenbrink L, White HD, for the PRISM Investigators—Platelet Receptor Inhibition in Ischemic Syndrome Management. Troponin concentrations for stratification of patients with acute coronary syndromes in relation to therapeutic efficacy of tirofiban. *Lancet* 1999;**354**:1757–1762.

7 Aviles RJ, Askari AT, Lindahl B *et al.* Troponin T levels in patients with acute coronary syndromes, with or without renal dysfunction. *N Engl J Med* 2002;**346**:2046–2052.

8 Frankel WL, Herold D, Ziegler TW, Fitzgerald RL. Cardiac troponin I is elevated in asymptomatic patients with chronic renal failure. *Am J Clin Pathol* 1996;**1**(6):118–123.

9 Wayand D, Hannsjorg B, Schatzle G, Scharf J, Neumeier D. Cardiac troponin T and I in end-stage renal failure. *Clin Chem* 2000:**46**(9):1345–1350.

10 Freda BJ, Tang HW, Van Lente F, Peacock WF, Francis GS. Cardiac troponins in renal insufficiency. Review and clinical implications. *J Am Coll Cardiol* 2002;**40**:2065–2071.

11 deFilippi C, Wasserman S, Rosanio S *et al*. Cardiac troponin T and C-reactive protein for predicting prognosis, coronary atherosclerosis, and cardiomyopathy in patients undergoing long-term hemodialysis. *JAMA* 2003;**290**:353–359.

12 Roppolo L, Fitzgerald R, Dillow J, Ziegler T, Rice M, Maisel A. A comparison of troponin T and troponin I as predictors of cardiac events in patients undergoing chronic dialysis at a Veterans Hospital. A pilot study. *J Am Coll Cardiol* 1999;**34**:448–454.

13 Apple FS, Murakami M, Pearce LA, Herzog CA. Predictive value of cardiac troponin I and T for subsequent death in end-stage renal disease. *Circulation* 2002;**106**:2941–2945.

14 Khan NA, Hemmelgarn BR, Tonelli M, Thompson CR, Levin A. Prognostic value of troponin T and I among asymptomatic patients with end-stage renal disease: a meta-analysis. *Circulation* 2005;**112**:3088–3096.

15 Antman EM. Decision making with cardiac troponin tests. *N Engl J Med* 2002;**346**(26):2079–2082.

16 McLaurin MD, Apple FS, Voss EM, Herzog CA, Sharkey SW. Cardiac troponin I, cardiac troponin T, and creatine kinase MB in dialysis patients without ischemic heart disease: evidence of cardiac troponin T expression in skeletal muscle. *Clin Chem* 1997;**43**:976–982.

17 Apple FS, Sharkey SW, Hoeft P, Skeate R, Dahlmeier BA, Preese LM. Prognostic value of serum cardiac troponin I and T in chronic dialysis patients. *Am J Kidney Dis* 1997;**29**:399–403.

18 Ricchiuti V, Voss EM, Ney A, Odland M, Anderson PAW, Apple FS. Cardiac troponin T isoforms expressed in renal diseased skeletal muscle will not cause false positive results by the second generation cardiac troponin T assay by Boehringer Mannheim. *Clin Chem* 1998;**44**:1919–1924.

19 Haller C, Zehelein J, Remppis A, Muller-Bardorff M. Cardiac troponin T in patients with end-stage renal disease: absence of expression in truncal skeletal muscle. *Clin Chem* 1998;**44**:930–938.

20 Muller-Bardorff M, Hallermayer K, Schroder A *et al*. Improved troponin T ELISA specific for cardiac troponin T isoform: assay development and analytical and clinical validation. *Clin Chem* 1997;**43**:458–466.

21 Wallace TW, Abdullah SM, Drazner MH *et al*. Prevalence and determinants of troponin T elevation in the general population. *Circulation* 2006;**113**:1958–1965.

22 Jeremias A, Gibson M. Narrative review: alternative causes for elevated cardiac troponin levels when acute coronary syndromes are excluded. *Ann Int Med* 2005;**142**:786–791.

23 Li D, Keffer J, Corry K, Vazquez M, Jialal I. Nonspecific elevation of troponin T Levels in patients with chronic renal failure. *Clin Biochem* 1995;**28**(4):474–477.

24 Fahie-Wilson M, Carmichael DJ, Delaney MP, Stevens PE, Hall EM, Lamb EJ. Cardiac troponin T circulates in the free intact form in patients with kidney failure. *Clin Chem* 2006;**52**:414–420.

25 U.S. Renal Data System. USRDS 2005 annual data report: atlas of end-stage renal disease in the United States, National Institutes of Health, National Institute of Diabetes and Digestive and Kidney Diseases, Bethesda, MD, 2005. Available at www.usrds.org.

26 Lauer MS. Cardiac troponins and renal failure: the evolution of a clinical test. *Circulation* 2005;**112**(20):3088–3096.

27 Wagner A, Mahrholdt H, Holly TA *et al.* Contrast-enhanced MRI and routine single photon emission computed tomography (SPECT) perfusion imaging for detection of subendocardial myocardial infarcts: an imaging study. *Lancet* 2003;**361**:374–379.

28 Ooi DS, Isotalo PA, Veinot JP. Correlation of antemortem serum creatine kinase, creatine kinase-MB, troponin I and troponin T with cardiac pathology. *Clin Chem* 2000;**46**:338–344.

29 Sharma R, Gaze DC, Pellerin D *et al.* Cardiac structural and functional abnormalities in end stage renal disease patients with elevated cardiac troponin T. *Heart* 2006;**92**:804–809.

30 Obialo CI, Sharda S, Goyal S, Ofili EO, Oduwole A, Gray N. Ability of troponin T to predict angiographic coronary artery disease in patients with chronic kidney disease. *Am J Cardiol* 2004;**94**:834–836.

31 Iliou MC, Fumeron C, Benoit MO *et al.* Factors associated with increased serum levels of cardiac troponins T and I in chronic haemodialysis patients. Chronic haemodialysis and new cardiac markers evaluation (CHANCE) study. *Nephrol Dial Transplant* 2001;**16**:1452–1458.

32 Lowbeer C, Ottosson-Seeberger A, Gustafsson SA, Norrman R, Hulting J, Gutierrez A. Increased cardiac troponin T and endothelin-1 concentrations in dialysis patients may indicate heart disease. *Nephrol Dial Transplant* 1999;**14**:1948–1955.

33 Mallamaci F, Zoccali C, Parlongo S *et al.* Troponin is related to left ventricular mass and predicts all-cause and cardiovascular mortality in hemodialysis patients. *Am J Kidney Dis* 2002;**40**:68–75.

34 Duman D, Tokay S, Toprak A *et al.* Elevated cardiac troponin T is associated with increased left ventricular mass index and predicts mortality in continuous ambulatory peritoneal dialysis patients. *Nephrol Dial Transplant* 2005;**20**:962–967.

35 Jeon DS, Lee MY, Kim CJ *et al.* Clinical findings in patients with cardiac troponin T elevation and end-stage renal disease without acute coronary syndrome. *Am J Cardiol* 2004;**94**:831–834.

36 Stewart GA, Foster J, Cowan M *et al.* Echocardiography overestimates left ventricular mass in hemodialysis patients relative to magnetic resonance imaging. *Kidney Int* 1999;**56**:2248–2253.

37 Mark PB, Johnston N, Groenning BA, Foster JE *et al.* Redefinition of uremic cardiomyopathy by contrast-enhanced cardiac magnetic resonance imaging. *Kidney Int* 2006;**69**(10): 1839–1845.

38 Aioki J, Ikari Y, Nakajima H, Mori M *et al.* Clinical and pathologic characteristics of dilated cardiomyopathy in hemodialysis patients. *Kidney Int* 2005;**67**:333–340.

CHAPTER 10

Cardiac biomarkers: detection of in-hospital myocardial reinfarction

Fred S. Apple

Case 1

This is the third admission for this 50-year-old black female with a history of hypertension. The patient states that she was awakened from sleep at approximately 230–300 AM this morning with crushing substernal chest pain that radiated to her back. This was associated with diaphoresis, nausea, and shortness of breath. She was brought to the emergency room (ER) by relatives. Her last pain of similar nature was 2 weeks prior to admission; her pain at that time was resolved by one sublingual nitroglycerin pill. In the ER, she was given morphine without relief of pain and was started on a nitroglycerine drip. Her initial ECG showed sinus bradycardia and T-wave inversions. She was admitted to the CCU to "rule out" for a myocardial infarction. The patient had continued chest pain, and a repeat ECG showed the interval development of ST elevation. She was treated with thrombolysis with the infusion of tissue plasminogen activator; during which time her ECG resolved to normal and felt to be indicative of successful reperfusion. On Day 4, the patient developed a recurrence of crushing chest pain with new ST elevations, which was relieved with nitroglycerine again. She was sent for cardiac angiography, which she was noted to have a 90% stenosis of her left anterior descending coronary artery. She was scheduled for an acute coronary artery bypass grafting procedure. Her biomarker laboratory results are shown as follows.

Time (h)	Total CK (U/L) (URL 200 U/L)	CKMB (ng/mL) (3.5 ng/mL)	cTnI (ng/mL) (<0.1 ng/mL)
0	105	2.0	<0.1
2	tPA administered		
6	5093	237	22.1
12	3866	107	19.0
26	2015	81	9.2
54	546	16.5	3.3
99	New onset chest pain		
99	150	8.0	0.5
105	198	9.8	1.1
112	345	28.0	3.9

Case 2

A 35-year-old male presents to the ER with severe chest pain following a week's history of lethargy and chronic renal insufficiency. The patient is on chronic hemodialysis. During the previous week the patient had developed an infection and now presents with a fever of 101°F. Within 40 minutes of presentation his systolic BP dropped to 40 mm. His ECG showed diffuse ST depression with a significant Q wave in the lateral leads. The initial results of his biomarker laboratory were: total CK 54,000 U/L, CKMB 411, and cTnI 3.5 ng/mL. In the cardiac catheterization laboratory his angiogram showed 75% occlusion of his left circumflex and 90% occlusion of his left anterior descending coronary arteries. A stent was placed in the LAD. He was medically followed in the hospital for the next 4 days with clinical improvement. His cTnI values decreased daily as follows: Day 2, 3.3 ng/mL; Day 3, 2.2 ng/mL; Day 4, 1.0 ng/mL, and Day 5, 0.7 ng/mL (upper reference limit 0.3 ng/mL). On Day 6, he had a new onset of severe chest pain that was only partially relieved by nitroglycerin. He was readmitted to the CCU and his point of care cTnI result 2 hours after the onset of new chest pain was 1.5 ng/mL, which increased to 4.8 ng/mL 4 hours later. His ECG now showed significant ST elevation. He returned to the catheterization laboratory, during which it was determined that he was a candidate for bypass surgery.

Time (h)	Total CK (U/L) (URL 300 U/L)	CKMB (ng/mL) (5.0 ng/mL)	cTnI (ng/mL) (0.3 ng/mL)
0	54,000	411	3.5
2	Stent placed		
Day 2	22,000	240	3.3
Day 3	8420		2.2
Day 4	2555	45	1.0
Day 5	550	18	0.7
Day 6	New onset chest pain		
Day 5 + 2 h	455	28	1.5
Day 5 + 6 h	666	38	4.8

Case 3

A 55-year-old male presented with worsening chest pain over the past 8 hours, starting at midnight. He presents at 0700 hours, describing a burning pain in his left shoulder, arm, and epigastrium. Pain was worsened while walking and eating, but there was some relief with sitting. In the ER, he receives some relief from nitroglycerin. He was admitted and hospitalized for a non-ST segment elevation myocardial infarction. The peak cTnI at 24 hours after onset of chest pain was 1.3 µg/L (peak CKMB 11.5 µg/L), followed-up with a normal 3-day post-event cTnI of 0.6 µg/L (CKMB was 5.0 µg/L). At 72 hours following the initial presentation the patient experienced new onset chest pain, again described as a burning pain in the left shoulder, arm, and epigastrium. While again nitroglycerin provided some relief, the ECG demonstrated only nonspecific T-wave abnormalities, not different from initial presentation. The initial cTnI on the suspected reinfarction day (Day 3) was increased at 1.4 µg/L (with a corresponding CKMB of 11.0 µg/L). Cardiac catheterization revealed new 85% distal left anterior descending stenosis, 95% mid right coronary artery narrowing, and an 80% occluded circumflex proximally. The patient was treated with successful stent placement in both the distal and proximal RCA. A summary of his cardiac biomarker laboratory results is shown.

Time (h)	CKMB (ng/mL) (URL 5.0 ng/mL)	cTnI (ng/mL) (URL 0.3 ng/mL)
0	4.2	0.7
4	11.5	0.9
12	6.8	1.3
72	Reinfarction symptoms	
72	5.0	0.6
76	11.0	1.4

Discussion of Cases 1, 2, and 3

Cardiac troponin monitoring for detection of myocardial injury has been designated the new standard for differentiating the diagnosis of unstable angina and non-ST elevation myocardial infarction (NSTEMI) in acute coronary syndrome (ACS) patients [1–4]. An increased cardiac troponin I (cTnI) or T (cTnT) in the clinical setting of ischemia is defined as an acute MI and has been endorsed by the European Society of Cardiology (ESC), American College of Cardiology (ACC), the American Heart Association (AHA), the International Federation for Clinical Chemistry (IFCC), and the Epidemiology World Council [1–5]. One of the challenges regarding cardiac troponin monitoring during a patient's hospitalization encompasses the clinical setting of myocardial reinfarction within a short time period following an initial MI. Since cardiac troponin can remain increased in the circulation for up to 5 days (cTnI) to 10 days (cTnT) after an acute MI [6], in theory the role for monitoring cardiac troponin during reinfarction has been questioned. The 2000 ESC/ACC document notes that in the clinical setting of a reinfarction creatine kinase MB (CKMB, mass assay recommended) may be more useful for monitoring for reinfarction than cardiac troponin because CKMB only remains increased for 2–4 days following an acute MI [2]. However, there is a little to no evidence to support this claim, especially when CKMB is compared head on with cardiac troponin I. There are now 11 case reports (two papers) in the literature that have readdressed the role of cardiac troponin monitoring in reinfarction [7, 8], which has led to a revised statement in the 2006 updated Global Task Force definition for reinfarction, predicated on monitoring serial changes using cardiac troponin.

The evidence-based findings, although small in number, in myocardial rein-farction patients demonstrate that CKMB analysis does not add clinically nec-essary information, and thus is not cost effective, in the differential diagnosis of myocardial reinfarction in ACS patients when cardiac troponin monitoring is available. It is time to dispel the theoretical rational for use of CKMB in addition to cardiac troponin testing; expediting the cost-effective adaptation favoring only cardiac troponin monitoring in testing for MI or reinfarction. In the case reports from the literature that utilize cardiac troponin, all reinfarc-tions occurred in-hospital within 24–96 hours of the initial index presentation. The mean time from onset of chest pain to initial presentation was 5.2 hours (median 4.0 hours; range 1–12 hours) [7, 8]. The serial cTnI and CKMB con-centrations versus time profiles for cases during both the initial MI presen-tation and reinfarction events show patients who presented initially with an STEMI and patients presenting with both increased cTnI and CKMB. At rein-farction, patients both demonstrate an increased baseline cTnI and increased CKMB. However, the rising and/or falling profiles of each biomarker paral-leled each other. In the patients where the last cTnI concentrations from the initial MI biomarker orders were increased, all reinfarctions demonstrated sub-stantial secondary increases of cTnI above the previous cTnI value [7, 8]. In the three cases presented in this chapter, similar observations are made with par-allel rising and falling biomarker patterns, with the key of following a second biomarker value within 4–6 hours after the initial value when a reinfarction is clinically suspected. Rising patterns were documented and confirmatory for cardiac troponin, paralleling CKMB mass findings, without the added concern that CKMB may be increased due to skeletal muscle contamination [9] from the documented skeletal injury in Cases 1 and 2.

The reported incidence rate of reinfarction appears to be lower than 20% [10]. A few studies have examined the secondary increases in cardiac biomarkers during an early recurrent infarction (reinfarction extension). In the largest se-ries of patients studied, Marmor *et al.* documented a secondary increase in CKMB activity occurred an average of 10 (SD 4) days after the initial infarct, but in only 17% of patients (34 of 200) [11]. Morrison *et al.*, examining release of CKMB to estimate infarct size in 35 MI patients, contended that the appear-ance of a second peak of CKMB before the return of the enzyme to baseline was not associated with an infarct extension [12]. Eisenberg *et al.* stratified 50 chest pain patients for MI based on a 50% change in CKMB levels, independent of whether CKMB was normalized between the initial or recurrent infarction [10].

No citations were identified following both MedLine and Pub Med searches for studies addressing cTnI and CKMB monitoring in myocardial reinfarction as diagnostic tools besides the two papers cited above [7, 8]. As cTnT demon-strates a longer time period for remaining increased following an initial MI (up to 10 days) [6], independent validation for cTnT should be carried out as a biomarker for reinfarction as all patients described in the literature document for cTnI after reinfarction. Given the limited financial resources in laboratories and healthcare, clinicians should consider just monitoring cardiac troponin

Table 10.1 Analytical characteristics as described by the manufacturer for the current generation cardiac troponin assays in the marketplace.

Assay	LLD	99th percentile	WHO-ROC	10%* CV
Abbott ARCH	0.009	0.012	0.3	0.032
Abbott AxSYM *ADV*	0.02	0.04	0.4	0.16
Abbott i-STAT[†]	0.02	0.08 (WB)	ND	0.1
Bayer Centaur	0.02	0.1	1.0	0.35
Bayer Ultra	0.006	0.04	0.9	0.03
Beckman Accu	0.01	0.04	0.5	0.06
Biosite Triage[†]	0.05	< 0.05	0.4	NA
Biomerieux Vds	0.001	0.01	0.16	0.11
Dade RxL	0.04	0.07	0.6–1.5	0.14
Dade CS[†]	0.03	0.07	0.6–1.5	0.06
DPC Immulite	0.1	0.2	1.0	0.6
MKI Pathfast	0.006	0.01	0.06	0.06
Ortho Vitros ES	0.012	0.032	0.12	0.053
Response[†]	0.03	< 0.03 (WB)	ND	0.21
Roche Elecsys	0.01	< 0.01	0.03	0.03
Roche Reader[†]	0.05	< 0.05 (WB)	0.1	ND
Tosoh AIA	0.06	0.06	0.31–0.64	0.06

*Per manufacturer.
[†]POC Assay, adapted from Ref. [13].

for the diagnosis of MI or in-hospital infarction. The choices of cardiac troponin assay availability have rapidly expanded. Since the first FDA cleared assay for cardiac troponin testing in 1996, the number of cardiac troponin I and T assays has increased to over 20, both in quantitative and qualitative formats, utilizing both central laboratory and point-of-care testing platforms (Table 10.1) [13, 14]. The use of cardiac troponin assays has become equal to and greater than either total CK and CKMB utilization in clinical practice per CAP surveys [15]. Implementation of quality assays for cardiac troponin testing in clinical practice based on the 99th percentile reference cutoff [13, 14, 16] will assist in the accurate and sensitive detection of an acute myocardial infarction, whether the initial index event or a secondary event indicative of in-hospital reinfarction.

References

1 Braunwald E, Antman EM, Beasley JW *et al.* ACC/AHA guidelines for the management of patients with unstable angina and non-ST-segment elevation myocardial infarction. *J Am Coll Cardiol* 2000;**36**:970–1062.

2 Joint European Society of Cardiology/American College of Cardiology Committee. Myocardial infarction defined—a consensus document of the Joint European Society of Cardiology/American College of Cardiology Committee for the redefinition of myocardial infarction. *J Am Coll Cardiol* 2000;**36**:959–969.

3 Jaffe AS, Ravkilde J, Roberts R *et al.* It's time for a change to a troponin standard. *Circulation* 2000;**102**:1216–1220.

4 http://www.americanheart.org/presenter.jhtml?identifier=3053#Heart_Attack.

5 Luepker RV, Apple FS, Christenson RH *et al.* Case definitions for acute coronary heart disease in epidemiology and clinical research studies. *Circulation* 2003;**108**:2543–2549.

6 Apple FS, Jaffe AS. Cardiac function. In: Burtis C, Ashwood E, Bruns DE, eds. *Tietz' Textbook of Clinical Chemistry and Molecular Diagnostics*, 4th edn. WB Saunders, Philadelphia, PA, 2005:1619–1670.

7 Falahati A, Sharkey SW, Christensen D *et al.* Implementation of cardiac troponin I for detection of acute myocardial injury in an urban medical center. *Am Heart J* 1999;**137**:332–337; letter to editor correction 1999;**138**:798–800.

8 Apple FS, Murakami MM. Cardiac troponin and creatine kinase MB monitoring during in-hospital myocardial reinfarction. *Clin Chem* 2005;**51**:460–463.

9 Apple FS. Tissue specificity of cardiac troponin I, cardiac troponin T, and creatine kinase MB. *Clin Chim Acta* 1999;**284**:151–159.

10 Eisenberg PR, Lee RG, Biello DR, Geltman EM, Jaffe AS. Chest pain after nontransmural infarction: the absence of remediable coronary vasospasm. *Am Heart J* 1985;**110**:515–521.

11 Marmor A, Sobel BE, Roberts R. Factors presaging early recurrent myocardial infarction ("extension"). *Am J Cardiol* 1981;**48**:603–610.

12 Morrison J, Coromilas J, Munsey D *et al.* Correlation of radionuclide estimates of myocardial infarction size and release of creatine kinase-MB in man. *Circulation* 1980;**62**:277–287.

13 Apple FS, Wu AHB, Jaffe AS. Implementation of the ESC/ACC guidelines for redefinition of myocardial infarction using cardiac troponin assays with special attention to clinical trial issues. *Am Heart J* 2002;**144**:981–986.

14 Apple FS, Quist HE, Doyle PJ, Otto AP, Murakami MM. Plasma 99th percentile reference limits for cardiac troponin and creatine kinase MB mass for use with European Society of Cardiology/American College of Cardiology consensus recommendations. *Clin Chem* 2003;**49**:1331–1336.

15 College of American Pathologist. Cardiac marker CAR-A survey participant summary report. 2004:1–30.

16 Panteghini M, Gerhardt W, Apple FS, Dati F, Ravkilde J, Wu AHB. Quality specifications for cardiac troponin assays. *Clin Chem Lab Med* 2001;**39**:174–178.

PART 2

Natriuretic peptides

CHAPTER 11

The future: interpreting new guidelines for myocardial infarction

Allan S. Jaffe

It is always difficult to predict, especially about the future; however, as new guidelines are being prepared, there are a multiplicity of issues that may contribute to changes in the way in which we ought to think about the use of troponin measurements. Accordingly, the present set of vignettes will attempt to focus on some of these complex issues.

Case 1

A 28-year-old man with a positive family history for coronary artery disease presents with typical central chest discomfort. He had not had a general physical for years, so was unaware of risk factors but was an active exerciser, running 20 miles per week and had never had similar symptoms. He was mildly diaphoretic and mildly short of breath, but his electrocardiogram was totally normal.

A troponin assay used locally had a limit of detection of 0.02 ng/mL. The 99th percentile value for that assay was 0.04 ng/mL, the 10% CV value was 0.06 ng/mL, and the ROC value was 0.5 ng/mL. The local laboratory had defined a cutoff value of 0.5 ng/mL as the cutoff value to be used to determine if patients had acute myocardial infarction.

When this patient had values of 0.06 ng/mL and then 0.45 ng/mL after 6 hours, the patient was sent home because the maximum value was below the recommended cutoff value used by the local laboratory. Twelve hours later, he represented with hypotension, ST–T wave changes in the anterior leads, and a troponin value of 1.62 ng/mL. He was taken emergently to the cardiac catheterization laboratory where an 80% LAD stenosis was identified and was stented. The QA committee at the hospital was then asked to address the issue whether this gentleman should have been sent home based on his troponin values. They decided that the use of the ROC value was no longer appropriate in the modern era.

Discussion of Case 1

This case highlights a critical issue related to how we use troponin assays. When troponin assays were initially approved, the FDA took the tact that clinicians would have difficulty and be confused if cutoff values were set far below what clinicians were used to using with CKMB. Accordingly, the so-called ROC value or receiver operator curve value was advocated for. This is the value at which troponin values are most often associated with CKMB values, which had been the previous gold standard. Using this cutoff value improved specificity because troponin is far more specific than CKMB but did not take advantage of the increased sensitivity with which troponin could be used. Subsequently, the ESC/ACC task force for the redefinition of MI embraced a more traditional laboratory-oriented approach. They indicated that the upper limit of normal should be defined by evaluating a reference population and defining the 95th or 99th percentile of a normal range for that particular test [1]. Individuals above that level would then be defined as having evidence of an elevation, which would define the presence of cardiac injury. This value was set at the 99th percentile because it would reduce the number of false positives that might exist, which was something that already was an area of sensitivity in the clinical community [2]. Subsequently, because of concerns that imprecision at the low end might influence these values, several individuals suggested the use of a value called the 10% CV value [3]. This was a value for an individual assay (in this situation of 0.06 ng/mL) where the imprecision was such that it could not be confounded by issues related to imprecision. This value was promulgated in many laboratories since laboratorians are sensitive to the concept of having values confounded by imprecision and concern that they might be generating analytical false positives. This approach has subsequently been rebuffed for four reasons. The first is the fact that imprecision as modeled recently by Apple *et al.* [4] should not in and of itself cause false positives. What imprecision does is to adversely affect the sensitivity of the assays. In addition, as we will discuss below, true normal values are substantially lower than the lower limit of most of our present assays. Thirdly, clinicians did not understand that although the 10% CV value was a value, which would not be analytically confounded, that it was not the upper limit of normal, and this led to confusion and, in some instances, to clinicians ignoring abnormal values. Finally, almost all of the studies in those with ischemic heart disease have documented that the 99th percentile identifies more individuals at risk [5] (Fig. 11.1) and because true normal values are so low, adds few if any false positives.

This individual who had a value substantially above the 99th percentile clearly had an elevation in his troponins. In addition, as we will discuss subsequently, his values were rising and he certainly should have been admitted to the hospital. At present, the recommended value that it is most likely guideline organizations will embrace is the 99th percentile. The 10% CV value because for the reasons cited above will no longer be suggested.

There is an additional issue that will affect the future. It is now clear from a multiplicity of studies that we may have in the past been incorrect about the 99th percentile calculation. These calculations are only as good as the assays involved and the populations studied. In most populations, there are individuals who have undetectable values (in the circumstance looked at above <0.02 ng/mL) and some who have values less than the 99th percentile

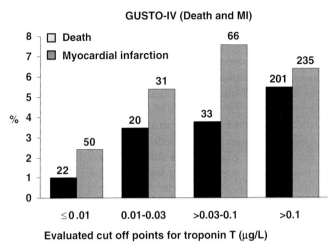

Figure 11.1 Prognostic importance of even low-level elevations in cardiac troponin from the GUSTO IV study. (Reproduced with permission from Ref. [5])

of 0.04 ng/mL but which still detectable (i.e., between 0.02 ng/mL and 0.04 ng/mL). Recent data have suggested that individuals in that range have an adverse prognosis whether when they present with acute chest discomfort or critically ill or when they have chronic stable disease or even in the absence of cardiovascular disease (Fig. 11.2) [6]. These findings from a multiplicity of studies suggest that the present calculation of the 99th percentile is confounded by a mixture of patients who have minor abnormalities and those who truly have nondetectable troponins. This synthesis of the data is totally consistent with recent information published utilizing a highly sensitive experimental assay [7] that suggests that normals have values that are at least a log unit lower than previously detected even with the more sensitive modern day assays.

Thus, in the future, we will find more elevations of troponin as assays become more sensitive. There are also data to suggest that many of these elevations are related to chronic structural heart disease [8, 9] and not to an acute presentation. This will make an additional aspect of this patient's troponin values even more important. That is to say, it is the rise of these values that suggests an acute problem [6]. If indeed rising values are observed, this likely is indicative of an acute cardiac injury whereas elevations that stay constant are indicative of chronic elevations associated with these constitutive structural changes. Most of these structural changes elicit only minor increases in the levels of troponin detectable in the circulation; however, there are subsets of individuals such as those with renal failure, some with LVH and heart failure who may have more chronic elevations even above the 99th percentile with the present iteration of assays [10]. Accordingly, utilizing a rising pattern in the troponin values will

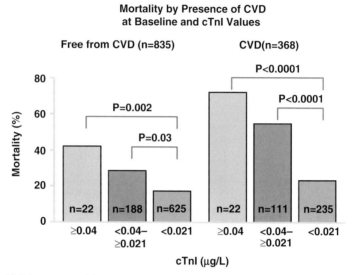

Figure 11.2 Importance of detectable levels of troponin below the 99th percentile of normal for patients with (right) and without (left) a history of cardiac disease. (Reproduced with permission from Ref. [8])

become more and more important in the future as we begin to unmask this trend. This patient had rising values, which should have been an alert to the astute clinician.

Of importance in thinking about how to define rising values is the issue of low-end precision. Imprecise assays make it more difficult to determine when changes have occurred [6]. Thus, a greater percentage change is likely to be required when one has values near the 99th percentile then when one has values that are higher. This will require some degree of individualization in regard to the assay used locally but will provide a potent ability to distinguish those more chronic elevations from those associated with acute disease. The latter obviously may require hospitalization whereas the former likely can be evaluated as outpatients.

Case 2

A 56-year-old gentleman with a known history of hypertension but without a history of coronary artery disease presents with left shoulder pain. He has been on hemodialysis for 3 years with excellent results because of polycystic kidney disease but his blood pressure has been difficult to control with hypertension when he is off dialysis and hypotension when dialyzing. He indicates that his left shoulder pain had on occasion migrated toward the center of his chest, but he had also been outside building a swing set for his children during the past weekend. His electrocardiogram showed LVH with secondary ST–T wave changes. His troponin T on admission was 0.09 ng/mL and 8 hours later was 0.10 ng/mL (99th percentile ≤0.01 ng/mL). The emergency department physician wanted to admit the patient because of the shoulder pain in the absence of a defined etiology and the fact that an elevated troponin defines high cardiovascular risk in this individual. The cardiologist was reluctant. You are called and asked for an opinion.

Discussion of Case 2

As indicated above, this gentleman presents with troponin values that are not changing [6]. Patients with renal failure and particularly when one is measuring cardiac troponin T can have elevations of cardiac troponin. Usually, they are modest, as in this case. Although this patient is clearly at increased risk long-term (Fig. 11.3) given the data from several groups [11, 12], the likelihood of a short-term problem related to his troponin is far less likely [6]. This is an example where structural heart disease may well be responsible for a troponin elevation, and this is a patient probably who could be evaluated as an outpatient given the relative benign nature of his presentation, the fact that another putative etiology for the discomfort is present (trauma while building the swing set). However, often when these patients are not admitted, their troponin elevations are ignored, and that is not appropriate. The Federal Drug Administration has approved the use of cardiac troponin T for risk stratification in patients like this who are on dialysis and the recent renal dialysis guidelines suggest that such an approach is appropriate [13]. Further research

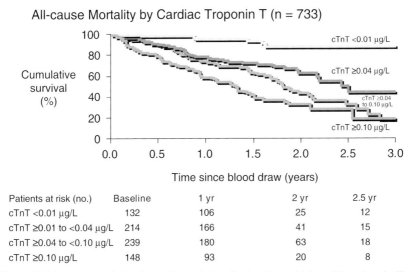

Figure 11.3 Importance of elevations of troponin in patients with renal failure. (Reproduced with permission from Ref. [11])

is necessary to define what the therapeutic implications of such an approach might be, but there are a large number of potential approaches one could take. It is known that patients who have hypertension that is poorly controlled and/or intra-dialysis hypotension are at increased risk for cardiovascular events, particularly if left ventricular hypertrophy is concomitantly present [14]. Thus, taking this gentleman's problem seriously would be terribly important, but it is not clear that could not be done in the outpatient setting.

If on the other hand, the values for cTnT had been rising, admission would have been advised. If subsequently, it appeared that the discomfort he had was likely cardiac in etiology, his prognosis, as with others who present with unstable ischemic heart disease and elevated troponins, would be adverse [15]. Obviously other acute causes for the elevations could also be present as described in other chapters.

Case 3

A 63-year-old man presented with 2 hours of the onset of new central chest discomfort to a rural hospital. His ECG showed inferior ST segment elevation, and he was given TNK and heparin and transferred to a tertiary referral center. His initial troponin value was normal, but it had risen to a value of 0.88 ng/mL (99th percentile of the assay used in this circumstance was 0.07 ng/mL) by 6 hours and to a high of 1.05 ng/mL at 15 hours. Then it declined to 0.76 ng/mL at 24 hours. The next day prior to the time when catheterization had been scheduled, he had recurrent chest discomfort and an immediate troponin result was obtained, which was 0.66 ng/mL. It subsequently rose to 0.98 ng/mL by 6 hours after stenting of the RCA for an 85% stenosis with some angiographically visible thrombus. A diagnosis of post-PCI injury was made by the attending physician, but the cardiac catheterization attending felt that the elevated troponins were due to acute reocclusion and recurrent infarction. You are asked to determine which of these individuals is correct.

Discussion of Case 3

This case is important from several perspectives. First of all, it indicates the modern day approach to making the diagnosis of recurrent infarction. The original concepts developed years before the reperfusion era when the mean time to reinfarction was 10 days [16, 17]. Accordingly, the concept evolved that any elevation of biomarkers (at that time CKMB) could be considered indicative of recurrent infarction. This obviously cannot be done with troponin, which continues to be elevated for a substantial period of time. However, with modern day interventional therapies, most patients go home 3–4 days after acute events. Thus, for many reinfarctions, which often occur early after admission and/or intervention, both troponin and CKMB may be elevated at baseline. If so, two results are necessary to make the diagnosis of recurrent infarction. An immediate result is necessary to provide a baseline value and a follow-up value is needed to document a rising pattern [18]. In this instance, the rise was substantial, over 33%, indicative of reinfarction. Whether that reinfarction was due to the procedure or due to urgent reocclusion will be addressed below. Nonetheless, given these circumstances, the use of troponin is at least equivalent for the diagnosis of reinfarction and given its other improved characteristics, this author would argue it is the analyte of choice for detection of reinfarction.

Of some importance is how to distinguish a real change from analytic variability related to the assay. If one does the calculations suggested for determining whether or not values are analytically different, they suggest that it is very unlikely to have a value more than three standard deviations of the variability of the measures when one is dealing with values that have similar variability around them [19]. For most troponin assays at values that are elevated as when reocclusion or recurrent infarction occurs, these values have a variability of 5–7%. Thus, an estimate of roughly a 20% change would be highly significant. Similar criteria could then be applied even on the down slope of the curve of someone who is having ST elevation infarction and has very high values. A similar approach can be taken with CKMB, but it is not clear given its lack of sensitivity that it would be nearly as sensitive and/or specific.

The second issue relates to whether this is reocclusion and reinfarction or related to the procedure itself is an important issue for the interpretation of post-PCI values. The issue of how to deal with baseline elevations in troponin has been ignored in most of the literature in this area. However, recent data suggest that if one adds the baseline troponin result to post-PCI values in defining prognosis that it is the baseline pre-PCI result that governs subsequent prognosis [20]. In this situation, elevations of neither troponin nor CKMB add information in regard to prognosis. This finding would provide a good explanation why previous studies, which did not take into account the baseline troponin, only the less sensitive baseline CKMB might have focused on post-PCI values as having prognostic significance. It is also clear that when one has elevations at baseline, the values that occur for both troponin and CKMB after PCI are much higher. In some instances, this may reflect the fact that the troponin is rising as in this patient, and it is very likely that the increase, which may have been augmented by the procedure, was largely due to reocclusion and reinfarction. In other patients, it may be that the troponin is simply a marker of an adverse anatomy, which is known to be associated with post-PCI values. Thus, in the presence of an abnormal baseline troponin, the ability to determine whether or not subsequent elevations are due to natural progression of the event occurring on admission or due to the procedure is impossible. Such elevations should not be designated as post-PCI elevations but should be related probably to the original event. If one has a stable but elevated baseline, the issue is more complex and unlikely one can utilize criteria for recurrent infarction in that circumstance.

In the patient who has a normal baseline troponin, subsequent elevations are generally very mild. Very few will reach the threshold suggested for CKBM of a

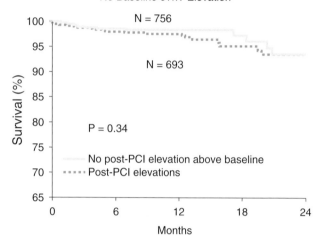

Figure 11.4 Significance of post-PCI C-troponin elevations when the baseline value is normal. (Reproduced with permission from Ref. [20])

multiple-fold increase, and there appears to be no prognostic significance associated with such elevations (Fig. 11.4) [20].

Nonetheless, it may be valuable from the point of view of quality control, quality assurance of new procedures, and/or the evaluation of various operators to evaluate post-PCI values. In addition, there may be an occasional marked elevation, which will in general correlate with in hospital complications [20]. However, it appears from the data cited above the prognostic significance whether it is of troponin or of CKMB is totally ablated when one factors the baseline troponin, a known risk factor into the equation.

These case vignettes characterize several elements of what are likely to become part of the new standards. No one can definitively anticipate the future, but these appear to be likely adjuncts to new criteria.

References

1 Myocardial infarction redefined—a consensus document of The Joint European Society of Cardiology/American College of Cardiology Committee for the redefinition of myocardial infarction. *Eur Heart J* 2000;**21**:1502–1513 and *J Am Coll Cardiol* 2000;**36**:959–969.

2 Jaffe AS, Ravkilde J, Roberts R *et al*. It's time for a change to a troponin standard. *Circulation* 2000;**102**:1216–1220.

3 Apple FS, Wu AH, Jaffe AS. European Society of Cardiology and American College of Cardiology guidelines for redefinition of myocardial infarction: how to use existing assays clinically and for clinical trials. *Am Heart J* 2002;**144**:981–986.

4 Apple FS, Parvin CA, Buechler KF, Christenson RH, Wu AH, Jaffe AS. Validation of the 99th percentile cutoff independent of assay imprecision (CV) for cardiac troponin monitoring for ruling out myocardial infarction. *Clin Chem* 2005;**51**:2198–2200.

5 James S, Armstrong P, Califf R *et al.* Troponin T levels and risk of 30-day outcomes in patients with the acute coronary syndrome: prospective verification in the GUSTO-IV trial. *Am J Med* 2003;**115**:178–184.

6 Jaffe AS. Chasing troponin—How low can you go if you can see the rise? *J Am Chem Soc* 2006;**48**:1763–1764.

7 Alan HB, Wu Noelle Fukushima, Robert Puskas, John Todd, Philippe Goix. Development and preliminary clinical validation of a high sensitivity assay for cardiac troponin using a capillary flow (single molecule) fluorescence detector. *Clin Chem* 2006;**52**: 2157–2159.

8 Zethelius B, Johnston N, Venge P. Troponin I as a predictor of coronary heart disease and mortality in 70-year-old men: a community-based cohort study. *Circulation* 2006;**113**:1071–1078.

9 Schulz O, Kirpal K, Stein J *et al.* Low-level cTnI in cardiovascular disease. *Clin Chem* 2006;**52**:1614–1615.

10 Wallace TW, Abdullah SM, Drazner MH *et al.* Prevalence and determinants of troponin T elevation in the general population. *Circulation* 2006;**113**:1958–1965.

11 Apple FS, Murakami MM, Pearce LA, Herzog CA. Predictive value of cardiac troponin I and T for subsequent death in end-stage renal disease. *Circulation* 2002;**106**:2941–2945.

12 deFilippi C, Wasserman S, Rosanio S *et al.* Cardiac troponin T and C-reactive protein for predicting prognosis, coronary atherosclerosis, and cardiomyopathy in patients undergoing long-term hemodialysis. *JAMA* 2003;**290**:353–359.

13 National Kidney Foundation. K/DOQI Clinical practice guidelines for cardiovascular disease in dialysis patients. *Am J Kidney Dis* 2005;**45**(suppl 3):S1–S154, S82.

14 Mallamaci F, Zoccali C, Parlongo S *et al.* Diagnostic value of troponin T for alterations in left ventricular mass and function in dialysis patients. *Kidney Int* 2002;**62**:1884–1890.

15 Aviles RJ, Askari AT, Lindahl B *et al.* Troponin T levels in patients with acute coronary syndromes, with or without renal dysfunction. *N Engl J Med* 2002;**346**:2047–2052.

16 Marmor A, Sobel BE, Roberts R. Factors presaging early recurrent myocardial infarction ("extension"). *Am J Cardiol* 1981;**48**:603–610.

17 Marmor A, Geltman EM, Schechtman K, Sobel BE, Roberts R. Recurrent myocardial infarction: clinical predictors and prognostic implications. *Circulation* 1982;**66**:415–421.

18 Apple FS, Murakami MM. Cardiac troponin and creatine kinase MB monitoring during in-hospital myocardial reinfarction. *Clin Chem* 2005;**51**:460–463.

19 Westgard JO, Klee GG. Quality management. In: Burtis CA, Ashwood ER, Bruns DE, eds. *Tietz Textbook of Clinical Chemistry and Molecular Diagnostics*, 4th edn. Elsevier, St. Louis, MO, 2006:498–499.

20 Miller WL, Garratt KN, Burrit MF, Lennon RJ, Reeder GS, Jaffe AS. Baseline troponin level: key to understanding the importance of post-PCI troponin elevations. *Eur Heart J* 2006;**27**:1061–1069.

CHAPTER 12

Basics of natriuretic peptides: practical aspects of assays, potential analytical confounders, and clinical interpretation

Alan H.B. Wu

Case 1: increased BNP in the presence of other confounding clinical variables

A 72-year-old white female is admitted to the emergency department (ED) with a chief complaint of dyspnea upon mild exertion. She has a history of acute coronary syndromes having suffered a non-ST-elevation myocardial infarction 10 years ago, but currently denies chest pain. A recent exercise stress test revealed the absence of ischemia. She has a prior history of hyperlipidemia. She is not a smoker, and has no prior history of heart failure, liver, pulmonary, or renal disease, hypertension, or diabetes. She regularly takes salicylates, a β-blocker, and a statin for high LDL cholesterol. The patient is 5 foot 9 inches tall and weighs 122 pounds (body mass index, BMI = 18.0). Laboratory results revealed a normal electrolyte panel, glucose 150 mg/dL (normal 70–99), creatinine 1.3 mg/dL (normal 0.6–1.2), estimated glomerular filtration rate (eGFR from the Modification of Diet in Renal Disease equation) 40 mL/min, urea nitrogen 36 mg/dL (normal 8–23), hemoglobin 12.5 g/dL (normal <12.0), cardiac troponin I <0.1 ng/mL at ED presentation and <0.1 ng/mL at 8 hours later (99th percentile <0.1), and B-type natriuretic peptide (BNP) 195 pg/mL (Biosite Triage <100 pg/mL). The patient is admitted to a non-ICU cardiology bed for further workup for possible heart failure. An echocardiogram revealed an ejection fraction of 50% (normal 45–55%). Based on this and other clinical and laboratory factors, a diagnosis of heart failure was ruled out. The patient was given diuretics that reduced the creatinine to 1.0 mg/dL and urea nitrogen to 22 mg/dL. The patient was discharged after 48 hours with a BNP of 84 pg/mL.

Discussion of Case 1

The absence of chest pain and a negative troponin at presentation and after 8 hours ruled out acute coronary syndromes during this admission. Although this patient has a BNP concentration that exceeded the cutoff concentrations, there were several other confounding variables that potentially contributed to the increased BNP concentration. It has been well established that among healthy individuals, BNP concentrations increase with age. Within an age group, women have higher BNP concentrations than men [1]. In studies conducted by the manufacturer of the BNP test used in this case, the median, 95th percentile, and range of values for women over the age of 75 years was 53.9, 179.4, and 5–218 pg/mL, respectively [2]. BNP concentrations are also affected by BMI and renal function. Among patients without heart failure, there is an inverse relationship between BMI and log BNP concentrations: lean individuals (BMI <18.5) have higher BNP concentrations than those who are overweight (BMI 25.0–29.9) or obese ($\geq$30.0) [3]. For patients with renal insufficiency, there is a direct relationship between eGFR and log BNP concentrations [4]. Regarding anemia, there is one study that showed a relationship between hemoglobin and log BNP, but only in men [5].

In this case, the patient had a history of acute coronary syndromes and was therefore at high risk for development of heart failure. However, she also had many of the confounders that increase BNP concentrations in the absence of heart failure, such as increased age, female gender, a lean BMI, and renal insufficiency. Although a cutoff of 100 pg/mL is typically used for diagnosis of heart failure, the clinical specificity at this cutoff is only 76% [6]. Thus, the BNP Consensus Panel has stated that a BNP concentration of >500 pg/mL for optimum specificity and positive predictive value [7]. In this case, a marginally increased BNP concentration was insufficient to rule in heart failure as the principal diagnosis. A normal ejection fraction also confirmed the absence of systolic heart failure.

Case 2: BNP and NT-proBNP concentrations in a patient who was transferred to another facility

A 55-year-old female presents to the ED with a diagnosis of decompensated heart failure. She was visiting a friend at a neighboring city when she became severely short of breath. She has a history of New York Heart Association (NYHA) Class II heart failure and has had several ED visits over the past year. The patient has hypertension, normal renal function, and has no history of coronary artery disease. An echocardiogram revealed an ejection fraction of 35% indicating mild systolic heart failure. Her B-type natriuretic concentration is 800 pg/mL (Biosite Triage <100 pg/mL). Her current medications included a β-blocker and an angiotensin converting enzyme (ACE) inhibitor. While in the hospital, she is treated with a diuretic resulting in an improvement in her breathing. Because she wanted to be closer to her home, she was transferred to the hospital where she had been previously treated. A new blood sample 5 days after her initial hospitalization revealed an NT-proBNP concentration of 600 pg/mL. The patient is discharged with a prescription for a higher ACE inhibitor dosage.

Discussion of Case 2

This case is complicated by the fact that the two hospitals that the patient was seen at used different analytes and assays for monitoring her heart failure.

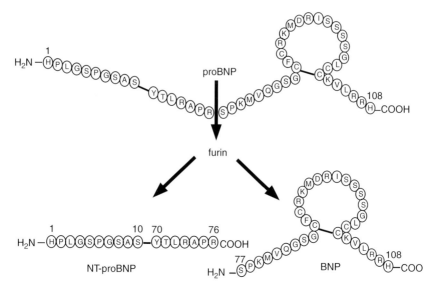

Figure 12.1 Release of BNP and NT-C from proBNP. (Used with permission from *European Journal of Heart Failure*, Elsevier Science)

Both BNP and NT-proBNP are released from proBNP (Fig. 12.1) as the result of increased ventricular filling pressures and volume overload [8]. In contrast to the biologically active BNP, NT-proBNP is inactive and has a longer half-life in blood (60–120 minutes versus 20 for BNP) [9]. BNP is cleared by natriuretic peptide receptors while NT-proBNP is largely cleared by renal function. Both are degraded in plasma by circulating proteases.

The clinical correlation between BNP and NT-proBNP testing has been shown to be essentially equivalent, particularly in patients without renal failure [10]. However, the analytical correlation between these two markers is not precise. In a published comparison of methods, the correlation between NT-proBNP (Roche Elecsys, y) and BNP (Biosite Triage, x) was: $y = 6.09x + 1132$ pg/mL, $r = 0.755$ [11]. Given the correlation coefficient that is not near unity, there is no conversion factor that can be applied to precisely convert one result to another. The manufacturer's recommended cutoff concentrations for BNP are 100 pg/mL (Biosite) and 125 pg/mL for NT-proBNP (Roche, for this patient's age). These cutoff concentrations are not consistent with the derived regression correlation between the two assays (i.e., slope of the equation), which showed that the NT-proBNP assay produced results that are roughly sixfold higher than for BNP. The pro-BNP Investigation of Dyspnea in the Emergency Department (PRIDE) study [12] showed that an NT-proBNP concentration of 450 pg/mL appears to be more congruent with 100 pg/mL BNP cutoff concentration derived from the Breathing Not Properly (BNP) Trial [6]. Using these respective cutoff concentrations, the diagnostic accuracy of these two tests is matched at 83%.

In this case report, the initial BNP concentration at 800 pg/mL was highly indicative of decompensated heart failure, as it is eightfold higher than the cutoff. While an absolute reduction in values from 800 to 600 pg/mL to NT-proBNP does not appear to be great, in actuality, there was a substantial reduction relative to the reference range, as this latter result for NT-proBNP is only marginally higher than the cutoff of 450 pg/mL. Thus, these data suggest that this patient had reached compensation to her heart failure with diuretic use and fluid clearance, consistent with clinical improvement of symptoms. The discharge NT-proBNP concentration was more consistent with her NYHA-II classification.

Case 3: decreased BNP in the presence of pre-analytic variables

A 45-year-old man with a history of NYHA Class III heart failure presents to the heart failure clinic for his bimonthly routine evaluation. The patient is on digoxin and an angiotensin II inhibitor. He has been seen in this clinic for the past year at 2-month intervals (Fig. 12.2). His plasma BNP concentration has been reasonably steady. Because he has been feeling better, he missed his last exam and is now 4 months from his last visit. In the past, his blood is collected into plastic tubes containing EDTA, the sample is centrifuged within 30 minutes, and the plasma is put into the –20°C freezer. The frozen sample is picked up by a courier in the evening, where it is delivered to a nearby reference laboratory and tested for BNP (the assay is unspecified). Today, a temporary nurse has collected the blood into a glass heparin tube, centrifuged, and the plasma is placed into the refrigerator. It is picked up by the usual courier tested approximately 6 hours after collection using the same assay as before. When the results return from the laboratory, the attending physician, unaware of the potential pre-analytical issues, tells the patient that a reduced dosage of angiotensin inhibitor was indicated.

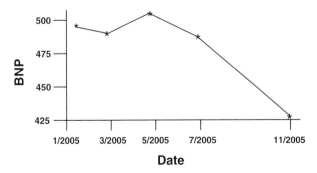

Figure 12.2 BNP concentrations in Case 3.

Discussion of Case 3

BNP is very unstable in blood and plasma and requires careful attention to pre-analytical conditions for optimum recovery of results. All manufacturers recommend that blood be collected in plastic EDTA tubes, as there is significant degradation of BNP due to the activation of the kallikrein system when glass is used [13]. EDTA is important as it inhibits serum proteases that are present at variable activities within blood [14]. Other inhibitors of arginine, serine, and kallikrein proteases can be used to further stabilize BNP in plasma, but are not available in existing blood collection tubes and must be inconveniently added after collection. While most manufacturers demonstrate BNP stability within 4 hours after collection, there are differences in the recommendations after 4 hours. Biosite states that plasma should be frozen at $-20°C$ if testing cannot be conducted within 4 hours. Abbott permits refrigerated (2–8°C) storage of whole blood or plasma but not room temperature, for up to 24 hours. Bayer suggests that whole blood samples are stable for up to 24 hours at either room temperature or refrigerated, and plasma is stable under refrigeration only. These differences in apparent stability relate to the mechanism by which BNP is degraded and the specific antibody combinations that are used for its measurement [15]. It may be possible that some antibody epitopes are lost during the degradation process while others are maintained.

In this case, the use of a glass tube and heparin as the preservative was inappropriate and likely compromised the BNP concentration that was found. It was inappropriate of the attending physician to lower the heart failure medication based on this erroneous result. Although there appeared to be a trend toward decreasing BNP concentrations during the last two visits, the result from the 7/2005 visit was well within the intra-individual biological variation of the test, estimated to be about 40% [16], while the result from the 11/2005 visit was probably falsely low as the result of the incorrect tube used. The delay from collection to testing may have also reduced the true BNP value (see Fig. 12.2).

Most attending physicians are unaware of pre-analytic variables affecting laboratory test results. Fortunately, the majority of analytes testing in the clinical laboratory have adequate stability and this is not a major issue. BNP is an exception and requires strict attention to sample handling details, particularly in an outpatient environment. Point-of-care testing within the physician office would reduce the pre-analytical variables associated with BNP testing. Alternatively, NT-proBNP testing could be used on an outpatient basis, as this analyte can be tested on heparinized plasma and serum, and has longer-term analyte stability [17]. It would not be appropriate, however, to use different tests within the same patient for longitudinal monitoring of heart failure therapy.

References

1 Wieczorek SJ, Wu AHB, Christenson R *et al.* A rapid B-type natriuretic peptide (BNP) assay accurately diagnoses left ventricular dysfunction and heart failure—a multi-center evaluation. *Am Heart J* 2002;**144**:834–839.

2 Package insert. *Triage BNP Test*. Biosite Diagnostics, San Diego, CA, 2004.

3 McCord J, Mundy BJ, Hudson MP *et al*. Relationship between obesity and B-type natriuretic peptide levels. *Arch Intern Med* 2004;**164**:2247–2252.

4 McCullough PA, Duc P, Omland T *et al*. B-type natriuretic peptide and renal function in the diagnosis of heart failure: an analysis from the breathing not properly multinational study. *Am J Kidney Dis* 2003;**41**:571–579.

5 Wu AHB, Omland T, Wold Knudsen C *et al*. Relationship of B-type natriuretic peptide and anemia in patients with and without heart failure: a substudy from the breathing not properly (BNP) multinational study. *Am J Hematol* 2005;**80**:174–180.

6 Maisel AS, Krishnaswamy P, Nowak RM *et al*. Rapid measurement of B-type natriuretic peptide in the emergency diagnosis of heart failure. *N Engl J Med* 2002;**347**:161–167.

7 Silver MA, Maisel A, Yancy CW *et al*. BNP Consensus Panel 2004: a clinical approach for the diagnostic, prognostic, screening, treatment monitoring, and therapeutic roles of natriuretic peptides in cardiovascular diseases. *Con Heart Fail* 2004;**10**(suppl 3):1–30.

8 Hall C. Essential biochemistry and physiology of (NT-pro)BNP. *Eur J Heart Fail* 2004;**6**:257–260.

9 Mair J, Friedl W, Thomas S *et al*. Natriuretic peptides in assessment of left-ventricular dysfunction. *Scand J Clin Lab Invest* 1999;**59**(suppl 230):132–142.

10 Hammerer-Lercher A, Neubauer E, Muller S *et al*. Head-to-head comparison of N-terminal pro-brain natriuretic peptide, brain natriuretic peptide and N-terminal pro-atrial natriuretic peptide in diagnosing left ventricular dysfunction. *Clin Chim Acta* 2001;**310**:193–197.

11 Sykes E, Karcher RE, Eisenstadt J *et al*. Analytical relationships among Biosite, Bayer, and Roche methods for BNP and NT-proBNP. *Am J Clin Pathol* 2005;**123**:584–590.

12 Januzzi JL, Jr, Camargo CA, Anwaruddin S *et al*. The N-terminal Pro-BNP investigation of dyspnea in the emergency department (PRIDE) study. *Am J Cardiol* 2005;**95**:948–954.

13 Shimizu H, Aono K, Masuta K *et al*. Degradation of human brain natriuretic peptide (BNP) by contact activation of blood coagulation system. *Clin Chim Acta* 2001;**305**:181–186.

14 Belenky A, Smith A, Zhang B *et al*. The effect of class-specific protease inhibitors on the stabilization of B-type natriuretic peptide in human plasma. *Clin Chim Acta* 2004;**340**:163–172.

15 Apple FS, Mair J, Ravkilde J *et al*. Quality specifications for B-type natriuretic peptide assays. *Clin Chem* 2005;**51**:486–491.

16 Wu AHB, Smith AC, Mather JF *et al*. Biological variation for NT-pro- and B-type natriuretic peptides and implications for therapeutic monitoring of patients with congestive heart failure. *Am J Cardiol* 2003;**92**:628–631.

17 van der Merwe D, Henly R, Lane G *et al*. Effect of different sample types and stability after blood collection of N-terminal pro-b-type natriuretic peptide as measured with Roche Elecsys system. *Clin Chem* 2004;**50**:779–780.

CHAPTER 13

Natriuretic peptides in clinical practice

Alan Maisel

Introduction

The explosion of natriuretic peptide levels in clinical practice has presented an opportunity to improve patient care with congestive heart failure (CHF), with regard to both diagnosis and treatment. However, natriuretic peptide determinations are nearly never straightforward, but must be interpreted in light of other clinical factors including the history and physical examination, other laboratory tests, along with understanding the nuances of natriuretic peptide levels. The following cases will help clear up some of these nuances and should make for a better understanding of their use in CHF.

Part I: BNP and diagnosis of CHF

Case 1

A 64-year-old patient comes to the emergency department (ED) with severe shortness of breath. He is new to the hospital system. On exam, he has poor air movement, normal JVP, and the question of a gallop. He has no edema. CXR is suboptimal. His BNP level comes back at 34 pg/mL.

A. The cause of this patient's dyspnea is likely to be CHF
B. The cause of this patient's dyspnea is likely not to be CHF
C. The cause of this patient's dyspnea is a mixture of CHF and pulmonary disease

The answer is B. The negative predictive value of BNP is one of the strongest features of the BNP assay. This was illustrated by Breathing Not Properly Study, the first large-scale, multinational prospective study using BNP levels to evaluate the cause of dyspnea. In this study of 1586 patients who came to the ED with acute dyspnea, patients' BNP levels were measured upon arrival, and the ED physicians (blinded to levels) were asked to assess the probability of the patient having CHF [1]. Two independent cardiologists also blinded to the BNP levels later reviewed all clinical data and standardized scores to produce a "gold standard" clinical diagnosis. BNP levels by themselves were found to be more accurate predictors of the presence or absence of CHF than any historical or physical findings or laboratory values. BNP levels were much higher in patients with subsequent CHF than with those of non-cardiac dyspnea (675 pg/mL versus 110 pg/mL). A BNP cutoff value of 100 pg/mL had a sensitivity of 90% and a specificity of 76% for differentiating CHF from other causes of dyspnea, and a cutoff level of 50 pg/mL had a negative predictive value of 96%.

Case 2

A 64-year-old comes to the ER with 2 hours of shortness of breath. The resident draws a BNP level which is only 75 pg/mL. Yet the patient is clearly in pulmonary edema with rales up to the clavicles, big neck veins, and pulmonary edema on chest X-ray. He excitedly pages the attending claiming the prize (attending) pays for dinner for two for the first patient with CHF and abnormal ventricular function, but who has a normal BNP. The attending comes down and examines the patient (doing one thing the resident forgot), and the patient is quickly herded off somewhere. The resident ends up having to buy the attending dinner. What did the attending find in the exam that made the resident pay up?

BNP levels should be elevated in all cases of congestive heart failure in which the ventricle is involved and the myocyte is stretched. This patient appears to have real congestive heart failure. The fact that the BNP is not elevated suggests a number of scenarios. Flash pulmonary edema occurs in such a short time that BNP levels may not have enough time to elevate. Also, if the heart failure is "upstream" from the left ventricle, as is the case here, BNP may not be elevated. In the present case, the patient had a silent inferior myocardial infarction 1 week previously and now presented with acute onset of mitral regurgitation secondary to papillary muscle rupture. All the heart failure is upstream from the left ventricle, which is why the BNP is not elevated.

Case 3

A 75-year-old patient presents to the ED with fatigue, mild shortness of breath, and dizziness. One week prior, he had URI symptoms with stabbing chest pain. On exam, his blood pressure is 90/60, pulse 95 and while he has no rales, he has JVP to the angle of the jaw. His BNP is only 36 pg/mL. What should be the next step?

A. Diuresis
B. Inotropes
C. Echo and pericardiocentesis
D. Immediate coronary artery angiography

In a patient who appears to have clear CHF, a normal BNP should alert the physician to several things. There are several conditions that mimic CHF but have normal BNP levels. Cardiac tamponade and constrictive pericarditis are probably those most important in this regard. In this case, the patient was subsequently found to have a large pulsus paradoxus and echocardiography revealed a large anterior pericardial effusion with diastolic collapse of the right ventricle. Subsequent pericardiocentesis alleviated the problems.

Case 4

You are called to a "code-blue" in dialysis clinic. You find a man who is being dialyzed but has a pressure of only 60 over 40. He has underlying LV diastolic dysfunction, but carries a pre-dialysis BNP level of around 600. As you revive him, the nurse mentions that a BNP before dialysis was only 240 pg/mL. Which of the following are likely to be true about the patient:

A. He no longer needs to be on dialysis.

B. BNP levels are not helpful in the setting of renal failure, so why bother.

C. The code-blue had nothing to do with the low BNP level.

D. When you later talk to the patient you find out he ate a frozen burrito from a fast food store and had 2 days of diarrhea. Thus, the lower BNP level likely represents decreased volume, even in the setting of renal failure. Therefore, less fluid should have been taken off the patient.

   The answer is D. There is confusion on how to use BNP levels in patients with renal dysfunction. The BNP Multinational Study was pivotal in establishing the correlations between eGFR and BNP in those with and without CHF [2]. This study pointed out that BNP values should not be interpreted in isolation, but should be integrated with other findings in the diagnostic evaluation. Importantly, chronic kidney disease (CKD) does appear to influence the optimum cutpoints for BNP in the diagnosis of CHF. In general, as the CKD stage advances, a higher cutpoint of BNP is implied. A cutpoint of ~200 pg/mL is reasonable for those with eGFR <60 mL/min/1.73 m². Using this approach, BNP would maintain a high level of diagnostic utility with an area under the receiver operating characteristic curve of >0.80 across all CKD groups. In the present case, the patient's baseline BNP included that from volume overload, when he became volume depleted because of the diarrhea, his BNP level was now representative of clearance and diastolic dysfunction, but not of excess volume.

Case 5

A 65-year-old patient with no previous cardiac or pulmonary disease comes in with progressive shortness of breath over 1 week. On exam, he has rales, normal JVP, and difficult to hear heart sounds. He has no edema. ECG shows nonspecific ST changes. His chest X-ray shows a normal heart size with alveolar pulmonary edema. One resident makes the diagnosis of CHF, the other of acute respiratory distress syndrome (ARDS). How can you differentiate? (More than one right answer)

A. PFT's

B. Echocardiogram

C. Swan–Ganz

D. BNP level

   The presence of these concomitant pulmonary disorders does not diminish the utility of the BNP test in distinguishing patients with heart failure from those without heart failure as long as one uses good clinical judgment along with appropriate ancillary testing.

Morrison *et al.* [3] demonstrated that rapid testing of BNP could help differentiate pulmonary from cardiac etiologies of dyspnea. Some types of pulmonary disease, such as cor pulmonale, lung cancer, and pulmonary embolism have elevated BNP levels, but these are not usually elevated to the extent as in patients with dyspnea from CHF. In a substudy of Breathing Not Properly [4], it was demonstrated that of 417 patients with a history of asthma or chronic obstructive pulmonary disease without a history of CHF, 21% were found to have newly discovered CHF. Only 37% were identified in the ED while a BNP >100 pg/mL identified 93%. Additionally, BNP levels greater than 100 pg/mL provided diagnostic information beyond that obtained from individual chest radiographic indicators (3,4).

Because BNP levels have been a useful surrogate of wedge pressure and are useful in differentiating heart failure from lung disease, they may be of value in differentiating noncardiogenic from cardiogenic pulmonary edema [5]. BNP levels were obtained in 35 patients with ARDS and from 42 patients hospitalized for severe dyspnea with the diagnosis of CHF. The median BNP level in patients with CHF of 773 pg/mL was significantly higher than patients with ARDS (123 pg/mL; $p < 0.001$). The area under the receiver-operated characteristic curve using BNP to differentiate CHF from ARDS was 0.90 (0.83–0.98; $p < 0.001$). At a cutpoint of 360 pg/mL, there was 90% sensitivity, 86% specificity, 89% positive predictive value, and a 94% negative predictive value (accuracy = 88%) for ARDS versus CHF. Thus, BNP may be accurate enough to differentiate noncardiogenic from cardiogenic pulmonary edema such that invasive hemodynamic catheter placement may not always be necessary. BNP levels >360 pg/mL suggest CHF as the diagnosis.

A pulmonary embolism large enough to raise the pulmonary artery pressure due to right ventricular strain may raise BNP levels. If the above can be ruled out, it is much more likely that BNP levels between 100 and 400 pg/mL represent CHF. In fact, BNP levels, along with troponin levels are prognostic in patients with pulmonary embolism [6].

Finally, BNP levels are closely related to functional impairment of patients with primary pulmonary hypertension and parallel the extent of pulmonary hemodynamic changes and right heart failure [7]. It is speculated that serial measurements of BNP may help improve the management of these patients.

Case 6

A 75-year-old woman with hypertension comes in with progressive dyspnea on exertion. A stress test was normal and a MUGA showed an ejection fraction of 55%. Her BNP is 255 pg/mL. Which of the following is correct?

A. She does not have CHF

B. She has severe pulmonary disease

C. She likely has diastolic dysfunction

Diastolic dysfunction, which is a common cause of CHF in patients presenting with dyspnea, is also associated with high BNP levels [8, 9]. In the Breathing Not Properly Study, BNP levels were roughly half as high as patients with systolic dysfunction (60) and interestingly, were similar in magnitude to patients with the diastolic patients with "restrictive-like" filling patterns through the mitral valve. A number of studies have elucidated the value of BNP levels to detect diastolic dysfunction. Lubien *et al.* [8] assessed BNP levels in 294 patients referred for echocardiography. Patients diagnosed with evidence of abnormal LV diastolic function ($N = 119$) had a mean BNP concentration of 286 ± 31 pg/mL while the normal LV group ($N = 175$) had a mean BNP concentration of 33 ± 3 pg/mL. Patients with restrictive-like filling patterns on echo had the highest BNP levels (408 ± 66 pg/mL), and patients with symptoms had higher BNP levels in all diastolic filling patterns. The area under the ROC curve for BNP to detect any diastolic dysfunction was 0.92 (0.87–0.95, $p < 0.001$). A BNP value of 62 pg/mL had a sensitivity of 85%, specificity of 83%, and an accuracy of 84% for detecting diastolic dysfunction when systolic function was normal.

Case 7

An obese man presents to the emergency room with progressive sob over the past month. He now has severe SOB at rest. On exam, he is breathing 390 times per minute JVP cannot be determined. Rales are not present and heart sounds are very distant. His CXR is of poor quality. His BNP is 250 pg/mL.

1 Most patients with CHF this sick will have BNP levels over 1000 so that this is not CHF

2 Pulmonary disease is the clear culprit

3 CHF is likely

CHF is indeed likely here. Obesity appears to be a marked risk factor for the development of CHF [9]. Yet obesity can interfere with our usual diagnostic approaches to CHF, including the physical exam, chest X-ray, and echocardiography [10, 11]. Thus, BNP levels may play in important role as an adjunct, certain caution is warranted.

Mehra *et al.* were the first to demonstrate that there is a significant inverse relationship between BMI (body mass index) and BNP levels [12]. The Breathing Not Properly Study supports Mehra's data. In patients presenting with heart failure and low BMI had BNP levels >1000 pg/mL 50% of the time. Patients with CHF and high BMI greater than 30 pg/mL had BNP levels >1000 pg/mL in only 8–24% of patients.

Part II: BNP in hospitalized patients

Case 1

A 78-year-old male is admitted for severe decompensated CHF. He has rales to the clavicles, a third heart sound, and JVP to the angle of the jaw. A Swan–Ganz catheter is placed and he has a filling pressure (wedge) of 33 mm Hg. His baseline BNP that is usually in the 200s is now 1600. Using diuretics and nitroprusside the wedge pressure falls to 22 mm Hg and he has a net urine output of 3 L. What can be said about the BNP level measured the following morning.

A. No change in BNP

B. Should show a marked decrease (up to 50 pg/mL/hour)

C. BNP levels will increase

   The answer is B. Since a major stimulus for the release of BNP is increased wall tension, one might expect that BNP levels would correlate with elevated LV filling pressures. Indeed, there is a body of data to support that supposition. However, in the clinical setting there are many occasions where high BNP level is not associated with high filling pressures. Some of these situations include BNP elevations from right-sided failure secondary to cor pulmonale, pulmonary embolism, or primary pulmonary hypertension; acute or chronic renal failure; and rapid lowering of the wedge pressure with diuretics and/or vasodilators before a Swan–Ganz catheter is placed.

   While in a given patient the BNP level does not always correlate to wedge pressure, in a patient admitted with CHF and high filling pressures secondary to volume overload, along with a high BNP level ("wet BNP," see below), a treatment-induced decrease in wedge pressure will almost always be associated with a rapid drop in BNP levels, as long as the patient is maintaining adequate urine output. Kazanegra *et al.* [13] measured wedge pressure, hemodynamic measurements (pulmonary capillary wedge pressure [PCWP], cardiac output, right atrial pressure, systemic vascular resistance [SVR]), and BNP levels every 2–4 hours for the first 24 hours and every 4 hours for the next 24–48 hours in patients admitted for decompensated CHF. PCWP dropped from 33 ± 2 mm Hg to 25 ± 2 mm Hg over the first 24 hours, while BNP dropped from 1472 ± 156 pg/mL to 670 ± 109 pg/mL.

Case 2

Please match "wet BNP levels" (decompensated) and "dry BNP levels" (euvolemic) with the following scenarios:

A. Anything significantly over baseline BNP level with symptoms

B. If a patient comes to the ED with dyspnea, often over 600 pg/mL

C. Usually falls rapidly with treatment

D. BNP level once euvolemia is reached

E. Correlates with functional class and prognosis

F. Falls slower with treatment

   The BNP level of a patient who is admitted with decompensated heart failure is comprised of two components: that of a baseline, euvolemic "dry" BNP level and that occurring from acute pressure or volume overload ("wet" BNP level). At the point of decompensation, a patient's BNP level will be a sum of their baseline BNP level plus what volume overload adds. Anything over the baseline BNP level with symptoms can be considered a wet BNP. In the emergency room, these will nearly always be over 600 pg/mL. Wet BNP levels fall toward baseline rapidly with effective treatment. Dry BNP levels fall slower with treatment and correlate to functional class and prognosis.

Case 3

A 75-year-old patient with previous hypertension, coronary artery disease, and COPD is admitted with pneumonia and is intubated due to progressive hypoxia and hypotension, presumably from sepsis. He improves on antibiotics, but is still difficult to wean from the ventilator. One morning after he fails a CPAP trial, someone orders a BNP. It comes back at 850 pg/mL.

The *incorrect* thing to do would be to:

A. Consider diuresis
B. Perhaps use Swan–Ganz guided therapy
C. Obtain echocardiography
D. Order a breathing treatment

The answer is D. The high BNP in this case strongly suggests that the difficulty in weaning may be secondary to lung water from high left ventricular diastolic pressure. CHF monitoring and treatment may be a benefit in this case.

Case 4

You are taking care of a patient who has just come out of the CCU where he was treated for severe CHF. With a swan in place, his BNP levels were lowered from 1400 to 325 over 48 hours. He comes to the floor on digoxin 0.25 mg, fosinopril 10 mg, and lasix 20 mg po. He can now lay flat in bed. The next day you are about to send him home. His BNP level comes back at 750 pg/mL. What should you do?

A. Outpatient follow-up
B. Back to the ICU—perhaps a swan
C. Up titrate beta-blocker
D. Consider in-patient titration of diuretics and ACE inhibitor

The lower the discharge "dry weight" BNP level is, the less likely the patient will be an early victim to rehospitalization. This is because a low BNP level (<200–300 pg/mL) represents an NYHA II patient and one that is more likely to be in a true euvolemic state. There are several possible reasons that a BNP level will rise following an initial rapid decline. First and foremost is that the oral medical regiment (diuretics and vasodilators) is not yet at the proper dose. These should be titrated depending on whether the major issue is fluid overload or increased afterload. If a patient is over-diuresed in the hospital, the subsequent renal impairment will cause a paradoxical increase in BNP levels.

Case 5

A patient comes in with apparent decompensated CHF. His BNP is 2300 pg/mL. He has no rales but his JVP is high and his blood pressure is only 95/65. He is given 80 mg of IV lasix and diuresis about 1 L. But his BNP level measured the following day did not drop. What are potential reasons for this: (more than one may be right)

A. Patient is already at his "dry weight" BNP level, which is a bad prognostic sign.
B. Patient is becoming pre-renal with the diuretics—which can actually decrease BNP clearance.
C. Patient might be getting rid of "third space" fluid, which is not the same as lowering the filling pressure.
D. Resident actually ordered "latex" instead of lasix. Patient still breathing rapidly but is now wearing rubber gloves.

There may be several explanations why elevated BNP levels do not fall with treatment in some patients with congestive heart failure. First and foremost, the high BNP level may actually be the patient's "dry" BNP level and will not be acutely lowered with diuretics or vasodilators. These patients tend to be NYHA class IV and have a poor prognosis.

Perhaps, patients who have high BNP levels that do not respond to treatment should be considered for other more invasive types of therapies such as cardiac transplantation or use of ventricular assist devices. Patients with a wide QRS might be considered for bi-ventricular pacing. In a recent trial of patients who received ventricular assist devices for end-stage heart failure, BNP levels appeared to fall as remodeling of the heart occurred, and an early decrease in BNP plasma concentration was indicative of recovery of cardiac function during mechanical circulatory support [14]. In any event, patients with high BNP levels at discharge are at increased risk, and if nothing else, are candidates for early follow-up and perhaps home nursing visits.

There are other reasons that a BNP level might not fall with treatment. It is possible that with parenteral diuretic treatment of the decompensated, pre-renal patient, further azotemia might occur. These will likely down-regulate BNP clearance receptors, and BNP levels will rise. In this setting nesiritide infusions might be indicated. Another possible scenario is that a patient with left along with right heart failure and significant ascites and/or edema, may often diurese many liters before BNP levels actually drop. This is possibly because rather than lowering wedge pressure, the urine output is occurring secondary to mobilization of third space fluid. Continuing diuresis and/or vasodilatation should eventually lower BNP levels. Finally, acute, severe pressure or volume overload might turn on the transcription of the messenger RNA for BNP to such a degree, that even upon initial lowering of the wedge pressure, BNP levels might sill be increasing.

Part III: monitoring BNP levels as an outpatient

Case 1

You are following a clinic patient with known CHF who has been stable NYHA class II, taking digoxin, fosinopril, and lasix. His BNPs have been stable in the mid-200s. He comes into clinic one day complaining of fatigue and shortness of breath. He is light-headed. He recently lost his wife due to breast cancer. On exam, he is tachypneic and slightly tachycardic (102 bpm) with no other findings. The best thing to do would be to:

A. Admit and treat for CHF.
B. Admit and put a swan in for diagnosis and treatment.
C. Up his outpatient regimen (increase diuretic).
D. Get a BNP level. If it's <200–300 pg/mL, it probably is not decompensated CHF.

   The answer is D. Perhaps, the best way to keep a person out of the hospital is not to let the discharge BNP level go up. Early after discharge, rise in BNP levels often are associated with volume overload and diuretics may need to be adjusted. As is the practice at several institutions [15] when a patient comes to the urgent care center with symptoms that could represent a decompensated state, a BNP level is drawn. If no different from baseline values, then decompensation is unlikely. How high a BNP level should be over baseline to call it decompensated is not known. As BNP is not a stand-alone test, it should be used in conjunction with other features of the exam. In our experience, clinical features of decompensation along with an increase of 50% or more from baseline are often associated with decompensation.

Case 2

You have someone you see in clinic that has long-standing CHF from myocarditis. He is on fosinopril 40 mg, lasix 40 mg, and you have begun to up-titrate carvedilol. Right now he is on 12. 5 mg bid. You would like to titrate up to at least 25 mg bid, but patient is reticent to try, as he felt weak with the last up-titration. Patient otherwise feels as if he is NYHA class II (can do most things he wants if he doesn't go too hard). The normal BNP for class II patients is about 200–300 pg/mL. His BNP is 450 pg/mL. What should you do?

A. Add a diuretic and forget about carvedilol
B. He's probably on enough beta-blocker now
C. Put him on transplant list
D. Reassure him about carvedilol because a BNP level this high might not be the best thing in the world

   The correlation between the drop in BNP level and the patient's improvement in symptoms (and subsequent outcome) during hospitalization suggests that BNP-guided treatment might make "tailored therapy" more effective in an outpatient setting such as a primary care or cardiology clinic. The Australia–New Zealand Heart Failure Group analyzed plasma neurohormones for prediction of adverse outcomes and response to treatment in 415 patients with left ventricular dysfunction randomly assigned to receive carvedilol or placebo [16]. They found that BNP was the best prognostic predictor of success or failure of carvedilol use. Recently, Troughton *et al.* randomized 69 patients to N-terminal BNP-guided treatment versus symptom-guided therapy [17].

Patients receiving N-terminal BNP-guided therapy had lower N–BNP levels along with reduced incidence of cardiovascular death, readmission, and new episodes of decompensated CHF. This study has spawned a number of larger studies including the multi-center Rapid Assessment of Bedside BNP in Treatment of Heart Failure (RABBIT) trial. But perhaps more importantly, is there an outpatient level of BNP we should aim for? This may be the "holy grail" for BNP testing, for if such an optimal BNP level exists, it may be the point we shoot for in titrating medications for patients. It is evident that patients with poor ejection fraction but with BNP levels that are under 200 pg/mL have a very good prognosis. A study of 452 ambulatory patients with an LV ejection fraction <35% found that, in patients with mild to moderate CHF (NYHA class I/II), BNP levels were independent predictors of sudden death, an important cause of mortality in these patients. They found that a cutoff BNP level of 130 pg/mL differentiated between patients with high and low survival rates of sudden death. Only 1% (1 of 110) of those patients with BNP levels below the cutoff point died suddenly, in comparison to a sudden death rate of 19% (43 of 227) among those patients with BNP levels above the cutoff point [18]. Using BNP levels to identify a patient population with a higher risk of sudden death can help to tailor their treatment and extend survival.

It also appears that ACE inhibitors, angiotensin receptor blocker agents, spironolactone, and perhaps beta-blockers drive BNP levels down, although it is unclear whether this is a true marker of clinical improvement. In the Valsartan Heart Failure Trial (Val-HeFT), changes in BNP over time induced by pharmacologic therapy were shown for the first time to correlate with morbidity and mortality [19]. Patients with the greatest percentage decrease in BNP and norepinephrine (NE) from baseline had the lowest morbidity and mortality, whereas patients with greatest percentage increase in BNP and NE were at greatest risk. The authors found BNP to be more predictive of morbidity and mortality than NE, or, in a separate analysis, than aldosterone.

Case 3

You are asked to see a 70-year-old patient with CHF. He had an MI 10 years ago. Though his ejection fraction is only 23%, you are surprised that he plays 1 hour of singles tennis everyday and never complains of shortness of breath. You are even more surprised when his BNP level comes back less than 100 pg/mL. What is going on?

A. The BNP level is wrong

B. The ejection fraction is wrong

C. The BNP reflects the fact that the heart has adapted nicely

D. The patient would have a high wedge pressure if swanned

The answer is C. There are many patients who have low ejection fractions but who also have low BNP levels. In most of these cases the heart and periphery has adapted. Most of these patients are asymptomatic or mildly symptomatic (NYHA I-II) and have an excellent prognosis. Remember that the obese patient will have lower levels of BNP than the non-obese patient.

Conclusion

The purpose of this paper was to illustrate using patient cases how BNP levels can be interpreted. The scenarios covered included the urgent care area, the hospital setting, and the outpatient setting. BNP levels are an exciting addition to the diagnosis and management of heart failure. They are not a stand-alone test but should be interpreted by integrating other historical, exam and laboratory tests. There is a learning curve for using BNP levels. It is the author's hope that the cases and discussion in this manuscript will further assist the health-care practitioner in their quest for improved medical delivery.

References

1 Maisel A, Krishnaswamy P, Nowak RM *et al.* Rapid measurement of B-type natriuretic peptide in the emergency diagnosis of heart failure. *N Engl J Med* 2002;**347**(3):161–167.

2 McCullough PA, Duc P, Omland T *et al.* B-type natriuretic peptide and renal function in the diagnosis of heart failure: an analysis from the breathing not properly multinational study. *Am J Kidney Dis* 2003;**41**(3):571–579.

3 Morrison KL, Harrison A, Krishnaswamy P *et al.* Utility of a rapid B-natriuretic peptide (BNP) assay in differentiating CHF from lung disease in patients presenting with dyspnea. *J Am Coll Cardiol* 2002;**39**:202–209.

4 McCullough PA, Hollander JE, Nowak RM *et al.* Uncovering heart failure in patients with a history of pulmonary disease: rationale for the early use of B-type natriuretic peptide in the emergency department. *Acad Emerg Med* 2003;**10**(3):198–204.

5 Berman B, Spragg R, Maisel A. B-type natriuretic peptide (BNP) levels in differentiating congestive heart failure from acute respiratory distress syndrome (ARDS). Abstracts from the 75th annual scientific meeting of the American Heart Association. *Circulation* 2002;**106**:S3191.

6 Kucher N, Printzen G, Goldhaber S. Prognostic role of brain natriuretic peptide in acute pulmonary embolism. *Circulation* 2003;**107**:2545–2547.

7 Leuchte HH, Holzapfel M, Baumgartner RA *et al.* Clinical significance of brain natriuretic peptide in primary pulmonary hypertension. *JACC* 2004;**43**(5):764–770.

8 Lubien E, DeMaria A, Krishnaswamy P *et al.* Utility of B-natriuretic peptide (BNP) in diagnosing diastolic dysfunction. *Circulation* 2002;**105**(5):595–601.

9 Krishnaswamy P, Lubien E, Clopton P *et al.* Utility of B-natriuretic peptide (BNP in elucidating left ventricular dysfunction (systolic and diastolic) in patients with and without symptoms of congestive heart failure at a veterans hospital. *Am J Med* 2001;**111**: 274–279.

10 Kenchaiah S, Eveans JC, Levy D *et al.* Obesity and the risk of heart failure. *N Engl J Med* 2002;**347**:358–359.

11 Eckel RH, Barouch WW, Ershow AG. Report of the National Heart, Lung, and Blood Institute—National Institute of Diabetes and Digestive and Kidney Diseases Working Group on the pathophysiology of obesity-associated cardiovascular disease. *Circulation* 2002;**105**:2923–2928.

12 Mehra MR, Uber PA, Park M *et al.* Obesity and suppressed B-type natriuretic peptide levels in heart failure. *JACC* 2004;**43**(9):1590–1595.

13 Kazanegra R, Cheng V, Garcia A *et al.* A rapid test for B-type natriuretic peptide correlates with falling wedge pressures in patients treated for decompensated heart failure: a pilot study. *J Card Fail* 2001;**7**:21–29.

14 Sodian R, Loebe M, Schmitt C *et al.* Decreased plasma concentrations of brain natriuretic peptide as a potential indicator of cardiac recovery in patients supported by mechanical circulatory assist systems. *J Am Coll Cardiol* 2001;**38**:1942–1949.

15 Maisel, A. Algorithm for using B-type natriuretic peptide levels in the diagnosis and management of congestive heart failure. *Crit Pathways Cardiol* 2002;**1**(2):67–73.

16 Richards AM, Doughty R, Nicholls MG *et al.* Neurohumoral predictors of benefit from carvedilol in ischemic left ventricular dysfunction. *Circulation* 1999;**99**:786–797.

17 Troughton RW, Frampton CM, Yandle TG, Espiner EA, Nicholls MG, Richards AM. Treatment of heart failure guided by plasma amino terminal brain natriuretic peptide (N-BNP) concentrations. *Lancet* 2000;**355**:1126–1130.

18 Berger R, Huelsman M, Strecker K *et al.* B-type natriuretic peptide predicts sudden death in patients with chronic heart failure. *Circulation* 2002;**105**:2392–2397.

19 Anand IS, Fisher LD, Chiang Y-T *et al.*, for the Val-HeFT Investigators. Changes in brain natriuretic peptide and norepinephrine over time and mortality and morbidity in the Valsartan Heart Failure Trial (Val-HeFT). *Circulation* 2003;**107**:1278–1283.

CHAPTER 14

Outpatient evaluation for cardiovascular diseases using natriuretic peptide testing

Aaron L. Baggish, James L. Januzzi

Introduction

Use of B-type natriuretic peptide (BNP) and its co-secreted amino-terminal pro-peptide (NT-proBNP) has been shown to be useful for the diagnostic evaluation of patients with acute dyspnea. These peptides can assist with correctly identifying or excluding acute destabilization of heart failure (HF) [1–3] and are also useful adjuncts for the triage and management of these patients [2, 4]. The role of BNP and NT-proBNP testing in areas outside of acute patient evaluation is only now becoming understood. There is great optimism that these markers will prove to be even more useful than originally anticipated.

This chapter will examine the role of natriuretic peptide testing in the outpatient setting across a wide variety of patient types: from the "apparently well" patient with no known heart disease to those with either symptomatic or previously documented heart disease. We will consider the role of BNP or NT-proBNP for numerous indications in this very large population of patients including early detection of HF in asymptomatic patients, risk stratification for cardiovascular events and mortality in patients with known heart disease (valvular, ischemic, congenital, and pulmonary arterial disease), and diagnosis and exclusion of HF in patients with symptoms suggestive of this diagnosis.

The challenge of early detection of HF in those previously not suspected of the diagnosis as well as comprehensive evaluation of those with known structural heart disease and the clinical syndrome of HF is relevant. HF and complications related to HF account for a staggering financial burden to the healthcare system and have a grave impact on patient quality of life, productivity, and mortality. In recognition of this fact, the American Heart Association recently redefined the stages of HF [5], placing particular emphasis on considering those "at risk" for HF (Stage A) or those with asymptomatic structural heart disease/HF in evolution (Stage B). It is thought that earlier applications of therapies known to benefit HF, such as agents modifying the angiotensin/aldosterone axis or beta adrenergic blockers might be expected to favorably alter the ultimate prognosis of patients at these earlier stages.

Natriuretic peptide testing: asymptomatic patients with no known heart disease

Case 1

A 71-year-old man is seen in a primary care clinic. He has a prior medical history of type II diabetes mellitus as well as hypertension. He is without symptoms, and has no sign of manifest cardiovascular disease, but he admits that he is not overly active. He has a family history for HF. His physical examination is normal. His electrocardiogram demonstrates mild nonspecific ST–T wave changes, but is otherwise unremarkable. What might natriuretic peptide testing offer in the evaluation of this patient?

Discussion of Case 1

HF is an increasingly important issue to the healthcare system and the burden of this syndrome is expected to rise as the general population ages. This is related to the age-dependent prevalence of risk factors for the development of HF, such as diabetes mellitus, hypertension, and coronary artery disease. By definition, the above-presented patient is likely to have either AHA Stage A or B HF and without echocardiography, this distinction is exceedingly difficult to resolve. As the prevalence rates of asymptomatic left ventricular (LV) systolic dysfunction in population studies may be as high as 3.0% [6–8], methods for earlier detection of those at risk for, or those with early stages of HF would be invaluable. It is neither logical nor cost-effective to perform two-dimensional echocardiography for universal evaluation of at-risk patients in primary care. Thus, the role of BNP and NT-proBNP testing for such patients is particularly relevant.

Numerous studies of BNP or NT-proBNP testing for detection of asymptomatic HF have addressed the potential utility of these assays for detecting patients at risk for the development of clinically overt HF (Table 14.1). In a head-to-head analysis of BNP and NT-proBNP, both assays were reasonably useful for the identification of AHA Stage B HF, with an edge in specificity for NT-proBNP (78% versus 69% for BNP, a difference that was statistically significant) [9]. Examining the role of these markers for population surveillance and screening, one trial obtained baseline NT-proBNP measurements in 672 subjects and then followed for a median period of two and a half years. NT-proBNP was reported as being 92% sensitive and 86% specific for the diagnosis of HF, and was also useful for stratifying risk patients for future cardiovascular events, including mortality, over the period of follow-up [10]. Similarly, BNP concentrations in excess of 18 pg/mL were strongly predictive of cardiovascular mortality over 4 years of follow-up in a random sample of over 1600 subjects in Glasgow [11], presumably due to incident ischemic heart disease events or HF. Similar findings relating hazard to concentrations of BNP in the population were demonstrated by Wang and colleagues among 3346 subjects from the population in Framingham, Massachusetts, in whom

Table 14.1 Summary of trials addressing the performance of natriuretic peptide (NP) testing (BNP and NT-proBNP) in asymptomatic patients without known heart disease.

Study	Natriuretic peptide (NP)	Study objective(s)	Conclusions	Findings support NP screening
McDonagh et al.	BNP	Assess the mortality of asymptomatic left ventricular systolic dysfunction and its association with NP levels in a random sample of the general population	Elevated NP levels were associated with the presence of asymptomatic LV dysfunction and were associated with increased mortality risk	Yes
De Sutter et al.	NT-proBNP	Study the predictive value of NP levels for coronary events in a middle-aged population of men	Over a 2.6 year follow-up, men with coronary events had significantly higher enrollment NP levels	Yes
Galasko et al.	NT-proBNP	To define the NP normal range and assess its cardiovascular screening characteristics in general population	Age and gender stratified NP levels have a 99% negative predictive value for excluding LV dysfunction, atrial fibrillation, and valvular heart disease	Yes
Ueda et al.	BNP	Estimate the prognostic importance of NP elevation in elderly (> 80 year old) patients without known heart disease	Risk of cardiovascular events and mortality rise in parallel fashion with NP levels in elderly patients without prior heart disease	Yes

Study	NP	Objective	Findings	
Wang *et al.*	BNP & NT-proBNP	Determine the prognostic significance of plasma natriuretic peptide levels in apparently asymptomatic persons	Elevated NP levels were associated with increased risk of mortality, new atrial fibrillation, stroke, heart failure, and aggregate cardiovascular events	Yes
Groenning *et al.*	NT-proBNP	Evaluate NP testing as a diagnostic and prognostic marker for systolic heart failure in the general population	Elevated NP levels above the median (32.5 pg/mL) were strongly associated with increased risk of mortality and hospitalization for heart failure	Yes
Wallen *et al.*	BNP	Determine whether prospective NP measurements NP predict mortality in the general elderly population	Increased risk of 5-year mortality was associated with elevated NP levels	Yes
Vasan *et al.*	BNP	Examine the usefulness of NP for screening for elevated LV mass and LVSD in the community	Area under the ROC curve for detecting elevated LV mass and LV systolic dysfunction was < 0.75. NP screening was concluded to be of limited usefulness	No
Redfield *et al.*	BNP	To determine whether NP might serve as a biomarker for preclinical ventricular dysfunction and guide the decision to pursue or forgo echocardiography	Low disease prevalence and suboptimal NP performance characteristics suggested NP screening to be suboptimal	No

concentrations of BNP were strongly predictive of incident cerebrovascular and cardiovascular complications [12], including incidence of death from any cause, major cardiovascular events, HF, atrial fibrillation, stroke or transient ischemic attack, and coronary artery disease. After adjustment for traditional cardiovascular risk factors, each increment of 1 standard deviation in the log of BNP levels was associated with a 27% increase in the risk of death ($p = 0.009$), a 28% increase in the risk of a first cardiovascular event ($p = 0.03$), a 66% increase in the risk of atrial fibrillation ($p < 0.001$), a 77% increase in the risk of HF ($p < 0.001$), and a 53% increase in the risk of stroke or transient ischemic attack ($p = 0.002$). In this relatively healthy population the measured BNP levels [medians = 6.2 pg/mL (men), 10.0 pg/mL (women); 80th percentile = 20.0 pg/mL (men), 23.3 pg/mL (women)] were well below the absolute values that have been established for the diagnosis of HF. These findings echo the results of other studies of populations at various levels of risk for the development of heart disease [13–15]. In each of these studies, elevated concentrations of BNP or NT-proBNP appeared to identify neurohormonal disarray (even in the absence of elevation in other markers of myocardial abnormalities such as activation of the renin–angiotensin system [16]) in otherwise normal-appearing patients and as such, may be useful for earlier detection or exclusion of HF. As well, both BNP and NT-proBNP consistently appear to strongly-predict hazard in these populations, even when adjusting for prevalent comorbidities [17, 18].

The data for population-based "screening" are not universally positive. A community-based prospective cohort study of 3177 individuals from the Framingham Study was performed to assess the performance of B-type natriuretic peptide for the screening of LV hypertrophy and systolic dysfunction. This study demonstrated relatively poor specificity of BNP [19], which was likely a reflection of the low baseline prevalence of disease in the studied population: hypertension (67%), established cardiovascular disease (16%), and diabetes (8%). Receiver operating characteristic curve (ROC) analysis of BNP testing for LV hypertrophy or systolic dysfunction revealed an area under the curve of <0.75 for both conditions. In addition to an evaluation of BNP testing used in isolation, the authors developed a multivariable model for predicting echocardiographic phenotype consisting of clinical variables. The addition of BNP testing to this model only marginally improved diagnostic accuracy and was only statistically significant in men. The authors concluded that BNP testing has limited usefulness as a screening tool for these diagnoses in lower-risk populations. In a similar fashion, a subsequent report from the Mayo clinic reported the performance of BNP as a biomarker for preclinical systolic and diastolic left ventricular dysfunction [20]. In this study, 2042 individuals without clinical HF but with underlying conditions including hypertension (29.5%), diabetes (7.5%), and coronary artery disease (12.2%) had an echocardiogram to assess for the presence of systolic and diastolic dysfunction and a concomitant measure of serum BNP concentration. The authors then used ROC curve analysis to determine the accuracy of BNP testing for the detection of echocardiographically determined diastolic and systolic dysfunction. In the overall cohort, BNP's ability to predict myocardial dysfunction revealed an AUC of 0.79 with an optimal BNP partition value of 25.0 pg/mL. Considering the relatively low prevalence of preclinical ventricular dysfunction (7.5%) and the modest observed specificity of BNP for this diagnosis (76%), a strategy relying on BNP testing as a guide for the need to pursue echocardiography was concluded to be suboptimal.

In aggregate, considering cardiovascular comorbidities with respect to testing for BNP or NT-proBNP levels, it is logical to expect that natriuretic peptide testing would be most useful for the evaluation of the "at-risk" population. Indeed, existing supports the use of these markers for stratifying the risk in such patients rather than the randomly selected general population.

As an example, hypertension is a primary risk factor for the development of LV hypertrophy and ultimately HF. NT-proBNP has been shown to predict LV mass in patients with hypertension [21, 22], and Hildebrandt and colleagues demonstrated values of NT-proBNP to be quite strongly prognostic in this patient population [21]. As well, when considering other prevalent risk factors for cardiovascular events in hypertensive subjects with LV hypertrophy, Olsen and colleagues actually demonstrated an exaggerated predictive value of NT-proBNP testing [23]. It is likely that BNP and NT-proBNP would also be expected to detect early abnormalities in diastolic function among patients with hypertension and data suggest potential utility for this application. In an analysis comparing BNP to NT-proBNP for the evaluation of preclinical cardiac impairment, Seino and colleagues demonstrated both markers to be useful for the detection of diastolic abnormalities [24], though NT-proBNP appeared to be superior to BNP in this regard, somewhat reminiscent of the superiority of NT-proBNP over BNP for evaluating symptomatic patients with non-systolic HF [25].

Another population at risk for incident cardiovascular events is patients with diabetes mellitus, now considered to be a coronary artery disease "equivalent." As has been shown in several studies, testing for either BNP or NT-proBNP is incrementally useful for identifying a risk for cardiovascular morbidity and mortality in diabetic individuals, even when considering other prevalent abnormalities, such as hypertension or ischemic heart disease and the presence or absence of symptoms suggestive of HF (Fig. 14.1) [26–32]. In keeping with observations from other studies, the prognostic value of natriuretic peptides appears to be amplified in diabetic subjects with other risk factors for structural heart disease, including those with microalbuminuria [30–34]. In patients with diabetes, it is likely that the signal detected predicting hazard is either subclinical diastolic (or systolic) abnormalities, related either to changes in myocardial structure/function related to the diabetic milieu, or the presence of subclinical ischemic heart disease. Indeed, elevated natriuretic peptides may reflect the presence of coronary artery disease in asymptomatic patients [35], and appear to be strongly prognostic in these patients (with and without diabetes mellitus) [29], implying a role for these peptides to stratify risk in patients at risk for, as well as those with established HF.

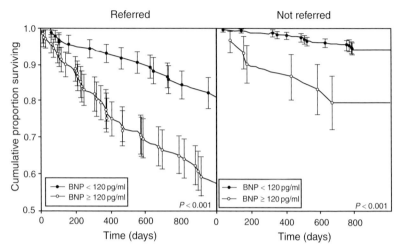

Figure 14.1 Kaplan–Meier survival curves of diabetic patients who died of all causes (including the cardiac death) with B-natriuretic peptide (BNP) values < 120 and (120 pg/mL in the patient groups referred for echo because of a clinical suspicion of heart failure (referred) and in those randomly selected from an ambulatory diabetic clinic (not referred). (Figure reprinted with permission from the *Journal of the American College of Cardiology*)

The relevant challenge is to identify the most logical application of the assays for BNP or NT-proBNP for the evaluation of the asymptomatic outpatient. It is now recognized that age and gender both modify the levels of these assays in otherwise apparently normal patients [18, 36]. Thus, optimal interpretation of the levels of natriuretic peptides in the general population should probably include consideration of both. As well, while the negative predictive value (NPV) of BNP or NT-proBNP is well established, the positive predictive value (PPV) is less secure for screening in general populations. Harnessing the high NPV, it has been suggested that use of BNP or NT-proBNP as a "gate-keeper" for more in-depth assessment of higher-risk subjects with echocardiography would be expected to improve the ability to more appropriately evaluate those patients more likely to benefit from further investigations [37, 38]. Conversely, integrating factors from clinical evaluation (such as history or physical examination findings consistent with a risk for HF) [18] or other abnormal laboratory finding (such as abnormalities on 12-lead electrocardiography) might be expected to further improve the PPV of these assays [39].

Natriuretic peptide testing: patients with asymptomatic heart disease

Given their relationship with diagnosis and prognosis in patients with symptomatic HF, there is great interest in the use of natriuretic peptide testing for the evaluation of patients without symptomatic HF but with established structural disease, such as valvular pathology, pulmonary artery hypertension, or coronary artery disease. It is generally held that the standard of care for the management of patients with asymptomatic valvular heart disease is to inter-vene at a time when the risk for morbidity and mortality rises. This "golden moment" for surgical intervention [40] is thought to largely depend on identi-fying the earliest stages of myocardial decompensation, either from pressure overload (such as in the case of aortic stenosis) or volume overload (such as in aortic or mitral regurgitation). While the timing for intervention has tradition-ally been to await sentinel signs, such as the development of symptoms, dila-tion of the LV on echocardiography, or the appearance of cardiac arrhythmia such as atrial fibrillation, there is increasing enthusiasm for the use of natri-uretic peptide surveillance in patients with valvular heart disease to identify earlier signs of neurohormonal derangement in such patients. It is thought that the mechanism of elevation of such markers in patients with preserved LV function is likely reflective of the onset of diastolic abnormalities (reflected by moderate elevations of the markers) followed by more marked elevations in the markers in the subsequent onset of systolic dysfunction [41].

Aortic valve disease

Case 2
A 55-year-old female has a past medical history of a bicuspid aortic valve. She has severe aortic stenosis with moderate aortic regurgitation. She is without symptoms. What is the role of natriuretic peptide testing in the care of this patient?

Discussion of Case 2
Several studies now demonstrate an intimate relationship between elevations of BNP or NT-proBNP and symptom onset as well as ultimate prognosis in patients with asymptomatic aortic stenosis (Table 14.2) [41–47]. Early data [42, 48] suggested a close relationship between the severity of aortic stenosis and concentrations of both BNP and NT-proBNP. In fact, natriuretic peptide val-ues were more strongly associated with symptom onset than aortic valve area. Subsequent data demonstrate that among patients treated with or without aor-tic valve replacement, NT-proBNP concentrations were consistently related to myocardial performance and survival for those patients treated surgically as well as those patients treated conservatively [45–47]. Among a cohort of asymptomatic subjects from New Zealand, NT-proBNP elevation was the ear-liest harbinger of the onset of symptoms (the traditional cross-road for surgical intervention) [43, 46, 47]. While limited data exist, there appears to be a simi-lar, albeit less intimate relationship between levels of natriuretic peptides and aortic valve regurgitation [48–50].

Mitral valve disease

Case 3
A 62-year-old female with a past medical history of childhood rheumatic fever and subsequent mitral valve stenosis presents for a routine health maintenance visit. Her most recent echocardiogram, done 1 year prior to this visit, reported

Table 14.2 Summary of trials addressing the role of natriuretic peptide (NP) testing (BNP and NT-proBNP) in patients with valvular aortic stenosis.

Study	Year	Natriuretic peptide (NP)	Study objective(s)	Conclusions
Kupari et al.	2005	BNP and NT-proBNP	Assess NP levels as function of normal LV function, asymptomatic LV dysfunction, and heart failure	NP levels are significantly higher in AS patients with LV dysfunction and HF
Gerber et al.	2003	NT-proBNP	Evaluate NP levels as predictors of symptom onset in initially asymptomatic patients	On average, rise in NP level was greater in patients who developed symptoms over 1-year follow-up
Lim et al.	2004	BNP	Identify NP cutoff for differentiating symptomatic from asymptomatic patients and evaluate relationship between NP levels and mortality	BNP < 66 pg/mL was accurate for excluding symptomatic AS while a BNP > 97 pg/mL was associated with increased mortality
Nessmith et al.	2005	BNP	Evaluate prognostic role of NP in patients managed without surgery	NP levels are highly predictive of 1-year mortality. A BNP > 819 pg/mL is associated with a 60% 1-year mortality
Weber et al.	2004	NT-proBNP	Evaluate the relationship between NP levels and both aortic valve area and symptom severity	NP levels are tightly correlated with aortic valve area and NYHA functional class

a calcific and thickened mitral valve with a mean trans-mitral gradient of 8 mm Hg. She has no symptoms and is in sinus rhythm. What is the role of natriuretic peptide testing in this patient's assessment?

In patients with mitral stenosis, even though the left ventricle is theoretically "protected" from volume or pressure load, concentrations of natriuretic peptides still appear to be useful for tracking disease presence and severity. In a study of 29 patients with isolated mitral stenosis, Arat-Ozkan and colleagues demonstrated that NT-proBNP was related to echocardiographic findings and functional classification [51]. The mechanism of the elevation of natriuretic peptides in patients with mitral stenosis likely reflects atrial distension as well as right ventricular pressure and volume overload due to pulmonary hypertension. This hypothesis is supported by data from Shang and colleagues who demonstrated that BNP concentrations were related to high left atrial and pulmonary artery pressures, and were strongly predictive of the onset of atrial fibrillation [52]. Notably, among those patients undergoing percutaneous balloon valvulotomy, concentrations of BNP fell in parallel with the improvements in trans-valvular gradient and resolution of pulmonary hypertension in those in normal sinus rhythm, compared to those in atrial fibrillation where levels remained elevated.

The relationship between mitral valve regurgitation and natriuretic peptides is well established (Table 14.3) [53–55]. Although concentrations of natriuretic peptides generally parallel the severity of mitral regurgitation [54, 55], it is now thought that elevations of these peptides not only reflect the volume overload in such patients, but also the myocardial consequences of such volume load. Hence, it is not surprising that in patients with significant mitral regurgitation, concentrations of BNP parallel the likelihood for death (hazard ratio per 10 pg/mL = 1.23, 95% confidence intervals = 1.07–1.48, $p = 0.004$) or the composite of death and HF (hazard ratio per 10 pg/mL = 1.001–1.19, $p = 0.04$) [56].

Congenital heart disease and pulmonary hypertension

Case 4
A 22-year-old man with Down's syndrome and a congenital membranous ventricular septal defect is seen for a scheduled maintenance visit. He has no signs or symptoms suggestive of right HF or pulmonary hypertension. What is the role of natriuretic peptide testing in this setting?

Discussion of Case 4
The intimate relationship between natriuretic peptide concentrations and both left and right heart structure and function has led to an increased enthusiasm for the use of these markers for the longitudinal follow-up of patients with congenital heart disease. As demonstrated [57–60], levels of BNP are useful to sort out those patients with congenital heart disease complicated by right HF. Levels of natriuretic peptides are thought to be related not only to ventricular overload in congenital heart disease, but also to the degree of arterial oxygen

Table 14.3 Summary of trials addressing the role of natriuretic peptide (NP) testing (BNP and NT-proBNP) in patients with mitral valve regurgitation.

Study	Year	Natriuretic peptide (NP)	Study objective(s)	Conclusions
Brookes et al.	1997	BNP	Determine whether NP levels are elevated and predictive of LV dysfunction in asymptomatic patients	NP levels were significantly higher in patients with organic MR than in matched controls with normal valves
Sutton et al.	2003	BNP and NT-proBNP	Describe association between NP levels and severity and symptoms	NP levels increase with MR severity and are higher in symptomatic compared to asymptomatic patients, even when LV EF is normal
Mayer et al.	2004	BNP	Assess the relationship between functional MR and NP levels in patients with heart failure	In patients with both systolic and diastolic heart failure, the presence of MR is associated with increased NP levels
Detaint et al.	2005	BNP	Define the determinants and prognostic value of NP levels in patients with organic MR	NP levels were more strongly associated with ventricular and atrial consequences rather than degree of MR. Elevated NP levels were associated adverse events in patients managed conservatively with MR

desaturation in patients with cyanotic heart disease [61], implying a role of arterial oxygen content in the mechanism of natriuretic peptide release [62] for those patients with cyanotic congenital defects. Whether values of natriuretic peptides will be useful for longitudinal management and earlier detection of the onset of myocardial decompensation in patients with congenital heart lesions is unclear, but early data suggest a role for patients with tetrology of Fallot [63, 64] as well as in those with ventricular septal defects [65].

It is not surprising, in light of the understanding of the role played by the right ventricle in elevations of BNP or NT-proBNP [66–69] that syndromes selectively involving the right ventricle, such as pulmonary hypertension, may be associated with elevations in natriuretic peptides. Such elevations are related to the presence and severity of pulmonary hypertension, and may change in parallel with changes in pulmonary hemodynamics and patient functional capacity [70–72] as well as response to inhaled pulmonary vasodilators [73]. This data suggests a role for BNP or NT-proBNP testing to monitor disease progression and response to therapy in these patients. In addition, concentrations of natriuretic peptides are strongly prognostic in patients with primary pulmonary hypertension [70–72, 74, 75].

Ischemic heart disease

Case 5
A 67-year-old man with known coronary artery disease resulting in an inferior wall ST-segment elevation myocardial infarction is seen for a routine office visit 2 years after his event. Prompt cardiac catheterization at the time of his initial presentation culminated in successful stenting of his right coronary artery. A post-catheterization echocardiogram showed preserved left ventricular function. He has no symptoms or signs of recurrent ischemia or HF. What is the value of natriuretic peptide testing for this patient?

Discussion of Case 5
Although the relationship between BNP or NT-proBNP for predicting reinfarction in patients with acute ischemic coronary disease is less established, as noted above, there is a clear association between BNP and NT-proBNP and myocardial ischemia [76, 77]. This relationship between natriuretic peptide elevation and myocardial ischemia appears to be independent of LV systolic function. In patients with stable ischemic heart disease, elevated concentrations of BNP and NT-proBNP are strongly prognostic for left ventricular dysfunction and adverse outcomes over long periods of follow-up, implying a possible role for these markers in the surveillance of risk in patients with known ischemic heart disease [29, 78] (Fig. 14.2). The relationship between natriuretic peptides and risk in patients with stable ischemic heart disease may reflect the magnitude of coronary artery disease in these patients [79–82], and may correlate with asymptomatic ischemic burden [83]. Given these relationships between BNP and NT-proBNP and the magnitude of and inherent risk

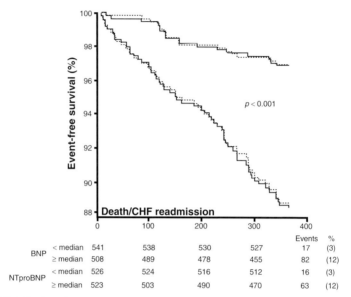

		Events	%
BNP	< median	541	538	530	527	17	(3)
	≥ median	508	489	478	455	82	(12)
NTproBNP	< median	526	524	516	512	16	(3)
	≥ median	523	503	490	470	63	(12)

Figure 14.2 Kaplan–Meier event-free survival curves for death or heart failure admission for 1049 patients with stable ischemic coronary artery disease with brain natriuretic peptide (BNP) (solid lines) and amino terminal pro-brain natriuretic peptide (NT-proBNP) (dotted lines) above (lower two lines) or below (upper two lines) the median level for the group. For both peptides, the separation of survival curves was highly significant ($p < 0.001$). CHF, congestive heart failure. (Figure reprinted with permission from the *Journal of the American College of Cardiology*)

attributable to coronary artery disease, there is interest for the use of these markers for the surveillance of patients following cardiac transplantation, where asymptomatic coronary atherosclerosis may develop consequent to transplant vasculopathy. As demonstrated by Mehra and colleagues, such a strategy of natriuretic peptide surveillance may be useful to detect not only allograft vasculopathy, but also identify a risk for graft failure and rising risk for death in these subjects [84].

Atrial arrhythmia

Case 6
A 42-year-old male with no previous medical history is found to be in atrial fibrillation at a pre-employment physical. At the time of his initial office visit he remains in atrial fibrillation, denies awareness of his atrial tachyarrhythmia, and has no signs of HF. Does natriuretic peptide testing have a role in this patient's initial assessment?

Discussion of Case 6
Independent of the relationship between atrial arrhythmia and structural heart disease, it is now established that natriuretic peptide concentrations are higher among patients with established atrial arrhythmias such as atrial fibrillation or flutter [85], and fall rapidly after restoration to normal sinus rhythm [86]. Importantly, it is now recognized that levels of natriuretic peptides may be

useful to differentiate those subjects more likely to have durable results from cardioversion than those at high risk for the recurrence of atrial arrhythmia, even in the absence of structural heart disease [87, 88]. In one study, median concentrations of NT-proBNP were higher among patients with "lone" atrial fibrillation destined for recurrent arrhythmia (166 pg/mL) versus those who did not (133 pg/mL, $p = 0.0003$ for difference) [88], while among subjects with atrial fibrillation from a various number of causes, BNP values were similarly higher in those who had recurrent fibrillation (293 pg/mL) than those who did not (163 pg/mL) [87].

Ventricular arrhythmia

Case 7

A 72-year-old man with coronary artery disease suffered a cardiac arrest from ventricular tachycardia. Coronary angiography revealed no acute culprit lesions and a trans-thoracic echocardiogram revealed a small inferior wall scar with a normal left ventricular ejection fraction. An implantable defibrillator was placed. He is seen for a routine visit 6 months after this episode. Is there a role for natriuretic peptide testing in this patient?

Discussion of Case 7

It is somewhat more difficult to define the independent relationship between ventricular arrhythmia and natriuretic peptide concentrations, as this arrhythmia is more likely to occur in patients with structural heart disease. As such, the relationship between BNP and sudden cardiac death related to arrhythmia is tenuous with some studies arguing for an independent relationship between BNP (but less so for NT-proBNP) and risk of sudden death [89] while others suggest the risk associated is more related to decompensation of HF rather than representing a direct signal of arrhythmic risk [90]. Nonetheless, studies among patients with implantable defibrillators showed that markedly elevated values of NT-proBNP (in excess of 9000 pg/mL) or BNP (in excess of 573 pg/mL) were strongly predictive of defibrillator discharge in subjects over a year of follow-up [91, 92], thus suggesting a role for these markers to stratify risk for potentially life-threatening arrhythmia.

Outpatient HF: systolic dysfunction

Case 8

A 70-year-old woman with a non-ischemic cardiomyopathy and stable NYHA (New York Heart Association) Class II failure is seen in clinic. She is at her dry body weight but slightly hypertensive with a blood pressure of 136/88. She has had no recent decline in her exertional capacity. What is to be gained from natriuretic peptide testing in this situation?

Discussion of Case 8

The role of natriuretic peptide testing is well established for predicting risk of death in chronic outpatient HF [93–95], appearing to supersede the risk of other known metrics for predicting death in this situation, including maximal oxygen consumption or NYHA Classification. Whether there is potential utility of natriuretic peptide testing for the *management* of patients with HF remains largely unclear, somewhat surprisingly.

There is logic in the use of either BNP or NT-proBNP measurement to guide therapy of patients with HF: higher levels of natriuretic peptides predict risk for death and a higher likelihood for re-hospitalization, while effective therapies for HF that lower the risk for morbidity or mortality (such as beta adrenergic blockers, angiotensin converting enzyme inhibitors, or angiotensin receptor blockers [94–98]) are associated with parallel reductions in the concentrations of natriuretic peptides in patients so treated. Quite remarkably, despite the logical relationship between natriuretic peptides and treatment response, as well as burden of HF patients in HF clinics world wide, there is a paucity of data supporting the use of biomarker-guided HF therapy. In one pilot study, HF management guided by NT-proBNP concentrations was superior to standard clinical judgment [99]. In this study, dosing of HF medication was intensified for patients in whom a concentration of NT-proBNP below the range of 1600 pg/mL was observed, even in the absence of decompensated symptoms. In this study, fewer adverse events were noted in those guided by NT-proBNP measurement, including fewer episodes of destabilized HF, less hospitalizations, and a near statistically significant reduction in mortality. The role of natriuretic peptide-guided HF management is currently under evaluation in several prospective clinical trials using both BNP and NT-proBNP. The main question or concern is which analyte would be best for this role, as BNP may be associated with a higher "false negative" rate among outpatient HF subjects [100] and NT-proBNP may be less responsive in the short run to therapeutic interventions [101]. Lastly, it remains unclear which target for therapy should be used (an absolute target or percent change in biomarker levels) [102].

Outpatient HF: diastolic dysfunction

Case 9
A 70-year-old woman with a past medical history of hypertension was recently hospitalized with a first episode of HF. After successful medical treatment, an echocardiogram showed mild left ventricular hypertrophy and an ejection fraction of 67% with no wall motion abnormalities. What is to be gained from natriuretic peptide testing in this situation?

Discussion of Case 9
The high prevalence and important clinical significance of HF in patients with preserved systolic function is becoming increasingly recognized [103, 104]. Our current understanding of this common clinical situation suggests that lusitropic abnormality (i.e., impaired ventricular relaxation) with a resultant rise in intraventricular filling pressure underlies this syndrome. Given the known link between natriuretic peptide release and elevations in cardiac filling

pressures, studies have begun to clarify the role of natriuretic peptide testing in patients so afflicted.

The impact of diastolic abnormalities in patients with concomitant systolic HF has been studied. Yu *et al.* evaluated the prevalence of diastolic dysfunction and its impact on natriuretic peptide levels in patients with symptomatic systolic dysfunction. They found that echocardiographic evidence of diastolic dysfunction was present in >90% of patients with reduced ejection fractions and that relaxation abnormalities were associated with higher levels of BNP [105]. In a similar analysis of patients with systolic HF, a strong positive correlation between echo indices of diastolic dysfunction and levels of BNP was reported [106].

In patients with preserved systolic function and the clinical syndrome of HF, natriuretic peptides appear to be useful for establishing a diagnosis of diastolic dysfunction. The correlation between elevated natriuretic peptide levels and echocardiographic signs of impaired relaxation has been reported in patients with preserved left ventricular function [107–109]. In an analysis of the PRIDE Study of patients with dyspnea attributed to acute destabilized HF, roughly half had systolic dysfunction and the other half isolated diastolic abnormalities. On average, both NT-proBNP and BNP were significantly higher in both HF groups than in dyspneic non-HF subjects. With regard to diagnostic accuracy of the both BNP and NT-proBNP, both peptides had similar power to diagnose HF in patients with systolic dysfunction while NT-proBNP outperformed BNP in patients with isolated diastolic dysfunction [25]. Thus, current data support a role for the use of the natriuretic peptides in the evaluation of patients with HF due to suspected diastolic dysfunction.

Natriuretic peptide testing: dyspneic outpatients without known structural heart disease

Case 10

A 62-year-old female, new to your practice, presents for a routine health visit. Her past medical history and cardiac risk factor profile are unremarkable. She leads a relatively sedentary life without regular exercise. Review of symptoms reveals exertional dyspnea that reproducibly occurs after climbing one or more flights of stairs. Physical examination reveals a blood pressure of 136/86 and an above-normal body mass index. Electrocardiogram reveals a sinus mechanism at a rate of 75, normal axis and intervals, and nonspecific ST-segment and T-wave abnormalities. A chest radiograph is unremarkable. What is the role of natriuretic peptide testing for this patient?

Discussion of Case 10

Mild dyspnea is a problem that is encountered frequently in the ambulatory setting, and is the cardinal manifestation of numerous distinct disease processes. Determination of the cause of dyspnea poses a formidable challenge as routine evaluation, including the complete medical history and a thorough physical exam, is often unrevealing. At its earliest stages, HF may be an insidious cause of dyspnea, and is a syndrome with distinct prognostic implications and beneficial disease-specific therapies. Unfortunately, the identification of those at risk for the ultimate development of clinically evident HF can be difficult, especially in the ambulatory setting where cardiac imaging is not readily available. Trans-thoracic echocardiography has thus become the test of choice for patients with dyspnea that is suspected to be due to myocardial abnormalities. The availability of echocardiography is limited by several factors including the need for trained sonographers, the availability of competent cardiologist interpreters, and the significant cost. This reality has led to intense interest in more effective methods for triaging patients for more intensive cardiovascular evaluation, or toward a non-cardiac evaluation.

Pilot trials specifically evaluating the role of natriuretic peptides as a tool for the diagnosis or exclusion of HF in the outpatient clinic have been promising: in one study, 305 patients presenting with dyspnea and/or lower extremity edema were evaluated by their primary care physician, and a provisional diagnosis was rendered. NT-proBNP concentrations were simultaneously measured and compared to the impression of the managing physician. In this study, knowledge of NT-proBNP values was useful, in particular, to exclude the diagnosis of HF, improving diagnostic accuracy by over 20% [110]. In a similar manner, among 306 patients in primary care, both BNP and NT-proBNP were useful for excluding HF in dyspneic subjects, with area under the ROC of 0.84 and 0.85, respectively [111]. In this study, NT-proBNP had a higher NPV (97%) than BNP (87%), suggesting a superior role for excluding HF in dyspneic outpatients. These data were confirmed in a study of 367 dyspneic primary care patients referred for evaluation using echocardiography, due to symptoms of dyspnea. In this study, NT-proBNP, using the manufacturer's recommended cutpoint for excluding HF (125 pg/mL) had an NPV of 99% for HF, with an overall area under the ROC of 0.87. In addition, dyspneic subjects with an NT-proBNP >125 pg/mL had a significantly higher risk of death over 2-year follow-up [112].

Even when the diagnosis of a dyspneic patient appears to be non-cardiac, the use of natriuretic peptides appears promising. Among 1186 dyspneic outpatients with obstructive airways disease and no prior history of HF, concentrations of NT-proBNP were useful to identify a diagnosis of "masked" HF (i.e., previously unsuspected comorbid HF in patients with pulmonary disease). In this study, adding NT-proBNP measurement to a predictive model (which included prior heart disease, high body mass index, lateral displacement of the apical impulse, and high pulse rate) significantly improved the diagnostic ability to identify previously unsuspected HF. This suggests a role for natriuretic peptide testing in the comprehensive evaluation of patients with lung disease with aims of further improving symptoms and prognosis [6].

Larger ongoing trials will further clarify the role of natriuretic peptides in the ambulatory evaluation of the dyspneic patient. At present, the optimal role of BNP or NT-proBNP testing in the outpatient setting is to exclude the presence of HF in symptomatic patients. For such patients who BNP or NT-proBNP levels are found to be below the suggested "rule out" cutpoints, an assiduous search for non-HF causes of dyspnea should be performed. While the NPV of BNP and NT-proBNP is unquestioned, the PPV is less established. For symptomatic outpatients with an elevated natriuretic peptide value, the diagnosis of HF is not definitively established. It is recommended that for such patients, the thoughtful application of echocardiography would be a logical next step. Available data suggest that this strategy may be both feasible and cost-effective [37, 38].

References

1 Januzzi JL, Jr, Camargo CA, Anwaruddin S *et al.* The N-terminal Pro-BNP investigation of dyspnea in the emergency department (PRIDE) study. *Am J Cardiol* 2005;**95**(8):948–954.

2 Maisel A, Hollander JE, Guss D *et al.* Primary results of the Rapid Emergency Department Heart Failure Outpatient Trial (REDHOT). A multicenter study of B-type natriuretic peptide levels, emergency department decision making, and outcomes in patients presenting with shortness of breath. *J Am Coll Cardiol* 2004;**44**(6):1328–1333.

3 Maisel AS, Krishnaswamy P, Nowak RM *et al.* Rapid measurement of B-type natriuretic peptide in the emergency diagnosis of heart failure. *N Engl J Med* 2002;**347**(3):161–167.

4 Mueller C, Scholer A, Laule-Kilian K *et al.* Use of B-type natriuretic peptide in the evaluation and management of acute dyspnea. *N Engl J Med* 2004;**350**(7):647–654.

5 Hunt SA, Abraham WT, Chin MH *et al.* ACC/AHA 2005 guideline update for the diagnosis and management of chronic heart failure in the adult: a report of the American College of Cardiology/American Heart Association task force on practice guidelines (Writing Committee to update the 2001 guidelines for the evaluation and management of heart failure): developed in collaboration with the American College of chest physicians and the International Society for Heart and Lung Transplantation: endorsed by the Heart Rhythm Society. *Circulation* 2005;**112**(12):e154–e235.

6 Rutten FH, Moons KG, Cramer MJ *et al.* Recognising heart failure in elderly patients with stable chronic obstructive pulmonary disease in primary care: cross sectional diagnostic study. *BMJ* 2005;**331**(7529):1379–1386.

7 Davies M, Hobbs F, Davis R *et al.* Prevalence of left-ventricular systolic dysfunction and heart failure in the Echocardiographic Heart of England Screening study: a population based study. *Lancet* 2001;**358**(9280):439–444.

8 McDonagh TA, Morrison CE, Lawrence A *et al.* Symptomatic and asymptomatic left-ventricular systolic dysfunction in an urban population. *Lancet* 1997;**350**(9081):829–833.

9 Mueller T, Gegenhuber A, Poelz W *et al.* Head-to-head comparison of the diagnostic utility of BNP and NT-proBNP in symptomatic and asymptomatic structural heart disease. *Clin Chim Acta* 2004;**341**(1–2):41–48.

10 Groenning BA, Raymond I, Hildebrandt PR *et al.* Diagnostic and prognostic evaluation of left ventricular systolic heart failure by plasma N-terminal pro-brain natriuretic peptide concentrations in a large sample of the general population. *Heart* 2004;**90**(3):297–303.

11 McDonagh TA, Cunningham AD, Morrison CE *et al.* Left ventricular dysfunction, natriuretic peptides, and mortality in an urban population. *Heart* 2001;**86**(1):21–26.

12 Wang TJ, Larson MG, Levy D *et al.* Plasma natriuretic peptide levels and the risk of cardiovascular events and death. *N Engl J Med* 2004;**350**(7):655–663.

13 Nielsen OW, Rasmussen V, Christensen NJ *et al.* Neuroendocrine testing in community patients with heart disease: plasma N-terminal proatrial natriuretic peptide predicts morbidity and mortality stronger than catecholamines and heart rate variability. *Scand J Clin Lab Invest* 2004;**64**(7):619–628.

14 Ueda R, Yokouchi M, Suzuki T *et al.* Prognostic value of high plasma brain natriuretic peptide concentrations in very elderly persons. *Am J Med* 2003;**114**(4):266–270.

15 Wallen T, Landahl S, Hedner T *et al.* Brain natriuretic peptide predicts mortality in the elderly. *Heart* 1997;**77**(3):264–267.

16 Mikkelsen KV, Bie P, Moller JE *et al.* Neurohormonal activation and diagnostic value of cardiac peptides in patients with suspected mild heart failure. *Int J Cardiol* 2006;**110**(3):324–333.

17 De Sutter J, De Bacquer D, Cuypers S *et al.* Plasma N-terminal pro-brain natriuretic peptide concentration predicts coronary events in men at work: a report from the BELSTRESS study. *Eur Heart J* 2005;**26**(24):2644–2649.

18 Galasko GI, Lahiri A, Barnes SC *et al.* What is the normal range for N-terminal pro-brain natriuretic peptide? How well does this normal range screen for cardiovascular disease? *Eur Heart J* 2005;**26**(21):2269–2276.

19 Vasan RS, Benjamin EJ, Larson MG *et al.* Plasma natriuretic peptides for community screening for left ventricular hypertrophy and systolic dysfunction: the Framingham heart study. *JAMA* 2002;**288**(10):1252–1259.

20 Redfield MM, Rodeheffer RJ, Jacobsen SJ *et al.* Plasma brain natriuretic peptide to detect preclinical ventricular systolic or diastolic dysfunction: a community-based study. *Circulation* 2004;**109**(25):3176–3181.

21 Hildebrandt P, Boesen M, Olsen M *et al.* N-terminal pro brain natriuretic peptide in arterial hypertension—a marker for left ventricular dimensions and prognosis. *Eur J Heart Fail* 2004;**6**(3):313–317.

22 Nishikimi T, Yoshihara F, Morimoto A *et al.* Relationship between left ventricular geometry and natriuretic peptide levels in essential hypertension. *Hypertension* 1996;**28**(1): 22–30.

23 Olsen MH, Wachtell K, Tuxen C *et al.* N-terminal pro-brain natriuretic peptide predicts cardiovascular events in patients with hypertension and left ventricular hypertrophy: a LIFE study. *J Hypertens* 2004;**22**(8):1597–1604.

24 Seino Y, Ogawa A, Yamashita T *et al.* Application of NT-proBNP and BNP measurements in cardiac care: a more discerning marker for the detection and evaluation of heart failure. *Eur J Heart Fail* 2004;**6**(3):295–300.

25 O'Donoghue M, Chen A, Baggish AL *et al.* The effects of ejection fraction on N-terminal ProBNP and BNP levels in patients with acute CHF: analysis from the ProBNP Investigation of Dyspnea in the Emergency Department (PRIDE) study. *J Card Fail* 2005;**11**(5 suppl):S9–S14.

26 Magnusson M, Melander O, Israelsson B *et al.* Elevated plasma levels of Nt-proBNP in patients with type 2 diabetes without overt cardiovascular disease. *Diabetes Care* 2004;**27**(8):1929–1935.

27 Bhalla MA, Chiang A, Epshteyn VA *et al.* Prognostic role of B-type natriuretic peptide levels in patients with type 2 diabetes mellitus. *J Am Coll Cardiol* 2004;**44**(5):1047–1052.

28 Igarashi M, Jimbu Y, Hirata A *et al.* Characterization of plasma brain natriuretic peptide level in patients with type 2 diabetes. *Endocr J* 2005;**52**(3):353–362.

29 Kragelund C, Gronning B, Kober L *et al.* N-terminal pro-B-type natriuretic peptide and long-term mortality in stable coronary heart disease. *N Engl J Med* 2005;**352**(7):666–675.

30 Tarnow L, Hildebrandt P, Hansen BV *et al.* Plasma N-terminal pro-brain natriuretic peptide as an independent predictor of mortality in diabetic nephropathy. *Diabetologia* 2005;**48**(1):149–155.

31 Yano Y, Katsuki A, Gabazza EC *et al.* Plasma brain natriuretic peptide levels in normotensive noninsulin-dependent diabetic patients with microalbuminuria. *J Clin Endocrinol Metab* 1999;**84**(7):2353–2356.

32 Asakawa H, Fukui T, Tokunaga K *et al.* Plasma brain natriuretic peptide levels in normotensive type 2 diabetic patients without cardiac disease and macroalbuminuria. *J Diabetes Complications* 2002;**16**(3):209–213.

33 Gaede P, Hildebrandt P, Hess G *et al.* Plasma N-terminal pro-brain natriuretic peptide as a major risk marker for cardiovascular disease in patients with type 2 diabetes and microalbuminuria. *Diabetologia* 2005;**48**(1):156–163.

34 Nagai T, Imamura M, Inukai T *et al.* Brain natriuretic polypeptide in type 2 NIDDM patients with albuminuria. *J Med* 2001;**32**(3–4):169–180.

35 Abdullah SM, Khera A, Das SR *et al.* Relation of coronary atherosclerosis determined by electron beam computed tomography and plasma levels of N-terminal pro-brain natriuretic peptide in a multiethnic population-based sample (the Dallas Heart Study). *Am J Cardiol* 2005;**96**(9):1284–1289.

36 Raymond I, Groenning BA, Hildebrandt PR *et al.* The influence of age, sex and other variables on the plasma level of N-terminal pro brain natriuretic peptide in a large sample of the general population. *Heart* 2003;**89**(7):745–751.

37 Nielsen OW, McDonagh TA, Robb SD *et al.* Retrospective analysis of the cost-effectiveness of using plasma brain natriuretic peptide in screening for left ventricular systolic dysfunction in the general population. *J Am Coll Cardiol* 2003;**41**(1):113–120.

38 Senior R, Galasko G. Cost-effective strategies to screen for left ventricular systolic dysfunction in the community—a concept. *Congest Heart Fail* 2005;**11**(4):194–198, 211.

39 Ng LL, Loke I, Davies JE *et al.* Identification of previously undiagnosed left ventricular systolic dysfunction: community screening using natriuretic peptides and electrocardiography. *Eur J Heart Fail* 2003;**5**(6):775–782.

40 Stewart WJ. Choosing the "golden moment" for mitral valve repair. *J Am Coll Cardiol* 1994;**24**(6):1544–1546.

41 Kupari M, Turto H, Lommi J *et al.* Transcardiac gradients of N-terminal B-type natriuretic peptide in aortic valve stenosis. *Eur J Heart Fail* 2005;**7**(5):809–814.

42 Gerber IL, Legget ME, West TM *et al.* Usefulness of serial measurement of N-terminal pro-brain natriuretic peptide plasma levels in asymptomatic patients with aortic stenosis to predict symptomatic deterioration. *Am J Cardiol* 2005;**95**(7):898–901.

43 Gerber IL, Stewart RA, Legget ME *et al.* Increased plasma natriuretic peptide levels reflect symptom onset in aortic stenosis. *Circulation* 2003;**107**(14):1884–1890.

44 Lim P, Monin JL, Monchi M *et al.* Predictors of outcome in patients with severe aortic stenosis and normal left ventricular function: role of B-type natriuretic peptide. *Eur Heart J* 2004;**25**(22):2048–2053.

45 Nessmith MG, Fukuta H, Brucks S *et al.* Usefulness of an elevated B-type natriuretic Peptide in predicting survival in patients with aortic stenosis treated without surgery. *Am J Cardiol* 2005;**96**(10):1445–1448.

46 Weber M, Arnold R, Rau M *et al.* Relation of N-terminal pro-B-type natriuretic peptide to severity of valvular aortic stenosis. *Am J Cardiol* 2004;**94**(6):740–745.

47 Weber M, Arnold R, Rau M *et al.* Relation of N-terminal pro B-type natriuretic peptide to progression of aortic valve disease. *Eur Heart J* 2005;**26**(10):1023–1030.

48 Gerber IL, Stewart RA, French JK *et al.* Associations between plasma natriuretic peptide levels, symptoms, and left ventricular function in patients with chronic aortic regurgitation. *Am J Cardiol* 2003;**92**(6):755–758.

49 Eimer MJ, Ekery DL, Rigolin VH *et al.* Elevated B-type natriuretic peptide in asymptomatic men with chronic aortic regurgitation and preserved left ventricular systolic function. *Am J Cardiol* 2004;**94**(5):676–678.

50 Ozkan M, Baysan O, Erinc K *et al.* Brain natriuretic peptide and the severity of aortic regurgitation: is there any correlation? *J Int Med Res* 2005;**33**(4):454–459.

51 Arat-Ozkan A, Kaya A, Yigit Z *et al.* Serum N-terminal pro-BNP levels correlate with symptoms and echocardiographic findings in patients with mitral stenosis. *Echocardiography* 2005;**22**(6):473–478.

52 Shang YP, Lai L, Chen J *et al.* Effects of percutaneous balloon mitral valvuloplasty on plasma B-type natriuretic peptide in rheumatic mitral stenosis with and without atrial fibrillation. *J Heart Valve Dis* 2005;**14**(4):453–459.

53 Brookes CI, Kemp MW, Hooper J *et al.* Plasma brain natriuretic peptide concentrations in patients with chronic mitral regurgitation. *J Heart Valve Dis* 1997;**6**(6):608–612.

54 Mayer SA, De Lemos JA, Murphy SA *et al.* Comparison of B-type natriuretic peptide levels in patients with heart failure with versus without mitral regurgitation. *Am J Cardiol* 2004;**93**(8):1002–1006.

55 Sutton TM, Stewart RA, Gerber IL *et al.* Plasma natriuretic peptide levels increase with symptoms and severity of mitral regurgitation. *J Am Coll Cardiol* 2003;**41**(12):2280–2287.

56 Detaint D, Messika-Zeitoun D, Avierinos JF *et al.* B-type natriuretic peptide in organic mitral regurgitation: determinants and impact on outcome. *Circulation* 2005;**111**(18):2391–2397.

57 Bolger AP, Sharma R, Li W *et al.* Neurohormonal activation and the chronic heart failure syndrome in adults with congenital heart disease. *Circulation* 2002;**106**(1):92–99.

58 Law YM, Keller BB, Feingold BM *et al.* Usefulness of plasma B-type natriuretic peptide to identify ventricular dysfunction in pediatric and adult patients with congenital heart disease. *Am J Cardiol* 2005;**95**(4):474–478.

59 Tulevski II, Dodge-Khatami A, Groenink M *et al.* Right ventricular function in congenital cardiac disease: noninvasive quantitative parameters for clinical follow-up. *Cardiol Young* 2003;**13**(5):397–403.

60 Tulevski II, Groenink M, van Der Wall EE *et al.* Increased brain and atrial natriuretic peptides in patients with chronic right ventricular pressure overload: correlation between plasma neurohormones and right ventricular dysfunction. *Heart* 2001;**86**(1):27–30.

61 Hopkins WE, Chen Z, Fukagawa NK *et al.* Increased atrial and brain natriuretic peptides in adults with cyanotic congenital heart disease: enhanced understanding of the relationship between hypoxia and natriuretic peptide secretion. *Circulation* 2004;**109**(23):2872–2877.

62 Nakanishi K, Tajima F, Itoh H *et al.* Changes in atrial natriuretic peptide and brain natriuretic peptide associated with hypobaric hypoxia-induced pulmonary hypertension in rats. *Virchows Arch* 2001;**439**(6):808–817.

63 Brili S, Alexopoulos N, Latsios G *et al.* Tissue Doppler imaging and brain natriuretic peptide levels in adults with repaired tetralogy of Fallot. *J Am Soc Echocardiogr* 2005;**18**(11):1149–1154.

64 Trojnarska O, Szyszka A, Gwizdala A *et al.* The BNP concentrations and exercise capacity assessment with cardiopulmonary stress test in patients after surgical repair of Fallot's tetralogy. *Int J Cardiol* 2006;**110**(1):86–92.

65 Suda K, Matsumura M, Matsumoto M. Clinical implication of plasma natriuretic peptides in children with ventricular septal defect. *Pediatr Int* 2003;**45**(3):249–254.

66 Pruszczyk P. N-terminal pro-brain natriuretic peptide as an indicator of right ventricular dysfunction. *J Card Fail* 2005;**11**(5 suppl):S65–S69.

67 Yap LB. B-type natriuretic peptide and the right heart. *Heart Fail Rev* 2004;**9**(2):99–105.

68 Yap LB, Ashrafian H, Mukerjee D *et al.* The natriuretic peptides and their role in disorders of right heart dysfunction and pulmonary hypertension. *Clin Biochem* 2004;**37**(10):847–856.

69 Yap LB, Mukerjee D, Timms PM *et al.* Natriuretic peptides, respiratory disease, and the right heart. *Chest* 2004;**126**(4):1330–1336.

70 Leuchte HH, Holzapfel M, Baumgartner RA *et al.* Clinical significance of brain natriuretic peptide in primary pulmonary hypertension. *J Am Coll Cardiol* 2004;**43**(5):764–770.

71 Leuchte HH, Holzapfel M, Baumgartner RA *et al.* Characterization of brain natriuretic peptide in long-term follow-up of pulmonary arterial hypertension. *Chest* 2005;**128**(4):2368–2374.

72 Leuchte HH, Neurohr C, Baumgartner R *et al.* Brain natriuretic peptide and exercise capacity in lung fibrosis and pulmonary hypertension. *Am J Respir Crit Care Med* 2004;**170**(4):360–365.

73 Souza R, Bogossian HB, Humbert M *et al.* N-terminal-pro-brain natriuretic peptide as a haemodynamic marker in idiopathic pulmonary arterial hypertension. *Eur Respir J* 2005;**25**(3):509–513.

74 Nagaya N, Nishikimi T, Uematsu M *et al.* Plasma brain natriuretic peptide as a prognostic indicator in patients with primary pulmonary hypertension. *Circulation* 2000;**102**(8):865–870.

75 Park MH, Scott RL, Uber PA *et al.* Usefulness of B-type natriuretic peptide as a predictor of treatment outcome in pulmonary arterial hypertension. *Congest Heart Fail* 2004;**10**(5):221–225.

76 Foote RS, Pearlman JD, Siegel AH *et al.* Detection of exercise-induced ischemia by changes in B-type natriuretic peptides. *J Am Coll Cardiol* 2004;**44**(10):1980–1987.

77 Sabatine MS, Morrow DA, de Lemos JA *et al.* Acute changes in circulating natriuretic peptide levels in relation to myocardial ischemia. *J Am Coll Cardiol* 2004;**44**(10):1988–1995.

78 Richards AM, Nicholls GM, Espiner EA *et al.* Comparison of B-type natriuretic peptides for assessment of cardiac function and prognosis in stable ischemic heart disease. *J Am Coll Cardiol* 2006;**47**(1):52–60.

79 Ndrepepa G, Braun S, Mehilli J *et al.* Plasma levels of N-terminal pro-brain natriuretic peptide in patients with coronary artery disease and relation to clinical presentation, angiographic severity, and left ventricular ejection fraction. *Am J Cardiol* 2005;**95**(5):553–557.

80 Omland T. Clinical and laboratory diagnostics of cardiovascular disease: focus on natriuretic peptides and cardiac ischemia. *Scand J Clin Lab Invest Suppl* 2005;**240**:18–24.

81 Omland T, Richards AM, Wergeland R *et al.* B-type natriuretic peptide and long-term survival in patients with stable coronary artery disease. *Am J Cardiol* 2005;**95**(1):24–28.

82 Sahinarslan A, Cengel A, Okyay K *et al.* B-type natriuretic peptide and extent of lesion on coronary angiography in stable coronary artery disease. *Coron Artery Dis* 2005;**16**(4):225–229.

83 Weber M, Dill T, Arnold R *et al.* N-terminal B-type natriuretic peptide predicts extent of coronary artery disease and ischemia in patients with stable angina pectoris. *Am Heart J* 2004;**148**(4):612–620.

84 Mehra MR, Uber PA, Potluri S *et al.* Usefulness of an elevated B-type natriuretic peptide to predict allograft failure, cardiac allograft vasculopathy, and survival after heart transplantation. *Am J Cardiol* 2004;**94**(4):454–458.

85 Knudsen CW, Omland T, Clopton P *et al.* Impact of atrial fibrillation on the diagnostic performance of B-type natriuretic peptide concentration in dyspneic patients: an analysis from the breathing not properly multinational study. *J Am Coll Cardiol* 2005;**46**(5): 838–844.

86 Vinch CS, Rashkin J, Logsetty G *et al.* Brain natriuretic peptide levels fall rapidly after cardioversion of atrial fibrillation to sinus rhythm. *Cardiology* 2004;**102**(4):188–193.

87 Beck-da-Silva L, de Bold A, Fraser M *et al.* Brain natriuretic peptide predicts successful cardioversion in patients with atrial fibrillation and maintenance of sinus rhythm. *Can J Cardiol* 2004;**20**(12):1245–1248.

88 Ellinor PT, Low AF, Patton KK *et al.* Discordant atrial natriuretic peptide and brain natriuretic peptide levels in lone atrial fibrillation. *J Am Coll Cardiol* 2005;**45**(1):82–86.

89 Berger R, Huelsman M, Strecker K *et al.* B-type natriuretic peptide predicts sudden death in patients with chronic heart failure. *Circulation* 2002;**105**(20):2392–2397.

90 Shehab AM, MacFadyen RJ, McLaren M *et al.* Sudden unexpected death in heart failure may be preceded by short term, intraindividual increases in inflammation and in autonomic dysfunction: a pilot study. *Heart* 2004;**90**(11):1263–1268.

91 Manios EG, Kallergis EM, Kanoupakis EM *et al.* Amino-terminal pro-brain natriuretic peptide predicts ventricular arrhythmogenesis in patients with ischemic cardiomyopathy and implantable cardioverter-defibrillators. *Chest* 2005;**128**(4):2604–2610.

92 Verma A, Kilicaslan F, Martin DO *et al.* Pre-implantation B-type natriuretic peptide level is an independent predictor of future appropriate implantable defibrillator therapies. *Heart* 2006;**92**(2):190–195.

93 Gardner RS, Ozalp F, Murday AJ *et al.* N-terminal pro-brain natriuretic peptide. A new gold standard in predicting mortality in patients with advanced heart failure. *Eur Heart J* 2003;**24**(19):1735–1743.

94 Hartmann F, Packer M, Coats AJ *et al.* Prognostic impact of plasma N-terminal pro-brain natriuretic peptide in severe chronic congestive heart failure: a substudy of the Carvedilol Prospective Randomized Cumulative Survival (COPERNICUS) trial. *Circulation* 2004;**110**(13):1780–1786.

95 Hartmann F, Packer M, Coats AJ *et al.* NT-proBNP in severe chronic heart failure: rationale, design and preliminary results of the COPERNICUS NT-proBNP substudy. *Eur J Heart Fail* 2004;**6**(3):343–350.

96 Anand IS, Fisher LD, Chiang YT *et al.* Changes in brain natriuretic peptide and norepinephrine over time and mortality and morbidity in the Valsartan Heart Failure Trial (Val-HeFT). *Circulation* 2003;**107**(9):1278–1283.

97 Richards AM, Doughty R, Nicholls MG *et al.*, for Australia–New Zealand Heart Failure Group. Neurohumoral prediction of benefit from carvedilol in ischemic left ventricular dysfunction. *Circulation* 1999;**99**(6):786–792.

98 Richards AM, Doughty R, Nicholls MG *et al.*, Australia–New Zealand Heart Failure Group. Plasma N-terminal pro-brain natriuretic peptide and adrenomedullin: prognostic utility and prediction of benefit from carvedilol in chronic ischemic left ventricular dysfunction. *J Am Coll Cardiol* 2001;**37**(7):1781–1787.

99 Troughton RW, Frampton CM, Yandle TG *et al.* Treatment of heart failure guided by plasma aminoterminal brain natriuretic peptide (N-BNP) concentrations. *Lancet* 2000;**355**(9210):1126–1130.

100 Tang WH, Girod JP, Lee MJ *et al.* Plasma B-type natriuretic peptide levels in ambulatory patients with established chronic symptomatic systolic heart failure. *Circulation* 2003;**108**(24):2964–2966.

101 Wu AH, Smith A, Apple FS. Optimum blood collection intervals for B-type natriuretic peptide testing in patients with heart failure. *Am J Cardiol* 2004;**93**(12):1562–1563.

102 Wu AH, Smith A, Wieczorek S *et al.* Biological variation for N-terminal pro- and B-type natriuretic peptides and implications for therapeutic monitoring of patients with congestive heart failure. *Am J Cardiol* 2003;**92**(5):628–631.

103 Vasan RS, Larson MG, Benjamin EJ *et al.* Congestive heart failure in subjects with normal versus reduced left ventricular ejection fraction: prevalence and mortality in a population-based cohort. *J Am Coll Cardiol* 1999;**33**(7):1948–1955.

104 Devereux RB, Roman MJ, Liu JE *et al.* Congestive heart failure despite normal left ventricular systolic function in a population-based sample: the Strong Heart Study. *Am J Cardiol* 2000;**86**(10):1090–1096.

105 Yu CM, Sanderson JE, Shum IO *et al.* Diastolic dysfunction and natriuretic peptides in systolic heart failure. Higher ANP and BNP levels are associated with the restrictive filling pattern. *Eur Heart J* 1996;**17**(11):1694–1702.

106 Troughton RW, Prior DL, Pereira JJ *et al.* Plasma B-type natriuretic peptide levels in systolic heart failure: importance of left ventricular diastolic function and right ventricular systolic function. *J Am Coll Cardiol* 2004;**43**(3):416–422.

107 Lubien E, DeMaria A, Krishnaswamy P *et al.* Utility of B-natriuretic peptide in detecting diastolic dysfunction: comparison with Doppler velocity recordings. *Circulation* 2002;**105**(5):595–601.

108 Mak GS, DeMaria A, Clopton P *et al.* Utility of B-natriuretic peptide in the evaluation of left ventricular diastolic function: comparison with tissue Doppler imaging recordings. *Am Heart J* 2004;**148**(5):895–902.

109 Chen AA, Wood MJ, Krauser DG *et al.* NT-proBNP levels, echocardiographic findings, and outcomes in breathless patients: results from the ProBNP Investigation of Dyspnoea in the Emergency Department (PRIDE) echocardiographic substudy. *Eur Heart J* 2006;**27**(7):839–845.

110 Wright SP, Doughty RN, Pearl A *et al.* Plasma amino-terminal pro-brain natriuretic peptide and accuracy of heart-failure diagnosis in primary care: a randomized, controlled trial. *J Am Coll Cardiol* 2003;**42**(10):1793–1800.

111 Zaphiriou A, Robb S, Murray-Thomas T *et al.* The diagnostic accuracy of plasma BNP and NTproBNP in patients referred from primary care with suspected heart failure: results of the UK natriuretic peptide study. *Eur J Heart Fail* 2005;**7**(4):537–541.

112 Gustafsson F, Steensgaard-Hansen F, Badskjaer J *et al.* Diagnostic and prognostic performance of N-terminal ProBNP in primary care patients with suspected heart failure. *J Card Fail* 2005;**11**(5 suppl):S15–S20.

CHAPTER 15

Natriuretic peptides in patients with renal failure

Peter A. McCullough

Case 1

A 46-year-old Caucasian man with a history of type 1 diabetes mellitus (DM), hypertension (HTN), and coronary artery disease presents with a 24-hour history of progressively worsening dyspnea on exertion and at rest. The night before admission he had orthopnea and slept in a chair. He has noticed worsened leg swelling and increasing fatigue. He denied having chest pain or discomfort, syncope, or dizziness. His past medical history was notable for a 36-year history of type 1 DM, which has been managed with an insulin pump for the last 8 years. He has had treatment for retinopathy and has been diagnosed with lower extremity neuropathy. He related a history of mild diabetic nephropathy but has never been seen by a nephrologist or required dialysis. He has had HTN requiring multiple medications for 26 years. At age 40, he developed angina and was found to have two-vessel coronary artery disease requiring percutaneous coronary intervention (PCI) with stenting of the proximal right and the mid left anterior coronary descending arteries. His left ventricular ejection fraction (LVEF) at the time of PCI was 70% and he had no prior history of heart failure (HF). Baseline medications included: aspirin 81 mg p.o. qd, atorvastatin 40 mg p.o. qd, ramipril 10 mg p.o. qd, amlodipine 10 mg p.o. qd, atenolol 100 mg p.o. qd, insulin pump with daily average regular insulin utilization of 38 units, and gabapentin 600 mg p.o. tid. Vital signs were: blood pressure (BP) = 160/90 mm Hg, pulse (P) = 80 beats/minute, respiratory rate (R) = 24 breaths/minute, afebrile, height 5'8", weight 160 lbs, body mass index (BMI = 24 kg/m^2). He was mildly dyspneic at rest, was pale, and had elevated jugular venous pressure, bibasilar rales, a diffuse point of cardiac maximal impulse (PMI) which was not displaced, regular rate and rhythm, S1, S2, and a soft S3, with a 1/6 holosystolic murmur heard best at the base consistent with mitral regurgitation. The liver was mildly enlarged. There were no signs of ascites. There was 2+ pitting edema in the lower extremities to the knees and decreased posterior tibial pulses bilaterally. Admission laboratories revealed: sodium (Na) = 140 mEq/L, potassium (K) = 5.0 mEq/L, creatinine (Cr) = 2.1 mg/dL, estimated glomerular filtration rate (eGFR) = 36 mL/min/1.73 m^2, glucose (Glu) = 221 mg/dL, hemoglobin (Hb) = 11.0 g/dL, B-type natriuretic peptide (BNP) = 2541 pg/mL, N-terminal pro-BNP (NT-proBNP) = 27,432 pg/mL, and urine albumin:creatinine ratio = 281 mg/g. Cardiac troponin I was <0.04 ng/mL (negative). The electrocardiogram (ECG) was read as normal sinus rhythm, normal intervals, left axis deviation, left atrial enlargement, and left ventricular hypertrophy (LVH) with strain pattern. No Q-waves were seen. Chest X-ray showed cardiomegaly and pulmonary congestion with no effusions or frank pulmonary edema.

The patient was diagnosed with new onset heart HF with superimposed renal failure due to diabetic nephropathy. Baseline Cr, 6 months ago was found to be 1.6 mg/dL. He was treated with intravenous furosemide 40 mg every 12 hours and hydralazine 25 mg p.o. tid was added. Atenolol and amlodipine were discontinued. Carvedilol 12.5 mg p.o. bid and candesartan 16 mg p.o. qd were added to his regimen. His LVEF was found to be 45% on echocardiography and outpatient cardiac stress imaging was planned. The patient steadily improved over the course of 4 days and released from the fifth hospital day. His laboratories on the day of discharge included BNP and NT proBNP levels, which were reduced to 680 pg/mL and 20,100 pg/mL, respectively.

Discussion of Case 1

In this case a central diagnostic question is how much of the BNP and NT-proBNP elevation is attributable to HF and how much is due to renal failure. While the fate of BNP is not completely known, it is believed that approximately 70% of BNP clearance occurs in the renal parenchyma largely due to endocytosis and phagocytosis via the C-receptors in renal cells [1]. B-type natriuretic peptide is 4 kDa in size, and theoretically, can be filtered at the level of the glomerulus and then reabsorbed at the level of the renal tubule. Trace amounts of BNP have been found in the urine by a few investigators; however, this has not been a consistently replicated observation [2]. The other 30% of BNP is cleared via neutral endopeptidase and other proteases in the peripheral vascular system and potentially other solid organs [3, 4]. The amino terminal breakdown fragment of BNP, NT-proBNP, is 8.5 kDa in size and may dimerize in its circulation, and is small enough to be filtered at the level of the glomerulus but is large enough to be incompletely reabsorbed by the proximal tubule, and thus, large quantities of NT-proBNP can be found in the urine as the blood levels of NT-proBNP increase (Fig. 15.1) [5].

There is no clearance of NT-proBNP by C-receptors or neutral endopeptidase. Thus both BNP, and to a greater extent, NT-proBNP can be elevated in the setting of renal parenchymal disease manifested by an elevated serum CR and reduced eGFR. In general, when the eGFR is less than 60 mL/min/1.73 m^2, then the BNP can be expected to rise in the absence of HF into the 100–500 pg/mL range (Fig. 15.2) [6]. Since NT-proBNP is reliant on excretion in the urine as a major elimination pathway, the NT-proBNP blood levels are typically elevated much greater than the expected 5X level of BNP, and in this case were >10-fold higher than the BNP level. So in this case, even if a baseline BNP of 500 pg/dL could be ascribed to chronic kidney disease (CKD), the excess

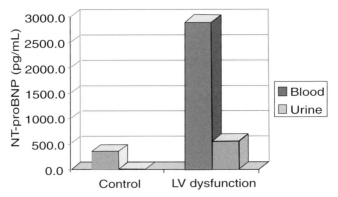

Figure 15.1 Blood and urine levels of NT-proBNP in patients with left ventricular (LV) dysfunction. (Data from Ref. [5])

of ~2000 pg/dL suggested superimposed, acute decompensated HF [6]. This case highlights the potential value of having a baseline BNP level in patients such as this who are at risk of HF.

Case 2

A 56-year-old African American man with a history of end-stage renal disease (ESRD) presented with progressive dyspnea at rest before and during hemodialysis. The dyspnea would improve slightly after the dialysis session but then would worsen a few hours later and progress to the point of moderate dyspnea at rest and complete orthopnea causing him to sleep bolt upright in a chair. His body weight has been maintained near his ideal or dry weight of

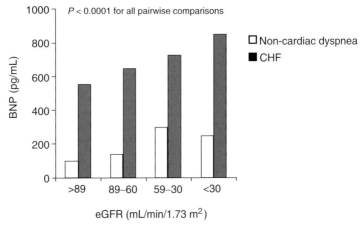

Figure 15.2 Levels of BNP stratified by estimated glomerular filtration rate (eGFR) in patients presenting to the emergency department with acute dyspnea in the BNP multinational study. (Reproduced with permission from Ref. [6])

172 lbs (80 kg) in the dialysis center. He denied any chest pain or discomfort, dizziness, or syncope. His past medical history was significant for hypertensive nephrosclerosis requiring hemodialysis for 3 years, anemia of chronic disease, and cigarette smoking. There was no prior history of heart disease. Baseline medications included lisinopril 40 mg p.o. qd, amlodipine 10 mg p.o. qd, clonidine 0.3 mg p.o. bid, metoprolol 50 mg p.o. bid, intravenous (IV) iron dextran 100 mg monthly, calcium acetate 667 mg tabs, 2 tabs p.o. ac, and darbepoetin 60 mcg IV monthly. His physical exam before his mid-week dialysis session revealed: BP 150/90 mm Hg, $P = 100$, $R = 28$, afebrile, height 5′10″, and weight = 180 lbs (BMI = 26 kg/m^2). There was markedly elevated jugular venous pressure, rales in the posterior lower one-third lung fields, a normally placed but diffuse PMI, S1, S2, S3, and loud S4. A 2/6 systolic ejection murmur was heard over the upper right sternal border consistent with aortic sclerosis. There was 1+ lower extremity edema to the ankles. All peripheral pulses were intact. Laboratories revealed: Na = 136 mEq/L, K = 5.6 mEq/L, Cr = 8.1 mg/dL, Glu = 84 mg/dL, Hb = 10.0 g/dL, BNP = 4481 pg/mL. Cardiac troponin was not measured. The ECG was read as normal sinus tachycardia, left bundle branch block, left axis deviation, and biatrial enlargement. Chest X-ray showed cardiomegaly and pulmonary congestion with evidence of pulmonary edema in the lower lung fields. Small bilateral effusions were present.

The patient had been compliant with dialysis sessions and his weight had not appreciably increased, thus with the clinical findings and the BNP value, his presumptive diagnosis was new onset HF due to hypertensive heart disease. An echocardiogram showed severe LVH and global hypokinesis with an LVEF of 35%. He was admitted to the hospital and dialysis was performed every other day with slightly more fluid removal than his regular dialysis regimen. Metoprolol was discontinued. Carvedilol 25 mg p.o. bid and was advanced to 50 mg p.o. bid. Clonidine was tapered and then discontinued. Hydralazine 75 mg p.o. tid and isosorbide dinitrate 20 mg p.o. tid were started. The patient showed steady improvement and was discharged after 7 days. Three months later, a pre-dialysis BNP level was 820 pg/mL and this was found to decrease to 672 pg/mL after a 3-hour dialysis session. The patient was felt to be euvolemic and he had functional class 2 symptoms.

Discussion of Case 2

This case illustrates the potential use of BNP in patients with ESRD on dialysis. This patient had no renal clearance of BNP and was functionally anephric. Thus BNP produced by cardiomyocytes relied on systemic neutral endopeptidase for clearance. So a baseline BNP value of ~800 mg/dL is realistic for a patient with ESRD on dialysis with hypertensive heart disease (Table 15.1) [7]. Removal of fluid with hemodialysis causes a transient reduction in left ventricular wall tension and thus a ~25% reduction in endogenous BNP (Table 15.1) [7]. The BNP is not removed with hemodialysis. BNP values can be expected to rise over the interdialytic period and be at a peak before the next dialysis session. If BNP measurement is part of a dialysis care program (currently not

Table 15.1 Summary of studies that have measured the relative change in BNP with HD and where the BNPRR could be derived from the data published.

Author (reference)	Year	N	CVD	Duration	BNP pre	BNP post	Derived BNPRR (%)	Comments
Ishizaka [12]	1994	40	No	4–5 h	63.7 ± 11.8 pg/mL	36.3 ± 7.6 pg/mL	43.0	BNP drop correlated with change in wt, $r = 0.85$
Corboy [13]	1994	8	No	4.5 h	76.1 ± 15.2 pg/mL	66.1 ± 13.8 pg/mL	13.1	Acute change in vol. Affect ANP > BNP
Haug [14]	1994	30	No	~3 h	192.1 ± 24.9 pg/mL	167.2 ± 21.8 pg/mL	13.0	ANP/BNP were indicative volume status
Totsune [15]	1994	13	NS	NS	75.0 ± 10.0 fmol/mL	55.0 ± 5.0 fmol/mL	26.7	Values taken from figure
Ishizaka [16]	1995	14	No	4–5 h	694.8±219.7 pg/mL	289.3 ± 85.5 pg/mL	58.3	BNP isoform ratios not changed
Takahashi [17]	1996	18	No	4–5 h	183 ± 45.8 pg/mL	127 ± 32.4 pg/mL	30.6	Significant drop in BNP with HD
Nitta [18]	1998	32	Mixed	4 h	688.5 ± 154.5 pg/mL	617.3 ± 157.1 pg/mL	10.3	BNP not correlated with weight
Osajima [19]	2001	39	Mixed	4 h	713 ± 928 pg/mL	477 ± 702 pg/mL	33.1	BNP correlated with severity of CAD
Nishikimi [20]	2001	48	Mixed	4 h	1078 ± 1729 pg/mL	977 ± 1554 pg/mL	9.4	BNP better than ANP correlated with LV volume indices
Clerico [21]	2001	51	Mixed	~4 h	74.2 ± 97.2 pmol/L	57.1 ± 69.3 pmol/L	15.8	BNP and ANP but not N-terminal assays dropped with HD
Uetake [22]	2001	19 17	Yes	NS	300 pg/mL 1900	200 1300	33.3 (nL LVEF) 31.6 (low LVEF)	BNP values taken from figures
Safley [7]	2005	27	Mixed	3.6 h	556.3 ± 451.5	538.6 ± 488.3	17.6	BNP weakly correlated to HD indices
Mean							−27.9	

CVD, cardiovascular disease present; BNP, B-type natriuretic peptide; ANP, atrial natriuretic peptide; HD, hemodialysis; LV, left ventricle.

BNPRR = BNP Reduction Rotation = $\frac{BNP_{pre} - BNP_{post}}{BNP_{pre}} \times 100\%$

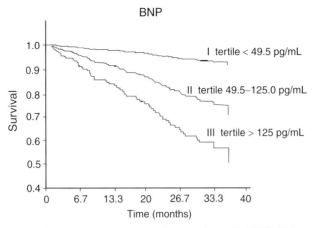

Figure 15.3 Baseline BNP values and overall survival in patients with ESRD. (Adapted from Ref. [9])

an approved indication for BNP) then a mid-week pre-dialysis value should be recorded. Research is ongoing to determine the optimal reduction of BNP that should occur with hemodialysis [8]. In addition, the value of BNP in the diagnosis of HF in a case such as this is yet to be determined. It is known, however, that patients with ESRD and chronically elevated BNP values, as in the case presented, are associated with increased left ventricular mass and are associated with higher all-cause mortality (Fig. 15.3), suggesting heart disease and potentially HF which could be managed with aggressive medical care as in this case [9–11].

Case 3

An asymptomatic 65-year-old Caucasian man presented to the office for routine medical care. He has a history of CKD secondary to polycystic kidney disease and well-controlled HTN. His current medications were perindopril 8 mg p.o. qd, amlodipine 10 mg p.o. qd, and hydrochlorothiazide 12.5 mg p.o. qd. There is no history of cardiovascular disease. His vital signs were: BP 124/70, P = 60, and R = 12. He was 5′8″ and weighed 145 lbs (BMI = 22 kg/m^2). He was well appearing and the physical examination was normal. Laboratories were notable for the following: Cr = 2.2 mg/dL (eGFR = 32 mL/min/1.73 m^2), BUN = 20 mg/dL, and BNP = 214 pg/mL. Additional examination was notable for an ECG, which showed normal sinus rhythm, left atrial enlargement, and LVH. A two-dimensional echocardiogram showed normal LV size, LVEF = 70%, mild LVH, and left atrial enlargement. Diastolic function was normal and there were no significant flow disturbances.

Discussion of Case 3

This case points out that CKD alone, in the absence of HF, can elevate the BNP into the 100–500 pg/mL range (Fig. 15.2). Results from the BNP Multinational

Study indicated that CKD can be a common explanation for BNP values in the 100–500 pg/mL range [6]. As this case points out, the left ventricle is rarely normal in CKD, and LVH as a manifestation of structural heart disease was present. However, since LVH without LV dilation does not lead to significantly increased wall tension, BNP is not markedly elevated due to LVH alone.

Case 4

A 75-year-old Hispanic female with a history of prior myocardial infarction and coronary artery bypass surgery is seen in the office for routine care. She has additional background history including lifelong obesity, type 2 DM, HTN, and CKD with a baseline Cr of 1.7 mg/dL. Her medications were aspirin 81 mg p.o. qd, lisinopril 20 mg p.o. qd, carvedilol 25 mg p.o. bid, and glargine insulin 40 units q.p.m. Vital signs revealed: BP 160/85 mm Hg, $P = 84$, $R = 16$. She was 5'2" and weighed 180 lbs (BMI $= 33$ kg/m^2). Physical exam was notable for clear lungs, a diffuse and laterally displaced PMI, soft S1 and S2, S4, no S3 and no murmurs. There was mild hepatomegaly and trace peripheral edema. Laboratories revealed: Cr $= 1.6$ mg/dL (eGFR $= 33$ mL/min/1.73 m^2), BUN $= 22$ mg/dL, and BNP $= 440$ pg/mL. The ECG showed normal sinus rhythm, Q-waves inferiorly, and left atrial enlargement. A two-dimensional echocardiogram found the LVEF $= 35\%$ with inferior akinesis, mild LVH, and left atrial enlargement. Diastolic function could not be fully assessed.

Discussion of Case 4

The elevated BNP in this case reflects both the presence of CKD and LV dysfunction (Table 15.2). Clinically, the patient was well treated for HF and was functional class 1. At this time it is unclear if additional treatment should be given for HF based on the BNP level. Multiple clinical trials are underway to assess this BNP-guided approach [23]. The patients' medications were not changed and the plan was to repeat the BNP levels if there was any change in the patient's status.

Table 15.2 Recommended cutpoints for BNP and NT-proBNP based on eGFR for the detection of LV dysfunction or HF.

EGFR (mL/min/1.73 m^2)	BNP cutpoint (pg/mL)	NT-proBNP cutpoint (pg/mL)
>90	70	450
89–60	100	1,200
59–30	200	1,800
<30	225	3,000
<15 or ESRD/dialysis	800	10,000

eGFR, estimated glomerular filtration rate; ESRD, end-stage renal disease; BNP, B-type natriuretic peptide; NT-proBNP, N-terminal pro-B-type natriuretic peptide.
Adapted from the following sources: McCullough *et al.* [6], Anwaruddin *et al.* [24], and Racek *et al.* [25].

Case 5

An asymptomatic 52-year-old African American man was referred to a cardiologist for a high BNP level of 869 pg/mL. The patient was asymptomatic but had a background history of obesity, type 2 DM, HTN, and chronic obstructive pulmonary disease. He was an active smoker and review of systems did reveal mild dyspnea on exertion attributed to obesity, deconditioning, and smoking. His chronic medications were metformin 500 mg p.o. bid, pioglitazone 45 mg p.o. qd, verapamil SR 240 mg p.o. qd, candesartan 32 mg p.o. qd, and albuterol and ipratropium inhalers. His vital signs were: BP 142/86, $P = 96$, $R = 20$. He was 5′9″ and weighed 240 lbs (BMI $= 36$ kg/m2). Physical exam was notable for smoking-related facial and voice changes, wheezes at the lung bases, a normal PMI, S1 S2, and a 2/6 holosystolic murmur at the right upper sternal border consistent with tricuspid regurgitation. The liver was mildly enlarged and there was no peripheral edema. Laboratories after the exam revealed a normal blood count, Cr $= 1.8$ mg/dL (eGFR $= 51$ mL/min/1.73 m^2), BUN $= 17$ mg/dL, and repeated BNP $= 651$ pg/mL. The ECG showed normal sinus rhythm, right and left atrial enlargement, right axis deviation, and a pulmonary disease pattern. The two-dimensional echocardiogram found the left ventricle was normal in size, there was mild LVH, LVEF $= 60\%$, bi-atrial enlargement, and mild TR with an estimated pulmonary artery pressure of 45 mm Hg. Diastolic function was normal.

Discussion of Case 5

This is an example of multiple factors contributing to the BNP elevation. Part of the elevation is due to reduced BNP clearance secondary to the reduction in renal parenchymal mass as reflected in the eGFR. Another source of the elevation is the right ventricular production of BNP in response to increased wall tension due to lung disease and slightly elevated right ventricular and pulmonary artery pressures. These factors working in combination yield BNP values in the 500–1000 pg/mL range in the clinic. Was the BNP change from 869 to 651 pg/mL on these two measurements significant? Almost certainly the answer is "no." There are technical attributes among the commercially available BNP assays that can cause differences of this magnitude in the same sample of blood. In addition, intra-individual variation can be as high as 50%. Thus a more than 50% reduction in BNP can be taken as a clinical sign of reduced wall tension and clinical improvement in some scenarios. In this case, the patients' medications were left unchanged and he will be followed over time with no plans for repeat BNP testing.

Cases 1 and 2 have the common comorbidity to both diabetic and nondiabetic CKD, that is, anemia of chronic disease. This form of anemia is due to reduced renal parenchymal mass and a relatively decreased production of erythropoietin, which is the major stimulus to the bone marrow that calls for the production of red blood cells from hemangioblasts [26]. Recently, BNP has been found to be modestly correlated to anemia (Fig. 15.4) [23]. The explanation for this

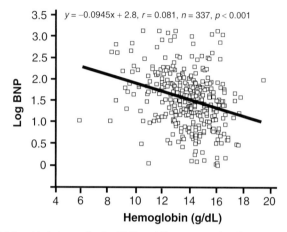

Figure 15.4 Relationship between the log BNP and Hb concentrations in men without HF from the BNP multinational study. (Adapted from Ref. [26])

relationship is probably the presence of increased left ventricular mass commonly associated with anemia, and thus, superimposed increased left ventricular wall tension, stimulating the synthesis and release of BNP at higher levels. It is currently unknown if therapeutic elevation of Hb with erythrocyte stimulating proteins (ESPs) (erythropoietin, darbepoetin) results in a reduction of BNP over time. Clinical trials are underway using ESPs in the treatment of anemia to impact rates of cardiovascular outcomes in patients with underlying CKD.

Another important comorbidity to consider in Cases 4 and 5 is obesity. Multiple studies in those who are asymptomatic and in those presenting with symptoms indicate that both BNP and NT-proBNP levels are depressed in the obese. Some studies indicate that levels can be reduced by 30–50% [27]. While these cases go through the exercise of explaining an elevated BNP in obese patients, it should be realized that the elevations in these patients may not be as high as comparable patients of normal body weight. Since the vast majority of patients are overweight or obese in clinical practice, this may not become a great concern for clinicians as they adjust to the many implications of the obesity pandemic.

In conclusion, CKD and associated reductions in renal parenchymal mass cause a predictable elevation of BNP due to reduced clearance of the peptide. In general, marked elevations of BNP in patients with CKD indicate the presence of superimposed HF [28]. In dialysis patients, BNP is commonly elevated and is reduced by 25% over the course of a hemodialysis session. While BNP in ESRD can be normal (<100 pg/mL), it is commonly observed to be >100 pg/mL and this finding is related to poorer long-term survival. Ongoing research aimed at understanding the relationship between the natriuretic peptides and renal function should give us better insights into diagnosis and management of patients with cardiorenal disease.

References

1 McCullough PA, Kuncheria J, Mathur VS. Diagnostic and therapeutic utility of B-type natriuretic peptide in patients with renal insufficiency and decompensated heart failure. *Rev Cardiovasc Med* 2003;**4**(suppl 7):S3–S12.

2 Totsune K, Takahashi K, Satoh F *et al.* Urinary immunoreactive brain natriuretic peptide in patients with renal disease. *Regul Pept* 1996;**63**:141–147.

3 Wegner M, Ganten D, Stasch JP. Neutral endopeptidase inhibition potentiates the effects of natriuretic peptides in renin transgenic rats. *Hypertens Res* 1996;**19**:229–238.

4 Ozaki J, Shimizu H, Hashimoto Y, Itoh H, Nakao K, Inui K. Enzymatic inactivation of major circulating forms of atrial and brain natriuretic peptides. *Eur J Pharmacol* 1999;**370**:307–312.

5 Ng LL, Loke IW, Davies JE *et al.* Community screening for left ventricular systolic dysfunction using plasma and urinary natriuretic peptides. *J Am Coll Cardiol* 2005;**45**(7):1043–1050.

6 McCullough PA, Duc P, Omland T *et al.* Breathing not properly multinational study investigators. B-type natriuretic peptide and renal function in the diagnosis of heart failure: an analysis from the breathing not properly multinational study. *Am J Kidney Dis* 2003;**41**(3):571–579.

7 Safley DM, Awad A, Sullivan RA *et al.* Changes in B-type natriuretic peptide levels in hemodialysis and the effect of depressed left ventricular function. *Adv Chronic Kidney Dis* 2005;**12**(1):117–124.

8 Dumler F, McCullough PA. Optimal dialysis for the end-stage renal disease patient with cardiovascular disease. *Adv Chronic Kidney Dis* 2004;**11**(3):261–273.

9 Zoccali C *et al.* Cardiac natriuretic peptides are related to left ventricular mass and function and predict mortality in dialysis patients. *J Am Soc Nephrol* 2001;**12**(7):1508–1515.

10 Naganuma T *et al.* The prognostic role of brain natriuretic peptides in hemodialysis patients. *Am J Nephrol* 2002;**22**(5–6):437–444.

11 Goto T *et al.* Increased circulating levels of natriuretic peptides predict future cardiac event in patients with chronic hemodialysis. *Nephron* 2002;**92**(3):610–615.

12 Ishizaka Y *et al.* Plasma concentration of human brain natriuretic peptide in patients on hemodialysis. *Am J Kidney Dis* 1994;**24**(3):461–472.

13 Corboy JC *et al.* Plasma natriuretic peptides and cardiac volume during acute changes in intravascular volume in haemodialysis patients. *Clin Sci (Lond)* 1994;**87**(6):679–684.

14 Haug C *et al.* Changes in brain natriuretic peptide and atrial natriuretic peptide plasma concentrations during hemodialysis in patients with chronic renal failure. *Horm Metab Res* 1994;**26**(5):246–249.

15 Totsune K, Takahashi K, Murakami O, Satoh F, Sone M, Mouri T. Elevated plasma C-type natriuretic peptide concentrations in patients with chronic renal failure. *Clin Sci (Lond)* 1994;**87**(3):319–322. Erratum in: *Clin Sci (Colch)* 1994;**87**(6):following xxv.

16 Ishizaka Y, Yamamoto Y, Tanaka M *et al.* Molecular forms of human brain natriuretic peptide (BNP) in plasma of patients on hemodialysis (HD). *Clin Nephrol* 1995;**43**(4):237–242.

17 Takahashi M *et al.* Plasma concentrations of natriuretic peptides in patients on hemodialysis. *Res Commun Mol Pathol Pharmacol* 1996;**92**(1):19–30.

18 Nitta K *et al.* Plasma concentration of brain natriuretic peptide as an indicator of cardiac ventricular function in patients on hemodialysis. *Am J Nephrol* 1998;**18**(5):411–415.

19 Osajima A *et al.* Clinical significance of natriuretic peptides and cyclic GMP in hemodialysis patients with coronary artery disease. *Am J Nephrol* 2001;**21**(2):112–129.

20 Nishikimi T *et al.* Plasma brain natriuretic peptide levels in chronic hemodialysis patients: influence of coronary artery disease. *Am J Kidney Dis* 2001;**37**(6):1201–1208.

21 Clerico A *et al.* Clinical relevance of cardiac natriuretic peptides measured by means of competitive and non-competitive immunoassay methods in patients with renal failure on chronic hemodialysis. *J Endocrinol Invest* 2001;**24**(1):24–30.

22 Uetake S, Takahashi M, Tamano K, Honda T, Kobayashi T, Horinaka S. Clinical significance of plasma atrial and brain natriuretic peptide levels during hemodialysis in hemodialysis patients with old myocardial infarction. *J Cardiol* 2001;**38**(2):61–71.

23 Wu AH, Omland T, Wold Knudsen C *et al.*, for The Breathing Not Properly Multinational Study Investigators. Relationship of B-type natriuretic peptide and anemia in patients with and without heart failure: a substudy from the Breathing Not Properly (BNP) multinational study. *Am J Hematol* 2005;**80**(3):174–180.

24 Anwaruddin S, Lloyd-Jones DM, Baggish A *et al.* Renal function, congestive heart failure, and amino-terminal pro-brain natriuretic peptide measurement: results from the ProBNP Investigation of Dyspnea in the Emergency Department (PRIDE) Study. *J Am Coll Cardiol* 2006;**47**(1):91–97.

25 Racek J, Kralova H, Trefil L, Rajdl D, Eiselt J. Brain natriuretic peptide and N-terminal proBNP in chronic haemodialysis patients. *Nephron Clin Pract* 2006;**103**(4):c162–c172.

26 McCullough PA, Lepor NE. Piecing together the evidence on anemia: the link between chronic kidney disease and cardiovascular disease. *Rev Cardiovasc Med* 2005;**6**(suppl 3):4–12.

27 Daniels LB, Clopton P, Bhalla V *et al.* How obesity affects the cut-points for B-type natriuretic peptide in the diagnosis of acute heart failure. Results from the Breathing Not Properly Multinational Study. *Am Heart J* 2006;**151**(5):1006–1012.

28 McCullough PA, Mueller C, Yancy CW, Jr. Overview of B-type natriuretic peptide as a blood test. *Congest Heart Fail* 2006;**12**(2):99–102.

CHAPTER 16

Congestive heart failure: treatment implications of natriuretic peptides

W. Frank Peacock

Case 1

Sherri Oregano is a 68-year-old woman who, after enjoying her usual morning coffee, went downstairs to get the morning newspaper. Upon her return, her husband noted that she was quite short of breath. Sherri had a long-standing history of congestive heart failure (CHF), and she always had difficulty climbing stairs, so this was not unusual for her. However, when she was still short of breath 15 minutes later, her husband became concerned and called an ambulance. On their arrival, they found her to be diaphoretic, with a respiratory rate of 32, a blood pressure of 92/69 mm Hg, and an irregular pulse at a rate of 123 beats/minute. They applied oxygen via a 100% non-rebreather mask, and this seemed to significantly improve her level of discomfort. Her oxygen saturation improved from an initial 86 to 93%. An intravenous line was started, and she was placed on the cardiac monitor that showed atrial fibrillation. Ms. Oregano was then taken uneventfully to Smedly Community Hospital. Vital signs repeated after hospital arrival were improved, and it was documented that her heart rate was 110 bpm, respiratory rate was 26, and the blood pressure was 112/79 mm Hg.

Shortly after her arrival at Smedly, Dr. Androponi met Ms. Oregano. At that time she stated that she was feeling improved. Dr. Androponi performed a history and physical, noting that Ms. Oregano had suffered with atrial fibrillation for many years. It was usually rate controlled, unless she over exerted herself. She specifically denied having any chest pain, or any prodromal illness in the weeks before her presentation.

Ms. Oregano's usual medication list included warfarin, carvedilol, enalapril, spironolactone, bumetanide, and potassium. She denied having any allergies, did not smoke or consume alcohol, and she did not know her family history, since she had been adopted at the age of 3.

The physical exam found Ms. Oregano to be persistently and significantly short of breath, although she stated that she felt improved compared to the period before EMS arrival. By auscultation she had a few rales in the bilateral lower lung fields, and no extra heart sounds were detectable. She had slight jugular venous distention, about 2 cm, and no dependent edema.

At the completion of his history and physical, Dr. Androponi ordered an electrocardiogram, cardiac troponin, CK-MB, a chest radiograph, B-type natriuretic peptide (BNP) concentration, and routine labs. He also requested the intravenous administration of 80 mg of furosemide. One hour later, Ms. Oregano had produced approximately 1200 cc of urine, but admitted to only a slight improvement in her respiratory status. Her BNP then returned from the lab and was reported to be 477 pg/mL. The chest film was interpreted as mild HF, and the remainder of all other testing was unremarkable.

At this point, Dr. Androponi admitted Mrs. Oregano to the hospital with a diagnosis of exacerbation of CHF. Dr. Androponi felt that the exertion had triggered the patient's symptoms, and this was supported by the elevated BNP finding.

One year later, Dr. Androponi received a subpoena for the wrongful death of Ms. Oregano. The salient features of the litigation stem from the issue that after admission to the hospital, Ms. Oregano was placed on a regular medical bed with intravenous furosemide monotherapy. At 6:30 AM, during their morning nursing rounds, Ms. Oregano was found to be in asystole. All resuscitative efforts failed, and Ms. Oregano was pronounced dead. At the subsequent autopsy, a large pulmonary embolus was identified as the proximate cause of her expiration. At no time during her hospitalization was the possibility of a pulmonary embolus considered, nor was any type of anticoagulation administered.

Discussion of Case 1

When interpreting BNP levels, the clinical scenario must also be considered. When the BNP result is less than 100 pg/mL, CHF is an unlikely diagnosis, and will be found in only a very small percentage of cases as the cause of the patient's dyspnea. At this level, BNP has an excellent negative predictive value [1, 2]. However, as BNP rises its sensitivity declines while its specificity improves. When the BNP level exceeds 500 pg/mL, CHF is very likely to be present. What is then left is a gray zone from 100 to 500 pg/mL. In this range CHF may be present, but confounding by a number of alternative diagnoses

Table 16.1 BNP levels in clinical use.

Low BNP (< 50–100 pg/mL)
   The symptoms are probably NOT due to HF
     Consider a different diagnosis (COPD, etc.)
Medium BNP (between 100 and 500 pg/mL)
   Consider the differential (PE, $1°$ Pulm HTN, etc.)
   Compare to prior BNP levels
High BNP (> 500 pg/mL)
HF likely, but must still consider alternative or concurrent diagnoses

PE, pulmonary embolus; $1°$ Pulm HTN, primary pulmonary hypertension; COPD, chronic obstructive pulmonary disease.
Adapted from Silver *et al.* [2].

must be considered. BNP can be increased by a number of non-HF pathologies (see Table 16.1). A partial reporting of an ever-expanding list includes being elderly, female gender, possibly those on hormone replacement therapy, patients with acute coronary syndromes (ACS), end stage cirrhosis, renal failure, pulmonary embolism, and primary pulmonary hypertension. Clinical acumen and the consideration of additional testing are needed when patients present with dyspnea and gray zone BNP levels.

In this case, Ms. Oregano's symptoms had appeared abruptly, did not resolve as expected, and were not improved despite effective therapy that would have been predicted to result in some clinical change. Even more importantly, had Dr. Androponi reviewed the medical record, he would have found that his patient had visited her physician just 7 days prior for a routine visit. At that time her BNP had been 710 pg/mL. While there are large variations in BNP concentrations across populations, within a given patient, changes in baseline BNP correlate reasonably well with changes in hemodynamics and symptoms. Since Ms. Oregano presented at a significantly lower BNP concentration than her established baseline, it would be expected that her CHF symptoms would be better. Since she was significantly more dyspneic, despite objective evidence of improved heart failure, the onus was upon the physician to consider alternative diagnoses to explain the patient's symptoms and to undertake additional diagnostic investigations. Comparing the "dry weight" BNP obtained in the outpatient clinic several days before, to the BNP in the ED and finding them to be similar suggests that some cause other than a heart failure exacerbation was the etiology for Ms. Oregano's presentation. This finding should have prompted a search for a non-HF cause of Ms. Oregano's dyspnea. The case did not go to trial, as Dr. Androponi settled for $800,000.

Case 2

Steven Alladay is a 79-year-old Korean war veteran. A guy who considers himself pretty tough, he has had to see his physician nearly weekly for the past 3 weeks. He lives with his wife, in a first story flat, only 3 blocks from Dr. Schmidt, who has been his physician for the last 23 years. Mr. Alladay is now pretty upset that he is short of breath with what he considers relatively minimal exertion. Although he was able to get up to Dr. Schmidt's second story office via the stairs, he still thinks he should go into the hospital so he "can be cured" of his long-standing chronic heart failure. He has had no URI symptoms, specifically denies any recent chest pain, and reports an unchanged weight.

Dr. Schmidt does a very careful physical examination. He notes that the vital signs are not in an immediately dangerous range, although there is some opportunity to increase his enalapril as the patient's blood pressure is 125/85 mm Hg. Dr. Schmidt notes that his patient has no jugular venous distention, but on auscultation he finds that an S4 is present and notices some slight scattered basilar rales that clear with coughing. He also documents that there was trace-dependent pitting edema, and that his weight is 1 pound heavier than his baseline of 1 month ago.

Reviewing his medical record, it is noted that Mr. Alladay is taking 40 mg of furosemide daily, in addition to enalapril, carvedilol, and occasionally viagra. Historically, he has always been compliant with both his medications and his diet requirements. He has an allergy to penicillin, is a non-smoker, social drinker, and has a family history significant only for breast cancer.

Dr. Schmidt is somewhat concerned about Mr. Alladay. He seems to have a degree of dysfunction that is unusual for this patient. He knows that Mr. Alladay's elderly wife has had markedly worsening Alzheimer's, and speculates that the stress of being the sole caregiver may be causing his patient's increased office visits, although his prior history of heart failure must be considered highly in the differential diagnosis of his presentation. Dr. Schmidt requests that his nurse perform an ECG, obtain a chest X-ray from the radiology suite one floor below, and draw blood for electrolytes, CBC, troponin, and a BNP level. Using their new point of care machine provides BNP results about 15 minutes later, and it is noted to be 178 pg/mL. The other labs are fairly unremarkable. His ECG shows normal sinus rhythm with a nonspecific intraventricular conduction delay, but is otherwise non-diagnostic for any pathology. His electrolytes all appear within the normal range, and his CBC is normal except for a mild normocytic normochromic anemia and a hemoglobin of 10.5 g/dL.

Discussion of Case 2

Based on the clinic presentation, which does not seem to warrant hospitalization for decompensated heart failure, Dr. Schmidt is unsure what guidance this BNP result in the diagnostic gray zone can provide. As discussed above, a BNP in the gray zone, between 100 and 500 pg/mL, requires the practitioner apply diagnostic skill and clinical acumen to determine the appropriate course of action. Table 16.1 is a graphical representation of the predictive range and therapeutic considerations.

One study has specifically addressed the importance of initial BNP and the necessity for hospitalization. In the REDHOT trial (Rapid Emergency Department Heart Failure Outpatient Trial) [3], a blinded BNP was obtained on 1743 patients presenting to a hospital emergency department (ED) with a chief complaint of dyspnea. Subsequent hospitalization and mortality was ascertained. The authors reported that 30-day survivors had much lower BNP concentrations compared to those who died during the same period (764 pg/mL versus 2096 pg/mL, respectively). Unfortunately, in the REDHOT study, patients who were discharged home had a mean BNP of 976 pg/mL. This compared to the cohort of patients who were felt to have a severity of illness sufficient to warrant in-hospital care who had a mean of BNP of 767 pg/mL.

When the REDHOT data were evaluated using logistic regression analysis, surprisingly an ED doctor's intention to admit or discharge a patient had no influence on 90-day outcomes, while the BNP level was a strong predictor of 90-day outcome. Of admitted patients, 11% had BNP levels <200 pg/mL (66% of which were perceived NYHA functional class III or IV). The 90-day combined event rate (CHF visits or admissions, and mortality) in the group of patients admitted with BNP <200 pg/mL and >200 pg/mL was 9% and 29%, respectively ($p = 0.006$).

This study clearly suggests that clinical grounds alone may be insufficient to effect an accurate decision on the need for hospitalization. In context of the case of Mr. Alladay, these data suggest that he is at low risk of adverse outcome from his heart failure over the next 90 days.

Other studies have evaluated outcome prediction using BNP and have reported that this simple lab test is able to predict clinical events in patients presenting to the ED. In one study, levels exceeding 480 pg/mL were associated with an increased risk of death or rehospitalization in the following 6 months [4].

Mr. Alladay's chest X-ray results returned and were found to have no suggestion of heart failure, except for cardiomegaly, which had been noted on successive previous films. In context with this data, Dr. Schmidt felt that an appropriate course of action would be to increase his patient's enalapril and arrange for bi-weekly visitation by the visiting nurse association. Although he did not hear from Mr. Alladay during the next month, he has received weekly communication from the visiting nurse indicating that he is doing much better, attending weekly meetings with an Alzheimer's support group, and is considering the placement of Mrs. Alladay into a nursing facility skilled in the care of demented patients.

Case 3

Sandy Elivar is a physician working at a veteran's hospital in near Cleveland, OH, where she has spent the last 20 years of her career. When she first began working there, it seemed that it was a relatively straightforward job. Patients tended to be younger, disease presentation fairly obvious, and the diagnostic course implicit. However, recent demographic changes have completely altered that perception. As the demography of America has aged, the complexity of the Emergency Department has increased. Whereas young patients who are suffering from shortness of breath will frequently have a single relatively easy differential diagnosis, the elderly represent a significant challenge. The reality of a lifetime of cigarettes and sedentary lifestyle result in diagnostic considerations that have complicated what once was fairly limited. Beyond demographics, age impacts other considerations. Not only are there multiple differential diagnosis considerations, there is also the fact that many pathologies share the final common pathway of dyspnea (see Table 16.2).

James Kirk is a 75-year-old veteran. He presents to the veterans administration ED from his nursing home where he lives due to his chronic dementia. The nursing home has sent accompanying papers that indicate he is more short of breath than usual. His past medical history, gleaned from a review of the computerized medical chart, shows that in the past 3 years, Mr. Kirk has been hospitalized for dyspnea due to emphysema, pneumonia, pulmonary

Table 16.2 A brief differential diagnosis of dyspnea in the elderly.

---

1 Respiratory compensation of metabolic acidosis
2 Aspiration
3 Anaphylaxis
4 Anemia
5 Anxiety
6 Chronic pulmonary disease examples
  a Asbestosis
  b Pulmonary fibrosis
7 Congestive heart failure
  a Intra-abdominal pathologies
  b Ascities
8 Myocardial infarction/ischemia
9 Panic attack
10 Pneumonia/bronchitis
11 Pneumothorax
12 Primary pulmonary hypertension
13 Pulmonary embolus
14 Renal failure with fluid overload
15 Sepsis

---

embolus, and CHF. Each time he was admitted via the ED with the diagnosis of dyspnea, he was treated with intravenous furosemide and azithromycin, aerosol bronchodilators of albuterol and ipratropium, and intravenous methylprednisolone. During his hospitalization he has received multiple work ups consisting of pulmonary function evaluation, several chest radiographs, arterial blood gases, numerous blood lab tests, cultures of both blood and sputum, several ECGs, and a helical CT scan with intravenous contrast. Unfortunately, following the performance of his last radiocontrast study, it was noted that his creatinine increased acutely to 3.5 mg/dL. Obviously, there are costs and consequences associated with the performance (and the non-performance) of clinical investigations.

At this visit, Dr. Elivar finds Mr. Kirk to be noticeably short of breath. His pulse oximetry reads 90%, and his respiratory rate is 22 breaths/minute. The respiratory therapist has already administered treatment with 2.5 mg of aerosol albuterol sulfate and 1.0 mg of ipratropium bromide, but this seems to have provided minimal benefit. Dr. Elivar orders serum lab testing that includes a BNP level, an electrocardiogram, and a chest X-ray. The ECG shows a left bundle branch block, similar to the prior ECG of 2 months earlier. The portable chest X-ray is interpreted as showing cardiomegaly and a small pleural effusion. The lab tests are unremarkable except for the creatinine of 3.2 mg/dL and a BNP of 1209 pg/mL.

In regard to Mr. Kirk, and considering his prior discharge BNP of 640 pg/mL from 6 weeks ago, the level of his BNP at presentation represents a significant increase. Dr. Elivar administers 80 mg of furosemide intravenously, then decreases his blood pressure by the oral administration of enalapril and topical

BNP and Renal $F(n)$

- BNP versus creatinine clearance in patients with and without HF

- Excluded CrCl<15 mL/min and dialysis patients

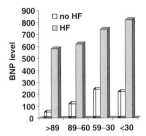

Estimated creatinine clearance (mL/min)

Figure 16.1 Renal function and HF diagnosis. (Adapted from McCullough *et al.* [5])

nitrates, and writes the order to admit him to a telemetry floor. He does not administer antibiotics, nor does he request any study for the exclusion of a pulmonary embolus. One hour later he leaves the ED.

After admission Mr. Kirk had diuresed 2 L urine by the time he was seen by Dr. Spango, his internal medicine physician, the next morning. At this juncture his respiratory rate was 16 breaths/minute, his blood pressure was 114/82, and his pulse oximetry was 91% on room air. He stated that he felt great, and asked Dr. Spango if he'd "like to go a few rounds." Dr. Spango declined, was pleased with Mr. Kirk's progress, and arranged for him to be discharged back to his nursing home the following morning.

Discussion of Case 3

Elevated BNP in the setting of renal failure can represent a diagnostic challenge. Because BNP can be elevated in renal failure, the level must be considered in the contextual setting of the patients past medical history, the level of the renal dysfunction, and the clinical presentation. One study [5] has suggested an alternative cutpoint of 200 pg/mL for considering the diagnosis of HF based upon the BNP level (see Fig. 16.1). In this analysis, patients were stratified based upon their estimated creatinine clearance. Even with extremely impaired renal function, a BNP in excess of 200 pg/mL suggests the presence of heart failure.

In the ED, BNP and NT-proBNP can both be used to diagnose CHF. They are most useful in those patients who are the most difficult to diagnose, e.g., those with the potential for many overlapping comorbidities. The value of BNP in this scenario has been studied. In dyspnea resulting from isolated chronic obstructive pulmonary disease, the level of BNP is usually less than 100 pg/mL, as compared to those whose symptoms are the result of CHF, where levels commonly exceed 1000 pg/mL. And a similar analysis of BNP in patients with edema found parallel results [1]. When signs and symptoms suggest CHF, a BNP level may contribute to an accurate diagnosis. The ability to accurately diagnose the cause of dyspnea has consequences in the institution of medical therapy, which has the potential to shorten hospitalization and improve patient outcomes.

Length of hospitalization is one of the greatest determinates of cost in the management of heart failure. And since HF patients tend to receive long hospitalizations, the costs can represent a financial burden to the hospital. In fact, the average US hospital loses $1288 for every single patient hospitalized with acute decompensated heart failure. One study has evaluated the impact of early BNP testing on hospital costs. In the European BASEL [6] trial, 452 patients presenting to an ED with dyspnea were randomized to receive either standard therapy, or rapid BNP testing with standard therapy. Patients were then followed to determine length of hospitalization and resource utilization. Those whose care was guided by the knowledge of an early BNP were discharged an average of 3 days sooner than when the physician's were blinded to the BNP results (8 days versus 11 days, respectively). The length of hospitalization differences translated into a savings of $1854 (US dollars) by the use of early ED BNP testing. Additionally, the BNP-guided group had a 10% lower hospitalization rate (85% versus 75%), and a 9% decrease in ICU admission (24% versus 15%). Although evaluated in the European health-care environment, with markedly longer HF hospitalization than in the US system, this study still demonstrates the principal of early diagnosis results in early treatment, both of which are important determinants of early discharge.

Case 4

Jason Marbury is a 25-year-old patient of Dr. Steve Kibble. Dr. Kibble works at the Urban Transplant Center and has been caring for Jason for about 2 years, following an initial referral for cardiomegaly and shortness of breath. Subsequently diagnosed with a viral cardiomyopathy, Jason is seen nearly monthly and has required frequent hospitalizations both for fluid overload, as well as dehydration occurring as a complication of excessive diuresis. Most recently, Jason has been doing well in managing the complexities of his disease. He is compliant with his self-assessment, weighing himself daily and adjusting his furosemide dose accordingly. Furthermore, despite a difficult up-titration, he is now compliant with his carvedilol and angiotensin converting enzyme inhibitor.

Today's presentation was a previously scheduled routine visit. The nurse has obtained his vital signs, which are blood pressure 92/68 mm Hg, heart rate 64 beats/minute, and a respiratory rate of 16 breaths/minute. The patient is afebrile and his pulse oximeter reads 93%. His weight is up 2 pounds since his visit of 1 month ago. He is complaining of increased dyspnea, worse on exertion, baseline orthopnea, and orthostatic symptoms that last for approximately 1 minute after standing. The patient is well known to you. He denies any smoking, but complains of a cough that has been present ever since starting the angiotensin converting enzyme inhibitor, although he now says he has occasional sputum production and increased fatigue, with some vague myalgias for the past several days. He specifically denies fever, chest pain, vomiting, other cardiorespiratory symptoms, and claims to have been compliant with his diet, medications, and fluid restriction.

On physical exam, you note that his neck veins are flat while he is sitting at about 45°, his lungs have basilar rales that clear with coughing, and he has a trace amount of pre-tibial edema. On cardiac auscultation, his rate is regular but you think you detect an S3. On evaluation of your prior notes, you notice that the S3 has been occasionally present, as are occasional basilar lung rales.

Discussion of Case 4

What is your course of action? Jason appears well enough that hospitalization is not currently considered, but he has signs that suggest his increased dyspnea may be the result of either worsening of his underlying heart failure, or conversely the superimposition of a concurrent viral syndrome. His orthostatic symptoms and flat neck veins suggest that he has intravascular volume depletion; however, his increased weight gain, and mild pre-tibial edema suggest excessive volume. Although the S3 and basilar rales can suggest excessive fluid, in this case of chronic heart failure and as reflected in your prior notes, these findings represent this patient's baseline.

A number of studies have suggested that BNP measurement can be helpful in determining the appropriate course of action in this patient. In the first, Maisel [4] evaluated BNP levels in patients presenting to the ED. They were able to demonstrate that BNP levels do predict future outcomes. In this analysis, patients with BNP levels less than 230 pg/mL had composite adverse outcomes of death or rehospitalization rates within the subsequent 6 months of less than 4%. In the same analysis, patients with BNP concentrations exceeding 480 pg/mL had adverse outcome rates (death or rehospitalization) of nearly 40%. Clearly, BNP elevation is associated with increased risk of adverse outcome. However, what this study did not address is the question of whether intervention has the potential to change the adverse outcome rate.

This has subsequently been investigated in an additional analysis in the office environment [7]. In a study of 69 patients randomized to treatment guided by BNP levels, versus usual care, physicians treating patients with the additional knowledge of BNP concentrations had better outcomes over the subsequent 9.5 months. Using a composite endpoint of death, hospitalization, and heart failure decompensation, the BNP group had 19 events, compared to 54 events in the standard therapy cohort ($p = 0.02$). When time to first cardiovascular event was analyzed, 27% of the cohort with BNP-guided therapy had an event within 6 months, compared to 53% of the standard therapy group ($p = 0.034$). Although this is a small study, it suggests that knowing the BNP result can be of clinical value when determining the appropriate course of action in the outpatient environment where symptoms and physical exam finding may more subtle than in the hospitalized cohort of heart failure patients.

In the office an ECG was performed which demonstrated no change as compared to baseline. A chest X-ray was also obtained. This was interpreted by the radiologist as demonstrating no acute pulmonary disease as compared to a film of 2 months ago. A BNP, performed that afternoon, found a level of 428 pg/mL. Reviewing the medical record of 6 months ago found a previously obtained routine BNP level of 365 pg/mL. Because there can be fairly large variation in BNP values, some claim as much as 30% without discernable clinical consequence, these two levels may be considered equivalent. Consequently, despite the undefined clinical presentation, the available investigations suggest that Mr. Marbury is most likely suffering from a viral syndrome. Consequently, you discharge him to home. About 10 days later you receive a call from a local ED that his cough has worsened and he has been running intermittent fevers for 3–4 days. A repeat radiograph demonstrates no interval change, and his BNP level was 485 pg/mL. After a discussion, the agreed up plan is that he will be discharged to follow-up with you within the next several days. Three days later, at the scheduled follow-up, Jason is feeling much better, and his symptoms have returned to baseline.

References

1 Maisel AS, Krishnaswamy P, Nowak RM *et al.*, for Breathing Not Properly Multinational Study Investigators. Rapid measurement of B-type natriuretic peptide in the emergency diagnosis of heart failure. *N Engl J Med* 2002;**347**:161–167.

2 Silver MA, Maisel A, Yancy CW, McCullough PA *et al.* BNP Consensus Panel 2004: a clinical approach for the diagnostic, prognostic, screening, treatment monitoring, and therapeutic roles of natriuretic peptides in cardiovascular disease. *Congestive Heart Fail* 2004;**10**(5):S3.

3 Maisel AS, Hollander JE, Guss D *et al.* Primary Results of the Rapid Emergency Department Heart Failure Outpatient Trial (REDHOT): a multicenter study of B-type natriuretic peptide levels, emergency department decision making, and outcomes in patients presenting with shortness of breath. *JACC* 2004;**44**(6):1328–1333.

4 Harrison A, Morrison LK, Krishnaswamy P *et al.* B-type natriuretic peptide predicts future cardiac events in patients presenting to the emergency department with dyspnea. *Ann Emerg Med* 2002;**39**(2):131–138.

5 Mccullough PA, Duc P, Omland T *et al.* B-type natriuretic peptide and renal function in the diagnosis of heart failure: an analysis from the breathing not properly multinational study. *Am J Kidney Dis* 2003;**41**(3):571–579.

6 Mueller C, Scholer A, Laule-Kilian K *et al.* Use of B-type natriuretic peptide in the evaluation and management of acute dyspnea. *N Engl J Med* 2004;**350**:647–654.

7 Troughton RW, Frampton CM, Yandle TG *et al.* Treatment of heart failure guided by plasma aminoterminal brain natriuretic peptide (N-BNP) concentrations. *Lancet* 2000;**355**(9210):1126–1130.

CHAPTER 17

Utilizing multimarker strategies in patients who present with congestive heart failure

Johannes Mair

Summary

Heart failure (HF) is not only a hemodynamic derangement of the ventricles, instead it is nowadays regarded as a progressive structural process altering the shape, volume, and cellular composition of the heart and the structure of the vasculature into which the left ventricle must empty. Thus, improvement in the contraction of left ventricle is not the sole focus of HF treatment any longer. Complex activation of neurohormonal systems is crucial for disease progression, and pharmacotherapy in HF should aim at antagonizing the detrimental effects of neurohumoral activation. Arterial underfilling activates neurohormonal effectors, such as sympathetic nervous system (SNS), renin–angiotensin–aldosterone system (RAAS), and vasopressin (VP). Over the long-term, these neurohormonal reflexes have deleterious effects and may enhance the loss of cardiomyocytes, which may lead to detectable cardiac troponin in blood samples of HF patients. As long as vasoconstriction and fluid retention are sufficiently counter-regulated by activation of vasodilatory and natriuretic substances, such as natriuretic peptides (NPs), HF patients stay asymptomatic. NPs gained attention as diagnostic and prognostic markers in HF patients. Several peptide growth factors and inflammatory cytokines appear to be involved in HF as well. High-sensitivity C-reactive protein (CRP) is a suitable routine marker to monitor the proinflammatory activity in HF. Given this pathophysiological background a multibiomarker approach appears to make sense in HF. In acute HF multimarker testing for diagnosis and differential diagnosis is supported by guidelines. First studies already have demonstrated the added value of troponin and BNP for risk stratification in chronic HF; however, the impact of multimarker measurement on clinical decision-making important for long-term management remains to be demonstrated.

Introduction

HF is a difficult disease to define, and no definition of this complex multisystem disorder is completely adequate and entirely satisfactory. Braunwald [1] defined this complex syndrome as a pathological state in which an abnormality of cardiac function is responsible for failure of the heart to pump blood at a rate commensurate with the requirements of the metabolizing tissues, or can do so only from an elevated filling pressure. HF usually develops from myocardial failure due to loss of a critical amount of functioning myocardium after damage to the heart (e.g., myocardial ischemia and infarction that alter regional function, and myocarditis, dilated, toxic or metabolic cardiomyopathies that alter global function) or due to chronically persisting hemodynamic changes leading to pressure or volume overload (e.g., heart valve diseases, systemic or pulmonary hypertension) which lead to hypertrophy and dilatation of the chamber. Nowadays the most common causes of HF in industrialized countries are coronary artery disease (CAD, approximately 60% of HF cases) and hypertension. To overcome the various difficulties in defining HF guidelines for its diagnosis have been developed by the cardiological societies [2, 3]. Essential features are the presence of clinical signs and symptoms of HF (e.g., breathlessness, fatigue, low arterial blood pressure, ankle swelling, pulmonary edema) and objective evidence for cardiac dysfunction, e.g., by echocardiography. In equivocal cases a response to treatment directed toward HF is helpful in establishing the diagnosis.

In the seventies, HF was perceived as a disease whose symptoms were closely allied to hemodynamic disequilibrium. This hemodynamic model suggested that increased ventricular wall stress is the principal cause of HF. It was thought that these abnormalities could be rectified by the use of vasodilating drugs, which lead to afterload reduction. These drugs in fact lowered left atrial pressure and increased cardiac output, and acute HF symptoms are rapidly improved by the use of drugs, such as diuretics, vasodilators, and morphine. This response relates largely to changes in central hemodynamics. However, it was soon realized that the administration of some of these afterload-reducing drugs was not associated with any clinical benefit on patient's outcome even after improvement in hemodynamic status has been achieved. The origin of symptoms in chronic HF (CHF) is not related in a simple manner to hemodynamic findings as well [4], and it has been shown that the degree of left ventricular dysfunction in CHF does not correlate with exercise tolerance or symptoms. These mismatches are explained by the complex interplay between central hemodynamic, pulmonary factors, and peripheral circulation, as well as by neuroendocrine adaptation, which led to the formulation of the neurohormonal hypothesis of the progression of HF [5].

Recent advances in the understanding of congestive HF: a primer for clinicians

The neurohumoral hypothesis of HF

In recent years, understanding HF has moved from a hemodynamic concept into accepting the importance of neuroendocrine pathophysiological changes in the progression of HF [6]. HF is characterized by a number of neurohormonal abnormalities, and it is nowadays regarded as a hemodynamic disorder due to impaired pump function with reduced cardiac output and subsequent venous congestion with complex neurohormonal activation aimed at improving the mechanical environment of the heart. Circulating and local hormones as well as proinflammatory cytokines play an important role in disease progression. In fact, in recent years the most important developments in the treatment of HF have been the introduction of first, the angiotensin-converting enzyme (ACE) inhibitors and then beta-blockers, which resulted in an almost 50% decrease in mortality in the last decade in therapeutic trials. The great benefits of these drugs on delaying the progression of HF are mainly attributable to their neurohumoral effects with beneficial effects on the remodeling of the failing heart.

The initial injury to the heart leads to low output with subsequent arterial un-derfilling. These hemodynamic changes are sensed by vascular baroreceptors. High-pressure receptors are located in the left ventricle, carotid sinus, aortic arch, and renal afferent arterioles and respond to decreases in arterial blood pressure, peripheral vascular resistance, or renal perfusion. They activate the vasomotor center in the medulla oblongata, and the SNS, RAAS, and VP are the activated principal neurohumoral effectors (see Fig. 17.1) [7]. Activation of carotid baroreceptors during arterial underfilling in HF is essential for non-osmotic VP release and overrides activation of atrial receptors. The immediate effects of SNS and RAAS activation as well as VP release are tachycardia, in-creased myocardial contractility, vasoconstriction with increased cardiac pre- and afterload, stimulation of thirst. Salt and water retention occur with a delay of several days. These hemodynamic mechanisms and baroreceptor-mediated reflexes are of clear benefit during the acute phase (acute HF) and initially

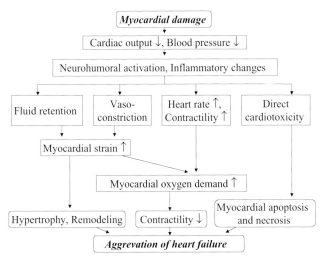

Figure 17.1 Pathophysiology of heart failure.

compensate for the failing heart and maintain perfusion of the brain and heart in the presence of severe reduction in cardiac output, but long-term neurohormonal activation is largely maladaptive and exacerbates the hemodynamic abnormalities by a vicious circle or causes myocyte hypertrophy and exerts a direct toxic effect on the myocardium (see Fig. 17.1). The clinical signs and symptoms of CHF largely result from neurohormonal activation leading to vasoconstriction and renal salt and water retention. Myocardial hypertrophy initially helps to reduce ventricular wall tension and unloads individual muscle fibers, but on the long-term it is a maladaptive process and increases myocardial oxygen demand. Activation of neurohormonal systems plays an important role in the alterations in ventricular architecture that occurs during the development of HF (cardiac remodeling). The degree of cardiac remodeling is influenced by left ventricular hemodynamic load, and ventricular remodeling involves the myocytes and interstitial myocardial components including collagen. Aldosterone is released systemically by the adrenal glands and locally in the myocardium itself. The whole aldosterone synthesis pathway is present in the myocardium and probably controlled by pathways similar to those of adrenalcortical cells (tissue ACE system). In addition to its vasoconstrictor effect, angiotensin II is an important mediator of cardiomyocyte hypertrophy. Increased local and circulating norepinephrine contributes to myocardial hypertrophy either directly or secondarily by activating the RAAS. Similarly, circulating aldosterone increases the production of collagen by fibroblasts and thereby the deposition of interstitial collagen in the failing ventricle (cardiac fibrosis). Both angiotensin II and aldosterone play a major role in the genesis of myocardial fibrosis. Interstitial myocardial fibrosis increases myocardial stiffness, reduces diastolic ventricular compliance, and is, therefore, important in the development of HF, in particular, diastolic dysfunction. Cardiac remodeling is on the long-term maladaptive, and it is therefore a key component of the progressive nature of HF [8]. The clinical efficacy of ACE inhibitors is closely related to their inhibition of ventricular remodeling by lowering angiotensin II and aldosterone. At the receptor level, angiotensin II receptor blockers and aldosterone receptor blockers (e.g., spironolactone) modulate the remodeling of the failing ventricle. Beta-blockers modify the hypertrophic and directly toxic effects of norepinephrine on the cardiomyocyte and also decrease the rate of apoptosis in HF.

Even in presence of myocardial hypertrophy and increased mitochondrial density, molecular and structural changes in the chronically failing human heart lead to an intrinsic contractile defect, i.e., a reduction in the velocity of shortening at any level of tension development. Important molecular changes at the levels of energetics, contractile responsiveness to SNS stimulation, and electromechanical coupling occur in all types of chronic HF, which finally lead to depressed myocardial contractility (see Table 17.1). Cardiomyocytes undergo phenotypic modifications and re-express several fetal genes (e.g., sarcomeric proteins, proteins of the calcium handling machinery, creatine kinase B subunits, and cytoskeletal proteins).

Table 17.1 Myocardial changes in chronic heart failure.

Molecular changes within cardiomyocytes
  Calcium homeostasis
    Sarcoplasmatic reticulum calcium content ↓, SERCA 2a activity ↓, plasmalemmal
  Na^+/Ca^{2+} exchanger activity ↑
  β-adrenergic responsiveness
    Receptor density ↓, impaired signal transduction
  Contractile and regulatory proteins
    Myosin and troponin isoform shifts, myosin ATPase activity ↓
  Energetics
    CK activity↓, CK-B ↑, creatine phosphate and ATP ↓
Structural changes
  Hypertrophy
  Dilatation
  Fibrosis
  Progressive loss of cardiomyocytes (necrosis or apoptosis)

CK, creatine kinase; ATP, adenosine triphosphate.

In summary, through a combination of ventricular dilatation and hypertrophy, and the activation of vasoconstrictor and vasodilator forces, a delicate hemodynamic and neurohormonal balance is achieved, which restores cardiac function toward that before myocardial damage at minimum energetic cost. Vasoconstrictive and sodium retentive actions by the RAAS, SNS, VP, thromboxane, and endothelin are completely counter-regulated by NPs, nitric oxide, bradykinin, adrenomedullin, and prostaglandins. In overt HF, the compensatory hemodynamic and neurohormonal mechanisms are overwhelmed or exhausted, which lead to development of the clinical signs and symptoms of HF and further deteriorates cardiac function.

The pathophysiological basis of a multimarker approach to HF
Cardiac NPs
More than 20 years ago, it was proven that the heart functions not only as a pump but also as an endocrine organ. De Bold *et al.* [9] demonstrated the existence of the long-predicted natriuretic factor, which is the endocrine link between the heart and the kidneys. This discovery finally led to the characterization of a whole family of structurally similar but genetically distinct peptides, the NPs [10]. These looped peptides are the main hormones in the body's defense against volume overload and hypertension. They are the naturally occurring antagonists of the hormones of the RAAS and the SNS. NPs inhibit the secretion of VP and corticotropin, and inhibit salt appetite and water drinking as well as sympathetic tone in the central nervous system, and peripherally they increase glomerular filtration rate and natriuresis to protect the heart from acute volume loads. The hemodynamic effects of NP comprise a decrease in systemic and pulmonary vascular resistance, systemic and pulmonary arterial pressure (afterload), plasma volume, venous return and right atrial, pulmonary

capillary wedge and left-ventricular end-diastolic pressures (preload), and dilatation of coronary arteries with increased coronary blood flow. As a result, the cardiac output increases and diastolic function improves. The naturally occurring antagonists of cardiovascular remodeling are also the NPs that limit the myocardial proliferative or hypertrophic and fibrotic response to damage and the remodeling of the heart and vessels (see Fig. 17.1).

Two members of the NP family, atrial natriuretic peptide (ANP) and brain or B-type natriuretic peptide (BNP), are mainly released in response to myocardial stretch induced by volume expansion and pressure overload of the heart. Additionally, neurohormones activated in HF, such as VP, phenylepinephrine, and endothelin, stimulate NP gene expression and release after binding to G-protein-coupled receptors. In a counterregulatory effort to maintain plasma volume homeostasis, ANP and BNP are highly activated in HF. Low-pressure baroreceptors, which are located in the atria, react to volume expansion or increasing stretch by enhancing NP release from the heart. Under physiological conditions, ANP and BNP are mainly expressed in and released from atrial myocardium. In left ventricular hypertrophy or chronic HF, both NPs are highly upregulated in ventricles and ventricular myocardium becomes the main source of circulating NPs, particularly BNP [10]. NPs have an important role in maintaining the compensated state of HF. However, in overt chronic HF, high-pressure baroreceptors override the low-pressure receptors since sodium and water retention occur despite elevated atrial pressures. Baroreceptor dysfunction is an important link between vasomotor and neuroendocrine dysfunction in HF.

A third member of the family, C-type natriuretic peptide (CNP), is produced by the vascular endothelium and may be important as a paracrine factor in the regulation of vascular tone, its exact role in HF remains unclear.

All mentioned neurohormones are increased in blood of patients with advanced HF, but increased plasma concentrations of NP are frequently found in asymptomatic left ventricular dysfunction as well. In recent years, it turned out that among all tested markers BNP and the N-terminal split product of its precursor proBNP (NT-proBNP) are the laboratory markers of choice for diagnosis, risk stratification, and disease monitoring in HF patients ([11], see Chapters 14 and 15).

Markers of myocardial necrosis

It is also recognized that myocyte loss or apoptosis may occur in the setting of HF and such myocyte disappearance also must be accompanied by collagen remodeling. Myocardial cell death is an important mechanism of HF. There are two principal causes, apoptosis and necrosis. As a consequence of cell dropout, the load on the remaining cardiomyocytes is increased. Neurohormonal–cytokine abnormalities cause apoptosis, which usually occurs in a spotty manner throughout the ventricles. Ischemic necrosis usually causes more localized myocardial scarring.

Cardiac troponins are the current criterion standard for the laboratory diagnosis of myocardial damage ([12], see Chapter 1), and increases in cardiac troponins have been reported in severe HF even in the absence of concomitant coronary artery disease [13, 14]. Troponin concentrations were related to disease severity and the reduction in left ventricular ejection fraction. The detection of circulating cardiac troponin was also identified as a risk indicator in HF patients [15, 16].

Inflammatory markers

Several peptide growth factors and inflammatory cytokines appear to be involved in HF [17]. These growth factors may mediate the structural changes in the failing heart. Activation of various cytokines may also contribute to cardiac dysfunction and to the clinical syndrome and disease progression by direct toxic effects on the heart and circulation ("cytokine hypothesis" of chronic HF), particularly in more advanced stages. Cytokines and nitric oxide may contribute to the reversible myocardial depression by mediating alterations in excitation–contraction coupling and ß-adrenergic desensitization. Neurohormonal–cytokine abnormalities also cause apoptosis, which usually occurs in a spotty manner throughout the ventricles. Proinflammatory cytokines play an important role in disease progression. It has now been well established that patients with HF exhibit elevated plasma concentrations of proinflammatory mediators, such as tumor necrosis factor alpha (TNF-α), interleukin-1, or interleukin-6. Many aspects of chronic HF can be explained by the known biological effects of TNF-α, e.g., TNF-α depresses myocardial function and induces apoptosis. Interleukin-6 and related cytokines are involved in the regulation of cardiomyocyte hypertrophy and apoptosis. Interleukin-6 and TNF-α plasma concentration have been reported to be independent prognostic marker of mortality in chronic HF patients [16]. Interleukin-6 and TNF-α stimulate the synthesis of CRP in the liver. CRP is widely measured in clinical routine using high-sensitivity assays. Increased CRP concentrations have been reported in HF patients and were related independently to patient's outcome particularly in case of ischemic etiology [17–20]. Thus, CRP appears to be a suitable routine marker to monitor the proinflammatory activity in HF patients. However, currently, it is not clear if CRP is merely a marker of inflammation with no particular role in the development of HF or if it directly also modulates the disease process.

Clinical cases
Case 1: 69-year-old male patient with acute HF
Clinical history
Present complaint: Increasing dyspnea after effort during recent weeks with acute dyspnea on the day of admission. The patient was transported by the emergency service to the local hospital. He was on digoxin and a diuretic drug, which were prescribed by his general practitioner.

Past history: Chronic back pain, three surgical interventions because of prolapsed intervertebral discs (laminectomies), left knee surgery (meniscectomy), total endoprosthesis of both hip joints, bladder cancer.

Physical examination on admission: Heart rate 96/minute; blood pressure 150/100 mm Hg, slightly reduced general appearance, orthopnea, dyspnea while talking; slight signs of jugular congestion; normofrequent, regular heart sounds, no murmurs; pulmonary auscultation: bronchial breath sounds with prolonged expiratory period; added sounds: dry rales; abdominal examination: regular; no peripheral edema.

Electrocardiogram on admission: Sinus rhythm, complete left bundle branch block, left anterior hemiblock; no ST segment or T-wave dynamics on serial recordings.

Chest X-ray on admission: Normal sized heart, slight signs of left-sided HF.

Echocardiography on admission: Dilated left ventricle, severely reduced systolic function (ejection fraction <30%), moderate diastolic dysfunction (Grad II, pseudonormal filling pattern), mitral valve regurgitation grade II–III, moderate pulmonary hypertension.

Laboratory data on admission
Erythrocytes: 4.45 G/L
Platelets: 246 G/L
Leucocytes: 6.2 G/L
CRP: 23 mg/L
Creatinine: 1.1 mg/dL
Troponin T: 0.215, 0.130 (1st day), 0.036 (2nd day), <0.01 μg/L (2 weeks later)
CK: 75, 74 (1st day), 46 (2nd day) U/L
NT-BNP: 3639 (1st day), 1097 ng/L (2 month later)
Liver enzymes, electrolytes, thyroid-stimulating hormone, lipids, HbA1c, urine within normal range.

Discussion of Case 1
After stabilization, the patient was transferred to the nearby University Hospital for cardiac catheterization, which excluded a clinically relevant coronary artery disease and confirmed severe left ventricular dysfunction (left ventricular ejection fraction 16%, left ventricular end-diastolic filling pressure 24 mm Hg).

Final diagnosis: Dilated cardiomyopathy without clinically relevant coronary artery disease with secondary mitral valve regurgitation and pulmonary hypertension with acute cardiac decompensation on the day of admission.

Clinical course after discharge: Under optimization of neurohumoral treatment of HF, NT-proBNP markedly decreased despite no change in echocardiographic parameters of systolic and diastolic left ventricular function. Two months later, the patient was clinically in New York Heart Association (NYHA) stage II.

Case 2: 55-year-old male patient with dilated cardiomyopathy and chronic obstructive pulmonary disease

This patient was first referred to our HF outpatient clinics in 2004 because of increasing dyspnea after effort. The careful examination revealed the following diagnosis:

1 Dilated cardiomyopathy
2 HF symptoms: NYHA III
3 Endomyocardial biopsy: borderline autoreactive, virus-negative myocarditis
4 Exclusion of clinically relevant coronary artery disease by coronary angiography
5 Severe left ventricular dysfunction (ejection fraction 20%, pulmonary capillary wedge pressure 35 mm Hg, cardiac index 1.4 L/min/m²)
6 Relative moderate to severe mitral valve regurgitation (MR II–III)
7 Pulmonary hypertension (mean pulmonary artery pressure 38 mm Hg)
8 Hypertension
9 Severe chronic obstructive pulmonary disease stage III–IV with severe pulmonary emphysema
10 History of severe smoking

Discussion of Case 2

The patient underwent an optimization of neurohumoral treatment and immunosuppressive treatment with azathioprine and cortisone for 1 year, which lead to a normalization of systolic function and a decrease of NT-proBNP into the normal range. After stop of immunosuppressive treatment, a slight worsening and a significant increase in NT-proBNP were found (see Table 17.2). The clinical symptoms of dyspnea and exercise capacity did not change very much because of severe concomitant chronic obstructive pulmonary disease. The time courses of clinical symptoms, echocardiographically determined ejection fractions, creatinine, CRP, NT-proBNP, and cardiac troponin T concentrations are shown in Table 17.2.

Table 17.2 Time courses in a chronic heart failure patient with dilated cardiomyopathy.

	Month/year								
	04/04	*06/04*	*08/04*	*10/04*	*01/05*	*03/05*	*05/05*	*09/05*	*12/05*
NYHA	III	III	II	III	II	II	III	II	II
EF (%)	17		27				50		37
CRP (mg/L)	5.8	2.9	3.4	5.3	2.1	9.1	6.0	7.3	3.9
Creatinine (mg/dL)	1.23	1.15	1.16	0.99	1.21	1.52	1.36	1.02	0.98
NT-proBNP (ng/L)	1048	1182	472	452	154	40	33	119	201
Troponin T (μg/L)		<0.01	<0.01			0.16			

NYHA, New York Heart Association; EF, ejection fraction; CRP, high sensitivity C-reactive protein; NT, N-terminal; BNP, brain or B-type natriuretic peptide.

In March 2005, the author was contacted for the interpretation of a documented increase in cardiac troponin T concentrations, which was difficult to
explain clinically. The clinical situation was as follows: The patient was admitted for a cardiopulmonary rehabilitation program in a nearby rehabilitation
center. On admission he did well and was clinically stable during recent weeks
and had no pulmonary infections. He, highly motivated, took part in the rehabilitation program without any complaints. Before the final exercise stress test
a resting ECG was recorded. Minor ST–T segment alterations were noted in
the chest leads, and, therefore, the exercise stress test was cancelled and it was
decided to determine cardiac troponin T. Retrospectively, it turned out that
this ECG recording was not different from previously recorded ECGs in our
department. Troponin T was detectable in two different samples (0.11 and 0.15
μg/L, respectively), whereas creatine kinase (155 and 152 U/L) and lactate de-
hydrogenase activities (181 and 221 U/L) were within the normal range. The
NT-proBNP was low with 40 ng/L and the creatinine concentration was increased (1.52 mg/dL). The patient was seen in our outpatient clinics. He had no
symptoms of angina pectoris or dyspnea, on the contrary he felt better than at
the beginning of the rehabilitation program. The test results of a blood sample
drawn at this visit were: creatinine 1.63 mg/dL, creatine kinase and myoglobin
within normal range (154 U/L and 67 μg/L, respectively), cardiac troponin T
0.162 μg/L, and cardiac troponin I not detectable (<0.02 μg/L). It was decided
to ignore the cardiac troponin T result not fitting to the clinical presentation
and to discharge the patient from the rehabilitation center as planned.

Discussion on the clinical application of the multimarker approach in HF

Multimarker approach in acute HF

Multibiomarker testing in patients presenting with acute HF is supported by
guidelines. The recently revised European Society of Cardiology guidelines
on the diagnosis and treatment of acute HF [21] include recommendations for
laboratory testing in patients hospitalized with acute HF. Parameters which
must be always measured include a complete blood count, coagulation (INR,
if the patient is anticoagulated), CRP, D-dimer (to exclude acute pulmonary
embolism, but a number of reasons for false-positive test results have to be
considered), urea, creatinine, electrolytes, blood glucose, and cardiac troponin
or creatine kinase isoenzyme MB. In severe HF or in diabetic patients, arterial
blood gases should be measured to assess oxygenation, respiratory adequacy,
and acid–base balance. Parameters to be considered include transaminases,
urinanalysis, and plasma BNP or NT-proBNP. Other specific laboratory tests
should be taken for differential diagnostic purposes or in order to identify
end-organ damage. Among the additional tests, thyroid stimulating hormone
testing is recommended to exclude thyroid dysfunction as a cause of HF. Goals
of the treatment of the patient with acute HF in the recent guidelines already
include laboratory testing as well. An improvement in renal or hepatic function

Table 17.3 Diseases with reported increases in natriuretic peptide concentrations.

Acute or chronic systolic or diastolic heart failure
Left ventricular hypertrophy
Inflammatory cardiac diseases
Systemic arterial hypertension with left ventricular hypertrophy
Pulmonary hypertension
Acute or chronic renal failure
Liver cirrhosis with ascites
Endocrine disorders (e.g., hyperaldosteronism, Cushing's syndrome, hyperthyroidism)
Anemia
Central nervous system diseases (e.g., subarachnoid hemorrhage, stroke)
Paraneoplastic syndrome

assessed as urea and creatinine and bilirubin and normalization of serum electrolytes and blood glucose are meaningful goals of treatment. A decrease in plasma BNP and NT-proBNP reflects hemodynamic or renal improvement and is therefore beneficial.

BNP and NT-proBNP: BNP in our patient was highly increased as it is usually found in acutely decompensated HF patients. Rare exceptions are only seen with very rapidly developing new-onset acute HF (e.g., flash pulmonary edema) when there was not enough time for up-regulation of BNP and increased BNP secretion from the heart. If elevated concentrations as in our case are found, further diagnostic tests are required because of the limited cardiac-specificities of both markers. Important non-cardiac causes of BNP and NT-proBNP increases are listed in Table 17.3 [22]. In our patient the diagnosis was established by echocardiography in the emergency department of the local hospital and NT-proBNP was not measured on admission. NT-proBNP, however, was measured on the first day after admission after stabilization of the patient. The value was still high and indicated a high risk of the patient, which was in accordance with echocardiographic findings. Under optimization of neurohumoral treatment of HF, NT-proBNP markedly decreased parallel to clinical improvement despite no change in echocardiographic parameters of systolic and diastolic left ventricular function. The decrease in NT-proBNP was marked and outside the reported high biological variability of NT-proBNP.

Cardiac troponin: Troponin measurements are recommended to exclude an acute myocardial infarction as the reason for acute worsening or first manifestation of HF. Troponin T concentrations in our patient were increased on admission and showed a subsequent decline into the normal range. Troponin release indicates myocardial necrosis without defining the cause of myocardial damage. There are numerous reasons for myocardial damage apart from an acute coronary syndrome, and troponin increases have been described in many diseases not related to myocardial ischemia (see Table 17.4; [12, 23]). As our patient did not undergo coronary angiography before, it was justified to refer him to our department for cardiac catheterization, which excluded clinically

Table 17.4 Troponin increases not related to an acute coronary syndrome.

---

1 Myocardial ischemia of other causes
  Coronary vasospasm: prolonged ischemia leads to myocardial necrosis
  Intracranial hemorrhage or stroke: excessive sympathetic nervous system activity
  Intoxication with sympathomimetic agents: direct adrenergic effects
2 Secondary myocardial ischemia (supply–demand mismatch)
  Sepsis/systemic inflammatory response syndrome: additional toxic myocardial depression
  Hypotension, hypovolemia, or prolonged supraventricular tachycardia: decreased coronary artery perfusion
  Severe left ventricular hypertrophy: subendocardial ischemia
3 Direct myocardial damage
  Traumatic: contusion, cardioversion, defibrillation
  Cardiomyocyte compression: infiltrative diseases (e.g., amyloidosis)
  Toxic: e.g., anthracyclines
  Inflammatory/immune-mediated: myocarditis, post-transplantation
4 Increased myocardial stretch or strain
  Severe heart failure
  Severe pulmonary embolism
  Severe chronic pulmonary hypertension
5 Unknown causes
  End-stage renal failure
  Post-ultraendurance exercise

---

relevant coronary artery disease and confirmed very severe ventricular dysfunction. Volume and pressure overload of the ventricles, as in acute HF, can lead to patchy, tiny myocardial necrosis as the result of excessive wall tension or myocardial strain with the subsequent release of cardiac troponin in the absence of myocardial ischemia as found in our patient. In addition, pulmonary congestion and edema impair the oxygenation of blood, which further facilitates the development of myocardial damage. Two weeks after admission, troponin T was no longer detectable, which excluded continuing myocardial necrosis in our patient.

CRP: CRP testing is recommended to exclude infection as a cause of worsening in acute HF patients. CRP is the classical acute phase reactant and increases in CRP after acute HF have already been reported many years ago [24]. The moderately increased values seen in our patients may be simply explained by an acute phase response after acute cardiac decompensation. CRP did not further increase in our patient, and there was no evidence for a severe bacterial infection as a trigger of acute cardiac decompensation. Clinical data on the use of CRP for risk stratification of acute HF patients without myocardial infarction are very limited and currently this application of CRP cannot be recommended for routine use.

Multimarker approach in chronic HF

The older, but recently revised, European recommendations for laboratory testing in chronic HF do not differ substantially from the guidelines for acute

HF patients [2, 3, 25]. The diagnostic value of NP determination was already realized in the former version [25], and BNP testing was recommended in untreated patients with the clinical suspicion of chronic HF for ruling out HF in patients with dyspnea in case of low concentrations, especially in primary care. In this context, it is important to stress that in patients with chronic HF on optimized treatment BNP concentrations may be low as well [26]. The role of BNP and NT-proBNP for risk stratification and disease monitoring is acknowledged in the European guidelines and recommendations [2, 27]. However, it must be stressed that currently these markers cannot be recommended for tailoring treatment.

Preliminary data demonstrated the added value of troponin and BNP for HF risk stratification, and CRP was reported to be an independent risk marker in chronic HF patients as well (see above). However, the impact of multimarker measurement for risk stratification or on in-hospital clinical decision-making regarding long-term management remains to be demonstrated. Thus, such a multimarker strategy is currently not supported by guidelines.

NT-proBNP: The added value of serial NT-proBNP determination is nicely demonstrated by our case. Clinical symptoms and exercise capacity were not reliable markers in our patient because of concomitant severe chronic obstructive pulmonary disease. NT-proBNP concentration changes nicely paralleled changes in ejection fraction, and with normalization of ventricular function under immunosuppressive treatment, NT-proBNP returned into the normal range. NT-proBNP stayed low even during a period of transient worsening of renal function (see Table 17.2). Although NT-proBNP concentrations are highly increased in end-stage renal failure [11], in moderate renal dysfunction ventricular function appears to de the dominant influence on NT-proBNP. This is further illustrated by the fact that with worsening of ejection fraction after stop of immunosuppressive treatment NT-proBNP markedly increased despite a normalization of creatinine concentrations.

CRP: Despite promising data from clinical studies on the use of this marker for risk stratification in chronic HF patients, this unspecific marker is often difficult to use in the individual patient due to numerous possible confounders of CRP concentrations. This is nicely illustrated by our case. Although CRP concentrations during periods of pulmonary infections or other infections during immunosuppressive therapy are not included in Table 17.2, there are substantial fluctuations of this marker even during periods without any clinical signs of infections, and it is very difficult to determine what is the real baseline CRP value in a patient, particularly in severely ill patients with severe HF as in our patient.

Cardiac troponin: Initially, cardiac troponin T was not detectable in our patient, but in March 2005, cardiac troponin T concentrations were increased, which was confirmed in two different laboratories. Detectable cardiac troponin in peripheral blood samples of chronic HF patients is a sign of a worse prognosis, but surprisingly cardiac troponin I was not detectable in the same sample, and the question arises whether there was really myocardial necrosis in this patient. All other tested cardiac markers were in the normal range as well, which supported the cardiac troponin I test result. Mismatches between cardiac troponins are sometimes seen and are frequently difficult to explain even for experts. Differences in biological half-lives and clearance mechanisms of both markers and differences in analytical interferences with troponin assays have been made responsible, but in most circumstances the reasons for such discrepancies remain speculative [12, 23]. Although mismatches between cardiac troponins are frequent in end-stage renal failure [12, 23], moderate renal dysfunction in our patient at the time of blood sampling is not a likely explanation for the observed mismatch between both markers. Recently, autoantibodies which interfere with the binding sites of antibodies used in cardiac troponin I assays have been described as causes of false-negative troponin I results [28]; however, our patient's serum was not tested for the presence of "troponin I inhibitory factor." Cardiac troponin increases have been reported in athletes after ultraendurance exercise [23], and the reasons for these increases are still not clear. Our patient underwent a carefully controlled rehabilitation program. It is very unlikely that the increase in cardiac troponin T may be attributed to too heavy physical exercise, particularly in case of a mismatch of cardiac troponin assay results. Finally there was no sound explanation for the troponin mismatch, and we decided to ignore the cardiac troponin T results and to rely on all the other cardiac markers tested which were in accordance with the clinical presentation of the patient. As there was later on no clinical indication for troponin measurement we did not subsequently measure troponin T to avoid further confusion for the physicians caring for this patient.

In summary, multimarker testing makes sense in patients with acute HF and is supported by guidelines. In patients with chronic HF, BNP and NT-proBNP are the only established markers which are supported by guidelines, and the clinical value for routine use of the panel BNP, troponin, and CRP remains to be demonstrated in chronic HF.

References

1 Colucci WS, Braunwald E. Pathophysiology of heart failure. In: Braunwald E, ed. *Heart Disease*. W.B. Saunders, Philadelphia, PA, 1997:394–444.

2 Swedberg K, Cleland J, Dargie H *et al.*, for the Task Force for the Diagnosis and Treatment of Chronic Heart Failure of the European Society of Cardiology. Guidelines for the diagnosis and treatment of chronic heart failure: executive summary (update 2005). *Eur Heart J* 2005;**26**:1115–1140.

3 Hunt SA. ACC/AHA guideline update for the diagnosis and management of chronic heart failure in the adult: a report of the American College of Cardiology/American Heart Association Task Force on Practice Guidelines (writing committee to update the 2001 guidelines for the evaluation and management of heart failure). *J Am Coll Cardiol* 2005;**46**:1–82.

4 Packer M. The neurohormonal hypothesis: a theory to explain the mechanism of disease progression in heart failure. *J Am Coll Cardiol* 1992;**20**:248–254.

5 Poole-Wilson PA, Buller NP. Causes of symptoms in chronic congestive heart failure and implications for treatment (review). *Am J Cardiol* 1988;**62**:31A–34A.

6 Braunwald E. Congestive heart failure: a half century perspective. *Eur Heart J* 2001;**22**:825–836.

7 Schrier RW, Abraham WT. Hormones and hemodynamics in heart failure (review). *N Engl J Med* 1999;**341**:577–585.

8 Gerdes AM, Capasso JM. Structural remodeling and mechanical dysfunction of cardiac myocytes in heart failure. *J Mol Cell Cardiol* 1995;**27**:849–856.

9 de Bold AJ, Borenstein HB, Veress AT, Sonnenberg H. A rapid and potent natriuretic response to intravenous injection of atrial myocardial extracts in rats. *Life Sci* 1981;**28**:89–94.

10 Vesely DL. Atrial natriuretic peptides in pathophysiological diseases (review). *Cardiovasc Res* 2001;**51**:647–658.

11 Mair J, Hammerer-Lercher A, Puschendorf B. The impact of cardiac natriuretic peptide determination on the diagnosis and management of heart failure (review). *Clin Chem Lab Med* 2001;**39**:571–588.

12 Mair J. Progress in myocardial damage detection: new biochemical markers for clinicians. *Crit Rev Clin Lab Sci* 1997;**34**:1–66.

13 Missov E, Mair J. A novel biochemical approach to congestive heart failure: cardiac troponin T. *Am Heart J* 1999;**138**:9–12.

14 Missov E, Calzolari C, Pau B. Circulating cardiac troponin I in severe congestive heart failure. *Circulation* 1997;**96**:2953–2958.

15 Sato Y, Yamada T, Taniguchi R *et al.* Persistently increased serum concentrations of cardiac troponin T in patients with idiopathic dilated cardiomyopathy are predictive of adverse outcomes. *Circulation* 2001;**103**:369–374.

16 Sugiura T, Takase H, Toriyama T, Goto T, Ueda R, Dohi Y. *J Card Fail* 2005;**11**:504–509.

17 Anker SD, von Haehling S. Inflammatory mediators in chronic heart failure: an overview. *Heart* 2004;**90**:464–470.

18 Lamblin N, Mouquet F, Hennache B *et al.* High-sensitivity C-reactive protein: potential adjunct for risk stratification in patients with stable congestive heart failure. *Eur Heart J* 2005;**26**:2245–2250.

19 Yin WH, Chen JW, Jen HL *et al.* Independent prognostic value of elevated high-sensitivity C-reactive protein in chronic heart failure. *Am Heart J* 2004;**147**:931–938.

20 Anand IS, Latini R, Florea VG *et al.* C-reactive protein in heart failure—prognostic value and the effect of valsartan. *Circulation* 2005;**112**:1428–1434.

21 Nieminen MS, Böhm M, Cowie MR *et al.*, for the Task Force on Acute Heart Failure of the European Society of Cardiology. Executive summary of the guidelines on the diagnosis and treatment of acute heart failure. *Eur Heart J* 2005;**26**:384–416.

22 Mair J. Monitoring of patients with heart failure. *Scand J Clin Lab Invest* 2005;**65**(suppl 240):99–106.

23 Jeremias A, Gibson MC. Narrative review: alternative causes for elevated cardiac troponin levels when acute coronary syndromes are excluded. *Ann Intern Med* 2005;**142**:786–791.

24 Pye M, Rae AP, Cobbe SM. Study of serum C-reactive protein concentration in cardiac failure. *Br Heart J* 1990;**63**:228–230.

25 Remme WJ, Swedberg K, for the European Society of Cardiology Task Force for the Diagnosis and Treatment of Chronic Heart Failure. Guidelines for the diagnosis and treatment of chronic heart failure. *Eur Heart J* 2001;**22**:1527–1560.

26 Packer M. Should B-type natriuretic peptide be measured routinely to guide the diagnosis and management of chronic heart failure? *Circulation* 2003;**108**:2950–2953.

27 Cowie MR, Jourdain P, Maisel A *et al.* Clinical applications of B-type natriuretic peptide testing (review). *Eur Heart J* 2003;**24**:1710–1718.

28 Eriksson S, Junikka M, Pettersson K. An interfering component in cardiac troponin I immunoassays—its nature and inhibiting effect on the binding of antibodies against different epitopes. *Clin Biochem* 2004;**37**:472–480.

Contemporary markers of risk

Clinical integration of C-reactive protein for primary and secondary risk factor stratification

Jesse E. Adams

Identification of patients at increased risk of cardiovascular events is a key part of titration of therapy, whether in primary or secondary prevention models. Our current diagnostic strategy focuses on so-called traditional risk factors: hyperlipidemia, hypertension, tobacco abuse, smoking, or obesity. However, approximately 20% of patients with coronary heart disease have none of these traditional risk factors, and many patients without atherosclerotic disease also can have one or more of these risk factors. Risk factors are not diagnostic tests, and as such would have appalling specificity if viewed in that manner. Thus, there has been tremendous interest in novel analytes that could improve the detection of individuals at risk of future cardiovascular risk. Over the last two decades, there has been an increased interest in so-called high-sensitivity C-reactive protein (hsCRP) as an additional contributor to the assessment of cardiovascular risk. CRP is a nonspecific acute phase reactant produced in the liver after stimulation by diverse cytokines, and numerous epidemiologic studies have demonstrated a graded relationship between the level of hsCRP and the subsequent risk of cardiovascular events in both men and women, with an approximately twofold increased risk in those patients in the highest tertile [1]. Patients can be categorized regarding their cardiovascular risk by levels of hsCRP into low (<1 mg/L), average (1–3 mg/L), and high (>3 mg/L) levels of hsCRP that roughly correspond to the tertile levels in the US population (see Table 18.1).

It is recommended that two measurements be obtained at least 2 weeks apart to help decrease the variability due to the nonspecific nature of this acute phase reactant.

Case 1

A 49-year-old male presents at his wife's insistence to his physician's office for evaluation. He has no history of cardiac or vascular disease and has no other significant medical problems. His wife is concerned, however, because his father died of a fatal myocardial infarction at age 52 and his older brother had a myocardial infarction at age 56. The patient has smoked in the past and now

Table 18.1 Relative risk category and average hsCRP level.

Low < 1 mg/L	
Average 1.0 to 3.0 mg/L	
High > 3.0 mg/ L	

only smokes "a few cigarettes a day." His blood pressure is 130/90 and he is overweight. He and his wife have recently started an exercise program, largely consisting of walking 3–4 days a week; prior to that he had no regular exercise habits. He has no history of diabetes mellitus. A fasting lipid measurement yields a total cholesterol of 182 mg/dL, HDL of 36 mg/dL, LDL of 116 mg/dL, and triglyceride level of 102 mg/dL. However, his wife inquires if there are any other tests that could help to further investigate if he is at risk for a future heart attack.

Discussion of Case 1

This case represents one of the primary roles of measurement of hsCRP in contemporary medicine. Appropriate treatment of individuals is currently predicated on an assessment of their future cardiac risk, with a calculation of 10-year risk being the standard recommended measure. This formula is widely available, and a number of tools are also available to provide assistance to clinicians, both via the internet as well as utilizing personal digital assistants (the National Cholesterol Education Program, under the auspices of the National Heart Lung and Blood Institute, provides a free 10-year cardiovascular disease risk calculator that incorporates age, gender, total cholesterol, HDL cholesterol, smoking status, systolic hypertension, and history of hypertension; it is available on the internet at http://hp2010.nhlbihin.net/atpiii/calculator.asp?usertype=prof). Based on the data provided in the case above the patient's 10-year risk is calculated at 12%. There are a number of obvious recommendations that can be made for this individual to lower his future frisk of cardiac disease. However, future cardiac risk is influenced by multiple variables and adequate assessment requires integration of the various independent risk factors. A basic principle of preventive cardiology is that the appropriate treatment and the degree of the intensity of the treatment should be titrated to the individual's absolute personal risk. Hypertension, diabetes mellitus, hyperlipidemia, obesity, male sex, and tobacco abuse have been viewed as the traditional risk factors. However, there is active research into additional markers of risk, due to the observation that many patients will have few of the "traditional" risk factors. For example, it has been reported that up to one third of patient who present with myocardial infarctions have normal or near-normal lipid levels. Over the past 15 years, a number of observational studies have identified hsCRP as a powerful independent marker of cardiac risk with a graded relationship to the magnitude of risk [2–4]. Much of the interest in hsCRP has been in the area of primary prevention and the apparent ability of levels of hsCRP to modulate clinical judgments when considering therapeutic options, especially in those patients whose 10-year risk is felt to be intermediate as in the case in question (10–20% 10-year risk of cardiovascular disease) [5].

Many studies have investigated the appropriate means of integrating hsCRP measurements into clinical practice. It appears that the optimum method of utilizing the results of an individual's hsCRP levels is through assignment tertiles (33%) of the population, then relating these segments to relative risk. Several studies have shown that, in apparently healthy adults, an hsCRP value that places an individual in the highest tertile of the otherwise "healthy" population is associated with a 2–3 times higher risk of atherosclerosis, stroke, myocardial infarction, or peripheral vascular disease. The relative risk for cardiovascular disease increases as the hsCRP level increases. Additionally, combining the risk-assignment quintiles from hsCRP levels and the total cholesterol/HDL cholesterol ratio (TC/HDLC) provides superior prediction of future cardiovascular disease [6]. Recommendations for the use of markers of inflammation in patients with coronary arterial disease was codified in a set of guidelines jointly released by the American Heart Association and the Center for Disease Control in 2003 [7]. A portion of the recommendation from these documents states that "Specifically, those patients at intermediate risk (e.g., 10–20% risk of coronary heart disease (CHD) over 10 years), in whom the physician may need additional information to guide considerations of further evaluation (e.g., imaging, exercise testing) or therapy (e.g., drug therapies with lipid lowering, antiplatelet, or cardioprotective agents), may benefit from measurement of hs-CRP" [7].

Interventions that lower hsCRP include diet, exercise, smoking cessation, aspirin, statin therapy, improved glycemic control, and potentially therapy with either ACE inhibitors or angiotension receptor blockers [8, 9]. In this patient, he was instructed on dietary compliance, smoking cessation, regular exercise, and weight loss. Follow-up was then scheduled to evaluate his success in these areas; consideration for statin therapy was deferred until the effect of the other modifications could be assessed.

Case 2

A 78-year-old man presents to a cardiologist's office for evaluation. He has a history of hypertension that is adequately treated with a combination of hydrochlorothiazide and lisinopril; he also takes one enteric-coated aspirin a day. He also has a history of hyperlipidemia and is on lovastatin daily with a fasting LDL of 78 mg/dL, total cholesterol of 156 mg/dL, HDL of 38 mg/dL, and triglyceride level of 112 mg/dL. The patient has no history of diabetes mellitus. He does have a history of severe rheumatoid arthritis and is currently treated with a combination of nonsteroidal agents and methotrexate with adequate pain control.

He recently went to a health fair at his church. Screening carotid and abdominal ultrasounds were unremarkable. However, he also had blood work drawn and was told that his CRP level was elevated at 16 and that he should have follow-up for this. Having just seen a show on television regarding the association of CRP and cardiac risk, he self-referred himself to the cardiologists for further evaluation and treatment.

Discussion of Case 2

This case highlights one of the primary limitations of hsCRP—the nonspecific nature of the analyte. The AHA/CDC guidelines from 2003 state that "Individuals with evidence of active infection, systemic inflammatory processes, or trauma should not be tested until these conditions have abated. An hs-CRP level of >10 mg/L, for example, should be discarded and repeated in 2 weeks to allow acute inflammations to subside before retesting" [7]. Some investigators have described that patients with hsCRP levels greater than 10 are at increased risk, and not all researchers agree with the AHA/CDC statement regarding hsCRP levels greater than 10 [10].

In this particular patient, a subsequent measurement of hsCRP yielded a nearly identical level. It was felt that due to his active rheumatoid arthritis that measurement of hsCRP was not of particular utility for the accurate determination of his future cardiovascular risk, and in addition, he was already being treated with all clinically available agents that have been shown to lower hsCRP levels and reduce risk. One could also argue that given his current treatment and identified risk factors that measurement of hsCRP would provide little additional incremental risk. He was instructed to continue his current regimen; no further measurements of hsCRP were planned. This decision would, of course, be reconsidered if novel treatments for hsCRP were identified in the future.

Case 3

A 32-year-old male presents to his physician's office for evaluation. He has no history of cardiac or vascular disease and has no other significant medical problems. He is concerned, however, because his friend's father just died of a fatal myocardial infarction. The patient has smoked in high school but not since. His blood pressure is 128/80 and he is not overweight. He plays basketball 1–2 times per week and also runs 1–2 miles at least once a week. He has no history of diabetes mellitus. A fasting lipid measurement yields a total cholesterol of 162 mg/dL, HDL of 46 mg/dL, LDL of 100 mg/Dl, and triglyceride level of 86 mg/dL. However, he had an hsCRP level obtained at a local health fair which yielded a result of 3.6; the accompanying letter stated that this placed him at "high risk" for a heart attack and he wants to know what to do.

Discussion of Case 3

This patient has a level of hsCRP that places him in the highest tertile of the population. However, it must be stressed that use of hsCRP is for those patients that are at intermediate risk (e.g., 10–20% risk of coronary heart disease over 10 years). There is no data to recommend screening of the population with hsCRP or to employ it routinely in those at very low risk (as is the case of the gentlemen here). A review of healthy lifestyle choices would be appropriate with this gentleman, but no other therapeutic actions should be considered. Specifically, this gentleman should not be started on any pharmacologic treatment. Also, there is no indication for subsequent hsCRP measurements, at least at this time. Ongoing studies are investigating the utility of hsCRP in low-risk individuals, and future recommendations may be altered predicated on those trials.

Case 4

A 55-year-old female presents to her primary care physician's office for an yearly physical. She has a history of hypertension, obesity, type II diabetes mellitus, and is postmenopausal. She is compliant with all recommendations that have been made to her in the past and is compliant with all medical therapies. During the interview she asks about other tests that could be performed to identify if she is at risk for future diseases. On her list is hsCRP that she had read about in a newspaper article. At the same time, the local newspaper had just run a series of articles on women (especially African American women) being underrepresented in clinical trials, and she asks if there is any evidence that hsCRP is affected by race or gender.

Discussion of Case 4

Because the assay for hsCRP is widely available, there are a number of studies that have allowed for it to be evaluated across various subsets of individuals. In contrast to many other situations, many of the initial epidemiological studies involved women, and there does not appear to be any difference in the levels of hsCRP between genders as long as the women are not receiving hormone replacement therapy; both have a 50th percentile point of approximately 1.5 mg/L [11]. Likewise, there is no significant alteration with age once patient weight is considered (levels of CRP increase with body size [12]). Studies that have included individuals across ethnic populations (including Caucasian, African American, Mexican American, Japanese, and Asian) have not found any significant differences regarding the distribution of hsCRP levels. Additionally, it can be noted that there are not significant variations of CRP for fasting versus fed; neither are there cirdadian variations. There are a number of factors that have been shown to reproducibly result in elevations of hsCRP levels (see Table 18.2).

Thus, you were able to reassure this individual that the results of any measurements of hsCRP would be valid for her, and additionally that the cutpoints for hsCRP (low is <1 mg/L, average is 1–3 mg/L, and high is greater than 3 mg/L) would apply to her as well.

Case 5

A 58-year-old male presents to the emergency department with a complaint of dull substernal chest pain. He has no cardiac history, but has noted for the last 6 months that he has been experiencing dull substernal chest pain with

Hypertension
Obesity
Metabolic syndrome
Diabetes mellitus
Hormone replacement therapy
Chronic infections
Chronic inflammatory diseases
Current tobacco abuse
Past history of tobacco abuse
Acute strenuous activity (short-term elevation)

Table 18.2 Factors associated with increases in hsCRP.

ambulation, activity, or stress. The duration of the chest discomfort (which he describes as a "dull weight") is typically 2–5 minutes and resolves with rest. The last 2 weeks the discomfort has started to be associated with left arm discomfort, and today he developed nausea and diaphoresis with the episode of discomfort, which prompted his presentation to the emergency department. He is pain-free on arrival. His electrocardiogram shows only mild nonspecific T-wave changes, and initial blood work (including cardiac troponin I and beta natriuretic peptide) were normal. However, a comprehensive lipid panel was drawn and sent on arrival, and the patient's lipids were: LDL of 156 mg/dL, total cholesterol of 228 mg/dL, HDL of 30 mg/dL, and triglycerides of 212 mg/dL. A measurement of hsCRP is included in the panel and returned with a value of 8 mg/L.

The patient underwent a stress cardiolyte the next morning after he ruled out for myocardial infarction with serial troponins and electrocardiograms. The stress cardiolyte was positive for inferior ischemia; a subsequent cardiac catheterization showed as 40% lesion in the mid-left anterior descending coronary artery and a 50% lesion in the proximal right coronary artery. Medical therapy and risk factor modification was recommended.

Discussion of Case 5

In this case, the patient has presented with an acute coronary arterial syndrome. The initial clinical focus is on determination if indeed this patient has underlying coronary arterial disease and if so what is the optimal strategy—medical therapy, catheter-based revascularization, or surgical revascularization. However, acute coronary syndrome is a heterogeneous classification with diverse etiologies. Improved identification of future risk in patients with this can powerfully augment the clinician's ability to individualize therapy. In addition to the analytic data provided by history, electrocardiographic data, and other blood-based markers (and discussed elsewhere in this text), investigations have demonstrated that measurement of CRP can provide important information to this clinical diagnosis. Most patients with stable coronary arterial disease demonstrate increased levels of CRP; indeed, this is in part why measurement of CRP has proven to be useful for the prognostication of patients with stable atherosclerotic lesions. However, studies have demonstrated that levels of CRP are significantly increased in the setting of plaque rupture, the most common pathobiologic event in patients who present with unstable angina pectoris [13]. Studies by multiple investigators have shown that increased levels of hsCRP have prognostic importance in patients who present to the hospital with unstable coronary syndromes [14, 15]. In the GUSTO IV ACS trial (with over 7000 patients enrolled), CRP was found to be highly predictive of 30-day mortality, with a 30-day incidence of over 6% in the highest quartile, compared with less than 2% in the lowest quartile. In the GUSTO IV ACS trial, there was no relationship between the levels of CRP and rate of subsequent myocardial infarction, although some (but not all) studies of this population have also found a relationship to subsequent myocardial injury [16]. In a small but very interesting study, Zouridakis and colleagues investigated 124 patients who were scheduled for elective angioplasty [17]. In this study, which was performed in the United Kingdom, the patients were on a waiting list for catheter-based intervention an average of 4.8 ± 2.4 months. Levels of hsCRP were obtained on enrollment into the trial, and the degree of stenosis was measured both on the original catheterization and then at the subsequent catheterization (at the time of the intervention). Twenty-eight percent of patients demonstrated progression of their lesion (defined as a 10% worsening in a lesion previously at least 50% stenosis, a greater than 30% worsening in a lesion previously less than 50% stenosis, development of at least a 30% stenosis in a previously normal segment, or progression of any lesion to total occlusion) in the interval between the two evaluations. The authors wrote that "The findings in the present study endorse previous suggestions that inflammation is a crucial factor in atherogenesis and CAD progression and that molecules such as CRP, neopterin, and CAMs [cellular adhesion molecules] may not be just markers of inflammation and cardiovascular risk but also are likely to play a pathogenic role in atheromatous plaque vulnerability and rapid coronary stenosis progression." The suggestion that CRP plays a role in the pathogenesis of atherosclerosis is supported by a number of studies but is still controversial [18].

The clinicians intercalated the results of the hsCRP on this patient, indicative of increased risk, and selected an appropriate combination of a lifestyle prescription, pharmacologic therapy, and close follow-up. Additionally, they discussed the results of his tests, including the results of the hsCRP, with this patient to allow him to understand the increased risk that he faced and the need for aggressive action on his part.

References

1 Libby P, Ridker PM, Maseri A. Inflammation and atherosclerosis. *Circulation* 2002;**105**:1135–1143.
2 Ridker PM, Rifai N, Rose L *et al.* Comparison of C-reactive protein and low-density lipoprotein cholesterol levels in the prediction of first cardiovascular events. *N Engl J Med* 2002;**347**:1557–1565.

3 Ridker PM, Hennekens CH, Buring JE *et al.* C-reactive protein and other markers of inflammation in the prediction of cardiovascular disease in women. *N Engl J Med* 2000;**342**:836–843.

4 Ridker PM, Buring JE, Cook NR *et al.* C-reactive protein, the metabolic syndrome, and risk of incident cardiovascular events: an 8-year follow-up of 14719 initially healthy American women. *Circulation* 2003;**107**:391–397.

5 Ridker PM. Clinical application of C-reactive protein for cardiovascular disease detection and prevention. *Circulation* 2003;**107**:363–369.

6 Rifai N, Ridker P. Proposed cardiovascular risk assessment algorithm using high-sensitivity C-reactive protein and lipid screening. *Clin Chem* 2001;**47**:28–30.

7 Pearson TA, Mensah GA, Alexander RW *et al.* Markers of inflammation and cardiovascular disease—Application to clinical and public health practice, a statement for healthcare professionals from the Centers for Disease Control and Prevention and the American Heart Association. *Circulation* 2003;**107**:499–511.

8 Ridker PM. Inflammation in atherosclerosis: how to use high-sensitivity C-reactive protein (hs-CRP) in clinical practice. *Am Heart Hosp J* 2004;**2**(4, suppl 1):4–9.

9 Yeh ETH, Willerson JT. Coming of age of C-reactive protein: using inflammation markers in cardiology. *Circulation* 2003;**107**:370–372.

10 Ridker PM, Cook N. Clinical significance of very high and very low levels of C-reactive protein across the full range of Framingham risk scores. *Circulation* 2004;**109**:1955–1959.

11 Rifai N, Ridker PM. Population distributions of C-reactive protein in apparently healthy men and women in the United States: implications for clinical interpretation. *Clin Chem* 2003;**49**:666–669.

12 Visser M, Bouter LM, McQuillan GM *et al.* Elevated C-reactive protein levels in overweight and obese adults. *JAMA* 1999;**282**:2131–2135.

13 Burke AP, Tracy RP, Kolodgie F *et al.* Elevated C-reactive protein values and atherosclerosis in sudden coronary death: association with different pathologies. *Circulation* 2002;**105**:2019–2023.

14 Liuzzo G, Biasucci LM, Gallimore JR *et al.* The prognostic value of C-reactive protein and serum amyloid A protein in severe unstable angina. *N Eng J Med* 1994;**331**:417–424.

15 Rebuzzi AG, Quaranta G, Luizzo G *et al.* Incremental prognostic value of serum levels of troponin T and C-reactive protein in patients with unstable angina pectoris. *Am J Cardiol* 1998;**82**:715–719.

16 James SK, Armstrong P, Barnathan E *et al. J Am Coll Cardiol* 2003;**41**:916–924.

17 Zouridakis E, Avanzas P, Arroyo-Espliguero R *et al.* Markers of inflammation and rapid coronary artery disease progression in patients with stable angina pectoris. *Circulation* 2004;**110**(13):1747–1753.

18 Scirica BM, Morrow DA. Is C-reactive protein an innocent bystander or proatherogenic culprit? *Circulation* 2006;**113**:2128–2134.

CHAPTER 19

Lipoprotein subfraction analysis using nuclear magnetic resonance spectroscopy

William C. Cromwell, Harold E. Bays, Peter P. Toth

Introduction

It is widely appreciated that the interaction of lipoprotein particles with the arterial wall impacts coronary heart disease (CHD) risk. In clinical practice, this risk is most commonly assessed by measuring the cholesterol in low-density lipoprotein (LDL) and high-density lipoprotein (HDL) particles, rather than the numbers of these atherogenic and antiatherogenic particles. However, there is little appreciation for how much the cholesterol content of lipoprotein particles, especially in LDL, varies from person to person. As a result, even the most accurate LDL cholesterol measurement will, for many individuals, provide an inaccurate assessment of the number of circulating LDL particles and their associated CHD risk [1]. Via an automated nuclear magnetic resonance spectroscopy (NMR) assay, lipoprotein particles may now be efficiently "counted." Several clinical outcome studies have reported superior CHD risk associations with NMR lipoprotein particle measures versus components of the standard lipid profile [2–7]. This chapter will discuss the potential utilization of NMR lipoprotein particle measures for the evaluation and management of CHD risk.

Lipoprotein particle quantification by NMR spectroscopy—a primer for clinicians

Fundamentally, two phenomena make NMR quantification of numbers of lipoprotein subclass particles possible: (1) lipoprotein subclasses of different size in plasma emit distinctive NMR signals whose individual amplitudes can be accurately and reproducibly measured; and (2) measured subclass signal amplitudes are directly proportional to the numbers of subclass particles emitting the signal, irrespective of variation in particle lipid composition [8].

The process begins with the measurement of a patient's whole plasma NMR spectra (Fig. 19.1). Highlighted is the spectral region at ~0.8 ppm, which contains the signals emitted by the methyl group protons of the four types of lipid in lipoprotein particles: phospholipid, unesterified cholesterol, cholesterol

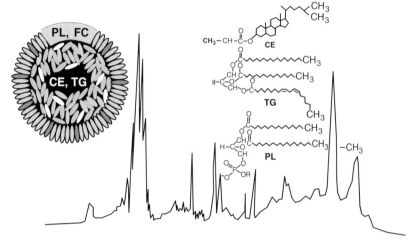

Figure 19.1 Typical NMR spectrum of plasma. Shown are the plasma methyl lipid signal (peak below large methyl group to the left) and a schematic representation of lipoprotein structure, depicted as a neutral lipid core of cholesterol ester (CE) and triglyceride (TG) surrounded by a shell consisting of phospholipid (PL) and free (unesterified) cholesterol (FC). (Reproduced with permission from Otvos [8])

ester, and triglyceride. Each lipoprotein subclass signal emanates from the aggregate number of terminal methyl groups on the lipids contained within the particle, with the cholesterol esters and triglycerides in the particle core each contributing three methyl groups and the phospholipids and unesterified cholesterol in the surface shell each contributing two methyl groups [8]. Since the methyl signals from these lipids are indistinguishable from each other, they overlap to produce a bulk lipid "particle signal." The amplitude of each lipoprotein particle signal serves as a measure of the concentration of that lipoprotein [9].

What makes it possible to exploit the methyl lipid signal for lipoprotein subclass quantification (without separating the subclasses first) is a magnetic property specific to lipoproteins that causes the lipids in larger particles to broadcast signals that are characteristically different in frequency and shape from the lipid signals emitted by smaller particles [10]. A clarifying analogy has been drawn between lipoprotein subclasses and bells of varying size (Fig. 19.2) [11]. We understand that bells of different size, although made of the same material, produce unique sound signals. For related reasons associated with the physical form of lipoprotein particles, different-size subclasses broadcast distinguishable lipid NMR signals. If we strike a group of bells with equalforce blows (similar to "exciting" the subclasses with a microsecond radiofrequency NMR pulse), we expect the amplitude (loudness) of the resultant sound signal to reflect the number of bells struck. By recording the composite signal produced by the simultaneous "ringing" of all of the lipoprotein subclasses in a plasma sample, it is possible to back-calculate the concentration of each

Each lipoprotein subclass broadcasts a unique NMR "Sound"

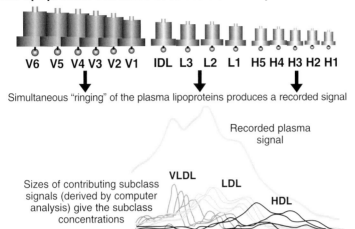

Figure 19.2 Each lipoprotein subclass broadcasts a unique NMR "sound." Lipoproteins subclasses behave like bells in the NMR analyzer. (Reproduced with permission from Otvos [8])

subclass using prior knowledge about the quantitative relationship between subclass concentration and signal amplitude.

It is important to note that the total number of methyl groups contained within a subclass particle is, to a close approximation, determined solely by the particle's diameter and is not affected by differences in lipid composition arising from such sources as variability in the relative amounts of cholesterol ester and triglyceride in the particle core, varying degrees of unsaturation of the lipid fatty acyl chains, or varying phospholipid composition. For this reason, the methyl NMR signal emitted by each subclass serves as a convenient and direct measure of the number of particles in that subclass.

The lipoprotein particle information from a single NMR test includes total LDL particle concentration (LDL-P), as well as the subclass particle concentrations of very low-density lipoprotein (VLDL) (large VLDL-P, medium VLDL-P, small VLDL-P), intermediate-density lipoprotein (IDL-P), LDL (large LDL-P, small LDL-P), and HDL (large HDL-P, medium HDL-P, small HDL-P). Although levels of total LDL, HDL, and VLDL have always been measured with high precision by NMR (variability <3%), recent modifications to the computational algorithm used in the analysis process have substantially improved the reproducibility of the quantification of individual LDL subclasses (variability <10%) [12]. This greater measurement precision makes it feasible for the first time for clinicians to address variations in risk due to LDL subclass heterogeneity by defining the issue as one of *quantity, not quality*.

Quantities of NMR-measured lipoprotein subclasses have been integrated with lipid parameters to produce the NMR LipoProfile Report. As shown in Fig. 19.3, this report consists of four distinct sections: (1) LDL Particle Numbers section reports total LDL-P and small LDL-P values, as well as potential goals for these values in high-risk and moderately high-risk patient populations; (2) Lipids section reports chemical total cholesterol and LDL-C calculated via the Friedewald formula using NMR-derived HDL-C and triglycerides; (3) Metabolic Syndrome Markers section contains three parameters (LDL size, large HDL-P, and large VLDL-P) closely associated with insulin resistance [13, 14] and incident type 2 diabetes mellitus [15]; (4) Subclass Particle Numbers section reports subclass particle concentrations of VLDL-P (large, medium, small), IDL-P, LDL-P (large and small), and HDL-P (large, medium, small).

Relationship of LDL cholesterol and LDL particle measurements

Traditionally, levels of LDL are assessed not by measuring the atherogenic cul-prit particles but by measuring the amount of cholesterol the particles contain (i.e., LDL-C). What is under-appreciated is that the amount of cholesterol car-ried inside LDL particles is highly variable among individuals with the same measured LDL-C. As a consequence of the magnitude and prevalence of this lipid compositional variability, even the most accurate LDL cholesterol mea-surements will, for many individuals, provide an inaccurate measure of the number of circulating LDL particles and the CHD risk they confer [12].

The metabolic origins of LDL compositional heterogeneity emanate from two independent sources of LDL cholesterol compositional variability, both related to plasma triglycerides (TG) or VLDL levels [1, 16]. The first is variability in *core lipid composition*, driven by reactions that modulate the relative amounts of cholesterol ester and triglyceride contained within the neutral lipid interior of the particles. The second is variability in *particle size*, due to the smaller physical volume of the lipid core in small versus large LDL particles.

When plasma TG levels are elevated, even modestly, a reaction catalyzed by cholesterol ester transfer protein (CETP) becomes important, in which triglyc-eride molecules from the core of triglyceride-rich lipoproteins (mainly VLDL) exchange one-for-one with cholesterol ester molecules in the core of LDL. As a result, large LDL particles become partially depleted in cholesterol and en-riched in triglycerides. In a physiologic attempt to reestablish the normal ratio of cholesterol/triglyceride in the particle core, these compositionally abnormal particles become a substrate for lipases (including hepatic lipase and endothe-lial lipase), which hydrolyze some of the core triglycerides. In response to the efflux of fatty acids from the core and remodeling of the surface shell, the parti-cles are transformed into smaller, denser LDL particles (Fig. 19.8). Depending on the TG level and CETP activity, small LDL particles may have a normal core lipid composition or become significantly cholesterol-depleted. As a result of these reactions, four different types of LDL particles are likely to be seen in indi-viduals depending on their metabolic circumstances (Fig. 19.4): large LDL with a normal core lipid content, large LDL with relatively cholesterol-deficient, triglyceride-rich lipid cores, small LDL with a normal lipid content, and small LDL with relatively cholesterol-deficient, triglyceride-rich lipid cores [12].

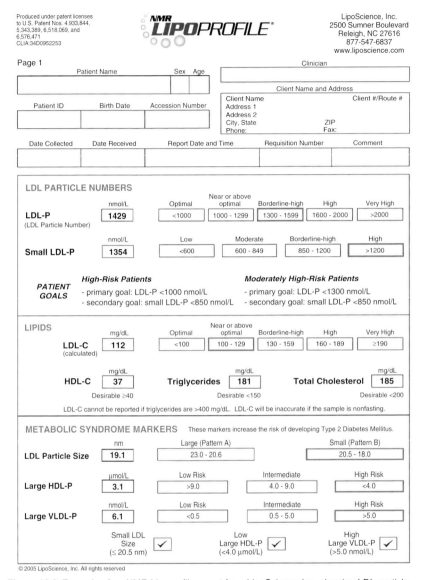

Figure 19.3 Example of an NMR Lipoprofile report from LipoScience Inc. showing LDL particle numbers, lipid profile, metabolic syndrome markers, and distributions of subclass particle numbers.

LDL size differences make an independent contribution to LDL cholesterol compositional variability. Although LDL diameters differ by a small amount, typically up to about 3 nm (~12%), the volume differences of the spherical lipid core are substantial because they scale according to the third power of the radius. For LDL particles differing by 3 nm in diameter, there is approximately 40% less core cholesterol in the smaller particle. As a result, individuals with

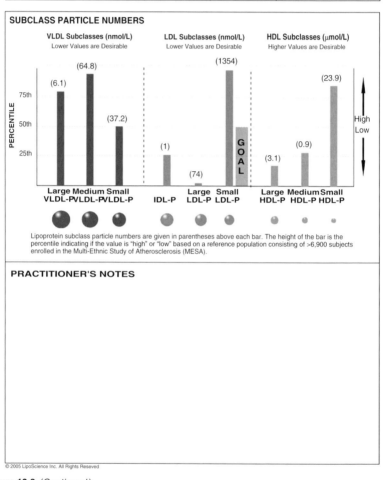

Figure 19.3 *(Continued)*

smaller LDL particles will require almost 70% more particles to carry the same amount of LDL cholesterol as the person with the larger particles [1].

Because of variations in LDL composition and size, LDL-P can vary up to 40% among individuals with the same LDL particle size. Moreover, among people with equal LDL-P, those with small LDL particles that are also compositionally cholesterol-poor and triglyceride-rich can easily have LDL-C values that are 50 mg/dL lower than people who have large LDL particles of normal lipid composition [1].

Less cholesterol per particle than "Normal"

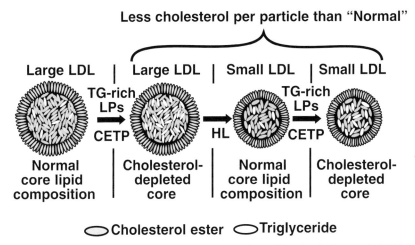

Figure 19.4 Schematic representation of the metabolic origins of low-density lipoprotein (LDL) particles containing less cholesterol than normal. CETP, cholesterol ester transfer protein; HL, hepatic lipase; LPs, lipoproteins; TG, triglycerides. (Reproduced with permission from Otvos *et al.* [1])

In the face of LDL cholesterol compositional variability of this magnitude, it is not difficult to understand why LDL cholesterol measurements do not always accurately reflect a patient's LDL particle number and associated risk of CHD [12].

Prevalence of quantitative LDL particle abnormalities

Data from the Framingham Offspring Study cycle 4 cohort ($n = 3437$) provide insight into the prevalence and clinical characteristics of individuals manifesting discrepancies between LDL-C and LDL-P values [1, 17]. The National Cholesterol Education Panel (NCEP) Adult Treatment Panel III (ATP III) guidelines recommend LDL cholesterol targets of <100 mg/dL for patients with CHD or CHD risk equivalents, <130 mg/dL for patients with ≥2 risk factors and a 10-year Framingham risk ≤20%, and <160 mg/dL for patients with 0–1 risk factors [18]. These targets correspond to the 20th, 50th, and 80th percentile values in the Framingham Offspring population. NMR data from the same samples indicate that the corresponding 20th, 50th, and 80th percentile values for LDL-P are 1100 nmol/L, 1400 nmol/L, and 1800 nmol/L, respectively [1]. Among those with LDL-C values <100 mg/dL (20th percentile), 34% of subjects manifested increased LDL-P >1100 nmol/L (20th percentile). Further analysis indicated that increased TG and decreased HDL-C were significantly associated with a "disconnect" between LDL cholesterol and LDL particle number (Fig. 19.5) [17].

Metabolic states characterized by high TG and low HDL-C would be expected to be associated with a relative excess of LDL particles relative to LDL-C. Garvey *et al.* [13] reported the NMR lipoprotein characteristics of non-diabetic

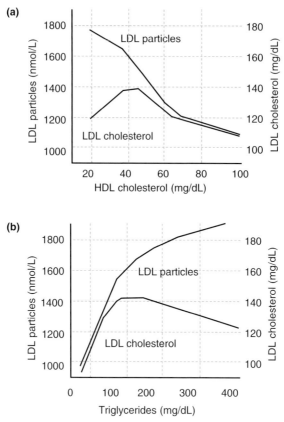

Figure 19.5 Relations in the Framingham Offspring Study of NMR measured LDL particles (LDL-P) and Friedewald calculated LDL cholesterol (LDL-C) to HDL-C and triglycerides. (Reproduced with permission from Otvos [17])

subjects with a wide range of insulin sensitivity measured by hyperinsuline-mic euglycemic clamp, as well as patients with type 2 diabetes mellitus. When compared with insulin sensitive (IS) subjects, the insulin resistant (IR) and diabetes subgroups exhibited the following significant LDL differences: (1) A twofold to threefold increase in the number of small LDL particles and a re-duction in the number of large LDL particles, resulting in a decrease in LDL particle size; (2) A progressive increase in overall LDL-P, despite no difference (IS versus IR) or a minimal difference (IS versus diabetes) in measured LDL-C. Additionally, lipoprotein subclass abnormalities present in IR subjects were moderately exacerbated in subjects with type 2 diabetes mellitus independent of glucose and glycemic control. Overall, the authors concluded that insulin resistance–induced changes in the NMR lipoprotein subclass profiles predict increased CHD risk that was not fully apparent with conventional lipid testing.

These data were extended by a recent study examining sex-specific relations of the metabolic syndrome with NMR measured LDL-P and small LDL-P in 2993 Framingham Heart Study offspring participants without known cardiovascular disease [19]. Overall, 27% of men and 17% of women met ATP-III criteria for metabolic syndrome. Age-adjusted total LDL-P was markedly higher in individuals with the metabolic syndrome than in those without (Fig. 19.6). This difference was the result of a compositional change in LDL, with numbers of small LDL particles increasing progressively in men and women having 0, 1, 2, 3, 4, or 5 components of the metabolic syndrome while numbers

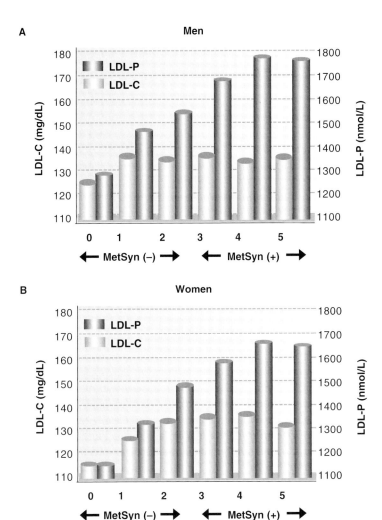

Figure 19.6 LDL-C and LDL-P in Framingham subjects (panel A men, panel B women) with increasing numbers of metabolic syndrome features. (Based on Kathiresan *et al.* [19])

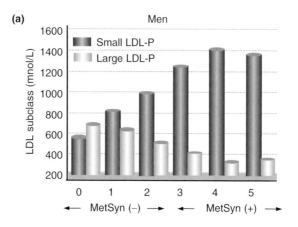

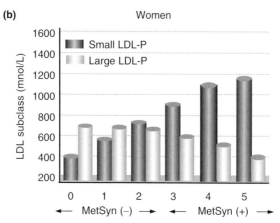

Figure 19.7 LDL subclasses in Framingham subjects (panel A men, panel B women) with increasing numbers of metabolic syndrome features. (Based on Kathiresan *et al.* [19])

of large LDL particles declined (Fig. 19.7). The combination of greatly increased small LDL-P (with less cholesterol per particle) and a numerically smaller decrease in large LDL-P (with more cholesterol per particle) resulted in LDL-C values that were not significantly different in men with and without the metabolic syndrome (136.4 versus 133.5 mg/dL, $P = 0.16$) and only modestly higher in metabolic syndrome women (136.2 versus 125.1 mg/dL, $P < 0.0001$). Increased total LDL-P and small LDL-P, but not LDL-C, were significantly associated with increasing triglycerides and decreasing HDL-C levels.

A substantial degree of LDL heterogeneity has also been documented in the ambulatory care setting. Split sample comparisons of Friedewald calculated LDL-C and NMR measured LDL-P were reported recently for 2355 patients with type 2 diabetes mellitus, seen in clinical practice, confirmed to have LDL-C

<100 mg/dL [20]. Patients were categorized according to their LDL-P values, using cutpoints corresponding to the 20th, 50th, 80th, and 95th percentile values of a reference population consisting of >6900 subjects enrolled in the Multiethnic Study of Atherosclerosis (MESA). A high percentage (61%) of patients with type 2 diabetes mellitus and optimal LDL-C values <100 mg/dL (20th percentile) had suboptimal LDL-P levels >1000 nmol/L (20th percentile). Even among patients with very low LDL-C <70 mg/dL (<5th percentile), a large number (40%) had LDL-P >1000 nmol/L (20th percentile). Collectively, these datasets provide a good illustration of how misleading LDL-C levels can be as a gauge of LDL excess.

Relationship of LDL particle size and number with CHD outcomes

Due to inherent limitations of serum lipids in predicting CHD across a wide range of lipid values and varying patient populations, lipoprotein subclasses have been studied with the aim of determining whether this higher level of information can improve CHD risk assessment and management. Recently, the relationships of CHD risk with LDL particle size and LDL particle number in more than 70 cross-sectional epidemiologic, prospective epidemiologic, and clinical intervention trials were reviewed [12].

With a few exceptions, small LDL particle size (pattern B) was found to be significantly associated with CHD risk in univariate analyses. However, the origin of this risk association remains controversial. Many authors cite indirect lines of evidence that implicate atherogenic properties of small-sized LDL particles. Various data indicate small LDL more easily enters the arterial wall, undergoes localized retention due to binding with arterial wall proteoglycans, exhibits enhanced oxidizability in several in vitro models, and directly participates in the production of subendothelial macrophage foam cells [21]. Collectively, these findings imply that small LDL is a potent atherogenic lipoprotein, the measurement of which may be useful to enhance CHD risk prediction and better evaluate response to lipid therapy [22–24].

However, small-sized LDL particles are most commonly present as a component of a broader pathophysiology characterized by high TG, low HDL-C, increased LDL particle number, obesity, insulin resistance, diabetes, and the metabolic syndrome [19, 25–27]. As a result, it is unclear if the increased risk associated with small LDL size in univariate analyses is a reflection of an increased atherogenic potential of small LDL particles, or simply a consequence of the broader pathophysiology of which small LDL is a part. Following multivariate adjustment for these confounding risk factors, qualitative LDL size was rarely found to be a significant, independent predictor of CHD risk.

An alternative explanation for the higher CHD risk observed among pattern B individuals is the increased quantity of LDL present in the individuals. Total plasma apolipoprotein B-100 (apoB) has been used historically to estimate the number of circulating LDL particles due to the presence of one apoB molecule per LDL, VLDL, and IDL particle, and the fact that approximately 95% of

Table 19.1 Associations of NMR-measured lipoproteins in recent cardiovascular outcome trials.

Study	CHD status	Atherosclerotic endpoint	NMR particle concentration associations*
Cardiovascular Health Study [5]	Primary prevention	Incident MI or angina	↑ LDL-P ↑ Small LDL-P
Women's Health Study [2]†	Primary prevention	Incident MI, CHD death, CVA	↑ LDL-P ↑ Small LDL-P
Framingham Heart Study [7]	Primary prevention	Incident MI or angina	↑ LDL-P ↑ Small LDL-P
VA-HDL Intervention Trial [6]†	Secondary prevention	Nonfatal MI or CHD death	↑ LDL-P ↑ Small LDL-P ↓ HDL-P ↓ Small HDL-P
PLAC-I [4]	Secondary prevention	Angiographic MLD	↑ LDL-P ↑ Small LDL-P ↑ Small HDL-P
Health Women Study [3]	Primary prevention	EBCT coronary calcium score	↑ LDL-P ↑ Small LDL-P

*Significant and independent after multivariate modeling.
†LDL particles significantly stronger versus apoB.

plasma apoB is bound to LDL particles. Using this assay, several prospective epidemiologic and clinical intervention trials demonstrate a significantly stronger association of cardiovascular events with increased LDL particle number versus LDL-C [12, 28]. The use of NMR spectroscopy to quantify lipoprotein particle subfractions provides further insight into the relationships of quantitative lipoprotein measures with CHD risk. Data from six recently published or presented outcome studies (Table 19.1) provide evidence that NMR measured LDL-P was a significantly stronger predictor of incident CHD events or disease progression versus LDL-C [2–7] or (in two studies in which it was measured) apoB [2, 6]. In all of these trials, CHD associations with LDL-P and small LDL-P were independent of the standard lipid variables. Although qualitative LDL particle size was univariately associated with CHD risk in 3 of 6 trials, it failed to be a significant predictor of CHD risk following multivariate adjustment for lipids or LDL particle number. In contrast, quantitative small LDL-P showed significant univariate and multivariate CHD risk associations in all trials.

Clinical utilization of NMR-measured LDL-P

Current NCEP recommendations advise clinicians to mange LDL-C as the primary target for lipid lowering therapy. Despite significant morbidity and mortality improvements noted in recent trials utilizing aggressive LDL lowering

Table 19.2 Population equivalent LDL-C and LDL-P goals.

Patient risk category	LDL-C goal	Population percentile cut-point	LDL-P goal*
Very high risk	<70 mg/dL (optional based on clinical judgment)		<1000 nmol/L
High risk	<100 mg/dL	20th percentile	<1000 nmol/L
Moderately high risk	<130 mg/dL	50th percentile	<1300 nmol/L

*Population equivalent values for a reference population consisting of >6900 subjects enrolled in the Multiethnic Study of Atherosclerosis (MESA) [20].

therapy, LDL-C levels have not been identified which confer optimal CHD risk reduction. Thus, clinicians are asked to use clinical judgment in determining which individuals are candidates for aggressive LDL lowering therapy and when an adequate therapeutic target has been reached.

Given the significant heterogeneity of LDL particle number among individuals at LDL-C goal levels, as well as clinical outcome data demonstrating that LDL-related CHD risk is most significantly associated with LDL particle number (not LDL size or the amount of cholesterol carried by a patient's LDL particles), the use of LDL-P as a clinical tool has been advocated [12].

While we await the results of clinical trials that may help to determine specific target levels of LDL particle numbers (with different targets possibly needed for large and small size particles), for patients in different CHD risk categories, some suggest utilization of LDL-P goals that mirror current NCEP ATP III targets at a population equivalent level (Table 19.2). Thus, for high-risk patients (CHD or CHD risk equivalents), the population equivalent LDL-P goal is LDL-P <1000 nmol/L (20th percentile). For moderately high-risk patients (multiple risk factors and a Framingham 10-year risk score <20%), the goal is LDL-P < 1300 nmol/L (50th percentile).

Once LDL-C and LDL-P values have been managed, secondary targets of therapy include (if indicated) increasing HDL-C and lowering triglycerides. This approach to clinical decision-making is illustrated in the case studies at the end of this chapter.

Triglycerides and very low-density lipoproteins

Unless serum triglyceride (TG) levels are profoundly elevated (~greater than 800 mg/dL), the major TG transporting lipoproteins in the preprandial fasting state are VLDL particles. In addition to TG, VLDL particles contain a core of lipophilic cholesterol esters, surrounded by an outer layer of water soluble phospholipids, unesterified cholesterol, and apolipoproteins, including apoB-100 which does not undergo exchange, as well as apoC and apoE which may be exchanged with other lipoproteins.

Fasting triglyceride levels are largely determined by a combination of genetically determined metabolic processes, underlying metabolic disorders (if present), concurrent drug therapy, as well as diet and physical exercise. For example, if the dietary intake of fats and carbohydrates exceed metabolic clearance, then these nutrients are often metabolized into TG, packaged into apoB containing VLDL particles, and subsequently released into the circulation. Once in the circulation, the TGs in VLDL particles may be exchanged for cholesterol esters found in HDL and LDL particles through the activity of cholesteryl ester transfer protein (CETP) (Fig. 19.8). In addition to exchange, endothelial lipoprotein lipase (LPL), mainly associated with muscle and adipose tissue, can hydrolyze triglycerides subsequent to activation by apoCII. Remnant VLDL particles (often also described as intermediate-density lipoproteins or IDL) are formed, which may then be taken up by the liver by hepatic apoB

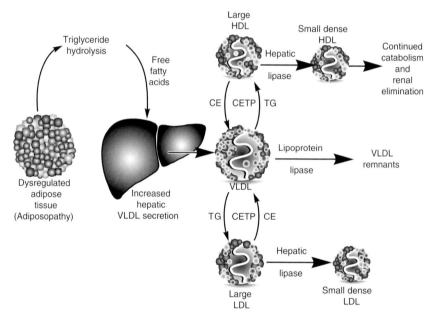

Figure 19.8 Lipoprotein metabolism in patients with metabolic syndrome (or insulin resistance). During positive caloric balance, excessive hypertrophy of individual peripheral adipocytes and/or accumulation and hypertrophy of visceral adipose tissue potentially reveals the pathogenic potential of adipose tissue (adiposopathy) resulting in a net increase release of free fatty acids into the circulation and portal vein. The increased delivery of free fatty acids to the liver increases the risk of hepatic steatosis. In an effort to dispose of excess of fatty acids, the hepatic parenchyma reassimilates triglycerides and incorporates them into VLDL particles which are then secreted into the central circulation. CETP catalyzes the net transfer of triglyceride from VLDL to HDL and LDL particles in exchange for cholesterol esters. As these smaller lipoproteins become progressively more enriched with triglyceride, they become more favorable targets for hepatic lipase, an enzyme that converts HDL2 into HDL3 and large, buoyant LDL into its smaller, denser, more atherogenic variant. Smaller HDL particles have greater thermodynamic inclination to dissociate from apoAI, which leads to further catabolism and reductions in circulating levels of this lipoprotein.

receptors. Alternatively, IDL's may undergo further catabolism via hepatic lipase and form LDL particles. Thus, one of the important end results of VLDL metabolism is the creation of LDL particles that are relatively depleted of TG, contain a core of cholesterol esters, and have an outer layer that contains such apoproteins as apoB-100 and apoE.

Elevated TG levels are associated with increased CHD risk [18, 29, 30], although the origin of this risk is unclear. Some data suggest that the increased atherogenicity associated with increased TG levels may be associated with chylomicron (CM) and VLDL remnants [31]. However, because of the larger pathophysiology of which remnant abnormalities are a part, it is unclear if CM and VLDL remnants are independently associated with CHD risk. Alternatively, elevated TG levels are an important component of the metabolic syndrome (Table 19.3), a clustering of risk factors thought to increase the risk of CHD [32–35]. Positive caloric balance in genetically and environmentally susceptible patients exacerbates the pathogenic potential of adipose tissue, leading to metabolic (such as a net increase in free fatty acids), endocrinologic, and immune processes which in pathologic partnership with other body tissues, contributes to abnormalities in glucose metabolism (such as insulin resistance and type 2 diabetes mellitus), high blood pressure and dyslipidemia, as well as endothelial function and possibly direct effects upon the development of atherosclerosis. A prominent consequence of these metabolic alterations is the development of the so-called "atherogenic lipid triad," including high TG, low HDL-C, and small LDL particle size despite normal or low LDL-C [36, 37]. The NMR lipoprotein characteristics that underlie the atherogenic lipid triad include increased large VLDL-P, increased LDL-P, increased small LDL-P, and decreased large HDL-P [13, 20]. Trials are currently underway that may help elucidate the risk attributable to these lipoprotein abnormalities.

Therapies directed primarily at decreasing TG levels include nicotinic acid [38], fibrates [39], and high dose supplementation with omega-3 fatty acids derived from marine fish oils, specifically eicosapentanoic acid and docosahexanoic acid (Table 19.4). In diabetic patients with significant insulin resistance and hypertriglyceridemia, the thiazolidinediones (pioglitazone, rosiglitazone) are also clinically useful in managing hypertriglyceridemia.

High-density lipoproteins

In contrast to LDL and VLDL, HDL particles are widely regarded as atheroprotective. A number of prospective epidemiologic investigations, including the Framingham Study [55], Multiple Risk Factor Intervention Trial [56], and the Prospective Munster Cardiovascular Study [57], among others, have all demonstrated an inverse, independent relationship between serum levels of HDL-C and risk for CHD. Low serum levels of HDL are found in approximately two thirds of patients with CHD [58, 59] and constitute an important risk factor for stroke, peripheral arterial disease, sudden death, and restenosis after angioplasty [60]. In one analysis by Gordon and coworkers, for every 1 mg/dL rise in HDL-C, risk for CHD decreased 2–3% [61]. Consistent with

Table 19.3 Comparison of NCEP ATP III and WHO criteria for metabolic syndrome [32].

NCEP ATP III
Three or more of the following must be present:

Waist circumference*	Men	> 102 cm (> 40 inches)
	Women	> 88 cm (> 35 inches)
Plasma TG	Men/women	≥1.7 mmol/L (≥150 mg/dL)
Plasma HDL cholesterol	Men	< 1.0 mmol/L (< 40 mg/dL)
	Women	< 1.3 mmol/L (< 50 mg/dL)
Blood pressure	Men/women	≥130/≥85 mm Hg
Fasting blood glucose	Men/women	≥6.1 mmol/L (≥100 mg/dL)

WHO
At least one of the following must be present:

Impaired fasting glycemia	Men/women	≥6.1 mmol/L (≥110 mg/dL) and < 7.0 mmol/L (< 126 mg/dL)
Impaired glucose tolerance	Fasting post-load	< 7.0 mmol/L (< 126 mg/dL) ≥7.8 mmol/L (≥140 mg/dL)
Diabetes	Fasting	≥7.0 mmol/L (≥126 mg/dL)
	Post-load	≥11.1 mmol/L (≥200 mg/dL)
Insulin resistance	Men/women	Glucose update below lowest quartile for background population under investigation

In addition, two or more of the following:

Arterial blood pressure	Men/women	≥140/90 mm Hg
Lipid abnormalities:		
Plasma TG	Men/women	≥1.7 mmol/L (≥150 mg/dL)
Or		
Plasma HDL cholesterol	Men	< 0.9 mmol/L (< 35 mg/dL)
	Women	< 1.0 mmol/L (< 39 mg/dL)
Central obesity:		
Waist:hip ratio	Men	> 0.9
	Women	> 0.85
Or		
BMI	Men/women	> 30 kg/m^2
Microalbuminuria:		
Urinary albumin excretion rate	Men/women	≥20 μg/min
Or		
Albumin:creatinine ratio	Men/women	≥30 mg/g

*In Asian populations, these values are commonly revised to a waist circumference in men and women of 90 cm and 80 cm, respectively.
†See *Lancet* 363, 157–163 (2004) for the WHO BMI definition for Asians.
BMI, body mass index; HDL, high-density lipoprotein; NCEP ATP, National Cholesterol Education Program Adult Treatment Panel; TG, triglyceride; WHO, World Health Organization.

this, in a recent analysis of data from the Nurses' Health Study, for every 17 mg/dL rise in HDL-C, risk for developing CHD decreased by 40% [62].

The mechanistic basis for HDL's antiatherogenic efficacy has been the subject of intensive investigation in recent years. Among the most important of its atheroprotective functions is reverse cholesterol transport, a series of reactions

Table 19.4 LDL particle number [6, 40–54] and lipid [39] altering efficacy of common lipid-altering agents.

Lipid-altering agent	Change in LDL particle number (%)	Change in LDL-C (%)	Change in triglyceride (%)	Change in HDL-C (%)
Statins	↓ 18–55*	↓ 18–55	↓ 7–30	↑ 5–15
Nicotinic acid (niacin)[†]	↓ 10–25	↓ 5–25	↓ 20–50	↑ 15–35
Fibric acids (fibrates)[†]	↓ 5–20*	↓ 5–20[‡]	↓ 20–50	↑ 10–20
Ezetimibe	↓ 15–25*	↓ 17–22	↓ 4–11	↑ 2–5
Bile acid sequestrants	↓ 15–30*	↓ 15–30	No change to increased	↑ 3–5
Fish oils[§]	Trials in progress	No change to increased	↓ 20–50	No change to increased
Phytosterols/phytostanols	Trials in progress	↓ 10–15	No change to decreased	No change to increased

*Combination of NMR and apoB Data.
[†]In patients with elevated numbers of small LDL particles, combination with statins usually decreases triglycerides, raises HDL cholesterol, and increases LDL size—causing LDL-P to be decreased more than LDL-C.
[‡]Fibrates may increase LDL-C blood levels in some patients with hypertriglyceridemia. This is the so-called beta-effect of fibrates and can occur secondary to a large increase in the conversion of VLDL to LDL as LPL is activated.
[§]The lipid-altering effects of oil listed are with administration of—5–9 g of omega-3 fatty acids per day.

by which HDL is able to promote the externalization of intracellular cholesterol from cell types such as foam cells in blood vessel walls, esterify and sequester the cholesterol into its hydrophobic core, and then transport the cholesterol to either the liver for elimination or to steroidogenic organs for steroid hormone biosynthesis [63] (Fig. 19.9). There is experimental support for the concept of reverse cholesterol transport in both animal models and in humans [64]. Some evidence suggests as the capacity for RCT in an organism increases, the risk for CHD decreases since the likelihood for the net accumulation of lipid in the vessel wall diminishes.

HDL also exerts a number of other antiatherogenic functions along the endothelial surface and within the blood vessel wall. HDL stimulates endothelial nitric oxide production and vasodilatation [66], reduces endothelial cell adhesion molecule expression by inhibiting sphingosine kinase [67], and inhibits endothelial cell apoptosis [68]. HDL has potent antioxidative capacity and carries paraoxonase and platelet activating factor acetylhydrolase, two enzymes capable of reducing oxidized fatty acids in oxidized LDL, the preferred substrate of scavenging macrophages in the subendothelial space [69, 70]. HDL has been shown to inhibit platelet aggregation and can promote endothelial cell production of prostacyclin, a prostaglandin with both vasodilatory and antithrombotic properties [71, 72].

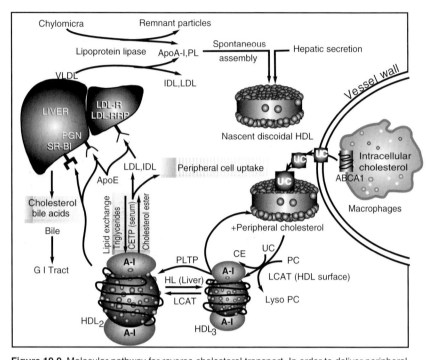

Figure 19.9 Molecular pathway for reverse cholesterol transport. In order to deliver peripheral cholesterol back to the liver or steroidogenic organs such as the adrenal glands, placenta, or ovaries, apoA-I and nascent discoidal HDL interact with cells such as macrophages in the subendothelial space of blood vessel walls. The HDL undergoes a series of cell receptor- and serum enzyme-dependent maturation reactions (i.e., "HDL speciation"). HDL can interact directly with a variety of hepatic cell receptors, the most important of which is SR-BI. The cholesterol ester in HDL can also be delivered back to the liver via a more indirect pathway for RCT, which is dependent upon CETP and the LDL and LDL-RRP receptors. Abbreviations: ABCA1, ATP-binding membrane cassette transporter A1; apoA-I, apoprotein A-I; apoE, apoprotein E; CE, cholesteryl ester; CETP, cholesterol ester transfer protein; HL, hepatic lipase; IDL, intermediate-density lipoprotein; LCAT, lecithin:cholesterol acyltransferase; LDL, low-density lipoprotein; LDL-R, low-density lipoprotein receptor; LDL-RRP, low-density lipoprotein receptor-related protein; lysoPC, lysophosphatidylcholine; PC, phosphatidylcholine; PGN, proteoglycans; PL, phospholipid; PLTP, phospholipid transfer protein; SR-BI, scavenger receptor BI; Trigly, triglyceride; UC, unesterified cholesterol; VLDL, very low-density lipoprotein. (Reprinted with permission from Toth [65])

When measuring HDL-C in a routine lipid profile, the NCEP has defined a level of < 40 mg/dL for this lipoprotein as a categorical risk factor for CHD [18]. Although NCEP does not suggest a target for HDL-C, it does recommend that patients with low HDL-C be treated with lifestyle modification (weight loss, step I diet, smoking cessation, aerobic exercise) and pharmacologic intervention as indicated. The Expert Group on HDL Cholesterol [73] and the European Consensus Panel on HDL-C [74] recommend that therapeutic effort be made to raise HDL to ≥40 mg/dL in patients with CAD and those at high risk for CAD (diabetes, metabolic syndrome, 10-year Framingham risk >20%).

The American Heart Association endorses a cutpoint for HDL-C >50 mg/dL as optimal in women [75]. In a recent update to its management guidelines for diabetics, the American Diabetes Association established HDL-C targets of ≥40 mg/dL in men and ≥50 mg/dL in women [76]. Expected changes in serum HDL in response to pharmacologic interventions are summarized in Table 19.4.

Low HDL is widely prevalent. In addition to having a high prevalence in patients with CAD, it is a defining feature of the metabolic syndrome and is characteristic of diabetic dyslipidemia. A large number of genetic polymorphisms play a role in determining any given individual's circulating level of HDL-C [77]. Consequently, HDL-C can prove very challenging to raise, especially in patients with a genetic predisposition toward low levels of this lipoprotein ("familial hypoalphalipoproteinemia secondary, for example, to low levels of expression of apoprotein AI or ABCA1 [78]). A common misconception about HDL is that the smaller, denser HDL particles are "proatherogenic" while the larger, more buoyant HDL particles are "antiatherogenic." All HDL particles can exert antiatherogenic effects. In fact, many of the antiatherogenic effects attributable to HDL, including the suppression of adhesion molecule expression and activation of prostacyclin expression, were discovered with HDL_3, the smaller, denser variant of HDL. Moreover, all subfractions of HDL participate in RCT, and it is the smaller HDL particles that likely function as the most avid traps for cellular cholesterol because they are less saturated with cholesterol than their larger lipid-laden counterparts. Although some studies have shown HDL_2 to be more protective against CHD than HDL_3, [79, 80] other studies such as the Physicians Health Study [81] and data from the Caerphilly and Speedwell cohorts [82] have shown the opposite. Moreover, in the VAHIT [83] and Lopid Coronary Angiography Trial [84], reductions in cardiovascular morbidity and mortality and rates of coronary and vein graft atheromatous plaque progression were predicted by fibrate-induced elevations in HDL_3. Consequently, it is elevations in total HDL mass that are important when treating low HDL, not necessarily the elevation of any one fraction over the other.

NMR spectroscopy quantifies five subfractions of HDL that are reported as particle concentrations (μmol/L) of small HDL-P, medium HDL-P, and large HDL-P (Fig. 19.3). Low levels of large HDL are a marker of insulin resistance and predict future development of diabetes mellitus, particularly in patients with concomitant elevations in large VLDL [13–15, 85]. In patients with insulin resistance, development of the atherogenic lipid triad is a manifestation of changes in the activity of lipolytic enzymes (Fig. 19.8). In patients with insulin resistance, LPL is inhibited [85]. LPL is responsible for hydrolyzing the triglycerides in VLDL and CMs. With reduced rates of catabolism, TG and VLDL levels rise. In the setting of insulin resistance, HDL levels decrease for at least three reasons: (1) There is an insulin response element in the gene for apoAI. With reduced sensitivity to insulin signaling, apoAI expression can decrease substantially. (2) As VLDL and CMs are hydrolyzed by LPL, surface coat constituents from these large lipoproteins are released, which can be used to assimilate HDL in serum. With reduced lipolytic activity, less surface coat mass is used to form HDL. (3) As TG levels rise, CETP transfers more triglyceride into HDL, rendering it a better target for lipolysis by HL. HDL catabolites and delipidated apoAI can be cleared from the circulation via the kidney (Fig. 19.8). HL also converts large, more buoyant LDL into smaller, denser LDL via this same mechanism. Consequently, among patients with low HDL and even modest elevation of triglycerides, patients commonly manifest increased LDL-P and small LDL-P despite having a normal LDL-C on routine lipid profiling.

Case studies for lipoprotein subfraction analysis

Case 1

CG is a 42-year-old man with family history of premature atherosclerotic cardiovascular disease and low HDL-C.

Selected health assessments include:

CHD history	No history of known CHD
Blood pressure	No history of elevated blood pressure
Cigarette smoking	No history of tobacco use
Diabetes mellitus	None
Exercise	30 minutes of elliptical walking 3 × weekly
Past medical history	Gastroesophageal reflux
Family history	Father fatal myocardial infarction (age 51), brother nonfatal myocardial infarction (age 45)
Medications	Ranitidine porn, ASA 81 mg daily
Height	74 inches
Weight	203 lbs
Body mass index	26 kg/m^2
Waist circumference	39 inches
Blood pressure	104/66 mm Hg
Physical exam	Non-contributory
Blood chemistries	Within normal limits
Thyroid blood tests	Within normal limits, including normal thyroid stimulating hormone
Creatinine blood level	Within normal limits
Urinalysis	Within normal limits, no protein
Fasting blood glucose	96 mg/dL
Hemoglobin A1c	5.8% (normal 4.5–6.3%)
Fasting insulin level	Normal, not elevated
Highly sensitive C-reactive protein	1.8 mg/L (CHD risk = <1.0 low; 1.0–3.0 average; 3.1–10.0 high; >10 mg/L may represent non-cardiovascular inflammation)

Standard lipid profile   Total cholesterol = 146 mg/dL
LDL cholesterol = 94 mg/dL
HDL cholesterol =24 mg/dL
Triglycerides =142 mg/dL
Framingham risk score   1% 10-year risk of CHD
NMR lipoprotein values   LDL-P = 1809 nmol/L
(High-risk goal <1000 nmol/L)
(Moderate high-risk goal <1300 nmol/L)
Small LDL-P = 1650 nmol/L
(Moderate- and high-risk goal <850 nmol/L)
LDL size = 19.2 nm
(Pattern B, high metabolic risk)
Large HDL-P = 1.6 μmol/L (Intermediate metabolic risk)
Large VLDL-P = 3.2 nmol/L (Intermediate metabolic risk)

Intervention: After discussing options with the patient he elected to engage therapeutic lifestyle changes by adopting a Step II American Heart Association (AHA) diet and increased elliptical walking to 60 minutes daily as tolerated.

Two weeks later he noted sudden onset of anterior chest pressure and diaphoresis. The patient presented to hospital where he was diagnosed with an acute coronary syndrome. On emergent cardiac catheterization he was found to have 95% mid-LAD and 40% mid-RCA lesions. The LAD lesion was treated with PTCA and stent placement. His hospital course was otherwise unremarkable. At discharge he was advised to continue Step II AHA diet, exercise as prescribed, and therapy with atorvastatin 20 mg daily was initiated. Laboratory studies were repeated 12 weeks post discharge.

Standard lipid profile   Total cholesterol = 125 mg/dL
LDL cholesterol = 84 mg/dL
HDL cholesterol = 27 mg/dL
Triglycerides = 96 mg/dL
NMR lipoprotein values   LDL-P = 1137 nmol/L
(High-risk goal <1000 nmol/L)
(Moderate high-risk goal <1300 nmol/L)
Small LDL-P = 1040 nmol/L
(Moderate- and high-risk goal <850 nmol/L)
LDL Size = 19.9 nm
(Pattern B, high metabolic risk)
Large HDL-P = 4.2 μmol/L
(Intermediate metabolic risk)
Large VLDL-P = 1.4 nmol/L
(Intermediate metabolic risk)

Intervention: On recheck the patient remained compliant with therapeutic lifestyle measures and atorvastatin without complaints. Extended release niacin 1000 mg prior to bedtime was added to the medical regimen. Repeat laboratory studies 12 weeks after institution of combination therapy were performed.

Standard lipid profile   Total cholesterol = 125 mg/dL
      LDL cholesterol = 79 mg/dL
      HDL cholesterol = 38 mg/dL
      Triglycerides = 42 mg/dL
NMR lipoprotein values   LDL-P = 905 nmol/L (Optimal)
      (High-risk goal <1000 nmol/L)
      (Moderate high-risk goal <1300 nmol/L)
      Small LDL-P = 120 nmol/L (Low)
      (Moderate- and high-risk goal <850 nmol/L)
      LDL Size = 20.6 nm
      (Pattern A, low metabolic risk)
      Large HDL-P = 4.8 μmol/L
      (Intermediate metabolic risk)
      Large VLDL-P = 0.8 nmol/L
      (Intermediate metabolic risk)

Discussion of Case 1

At presentation this patient would be felt by many clinicians to harbor increased CHD risk due to his strong family history of premature cardiovascular disease and, what appears to be at a lipid level, "isolated" low HDL-C. At a lipoprotein level, NMR values demonstrated the combination of significant LDL-P (1809 nmol/L) and small LDL-P (1650 nmol/L) elevations despite a low LDL-C value (94 mg/dL). This quantitative LDL excess is also qualitatively expressed as small LDL particle size. The discordance of LDL-P and LDL-C concentrations is consistent with data from the Framingham Offspring Study presented previously which demonstrate progressive increasing LDL-P and decreasing LDL-C as HDL-C values decline below 50 mg/dL. As a result, this patient harbors both LDL-related CHD risk (excess LDL-P and small LDL-P) and HDL-related CHD risk. Although his 10-year Framingham risk score at presentation was low (1%), this parameter is heavily age weighted. Consequently, CHD risk may be underestimated in younger patients despite findings that would imply higher clinical risk.

Lipoprotein management of this patient will require both reduction of his increased number of LDL particles and efforts to increase HDL-C. Integrating LDL-P into clinical decision-making is illustrated in Table 19.5. Overall, the priority of intervention is to first address LDL-related risk, followed by management of HDL-C and TG-related risk. Because LDL-P is often elevated

Table 19.5 Integrating lipoprotein particle number (LDL-P) and lipid management.

		LDL-P		
		At goal	Near goal	Not near goal
LDL-C	At goal	No further therapy	Further LDL lowering therapy	
	Near goal			
	Not near goal	Consider further LDL lowering therapy		
HDL-C	At goal	No further therapy	Further LDL lowering therapy	
	Near goal	Consider HDL raising therapy	Further LDL lowering therapy (priority 1)	
	Not near goal	Further HDL raising therapy	Further HDL raising therapy (priority 2)	
TG	At goal	No further therapy	Further LDL lowering therapy	
	Near goal	Consider TG lowering therapy	Further LDL lowering therapy (priority 1)	
	Not near goal	Further TG lowering therapy	Further TG lowering therapy (priority 2)	

among individuals at or near LDL-C goal, one cannot assume goal LDL-C values reflect goal LDL-P values. Thus, both LDL-C and LDL-P should be managed to successfully address LDL-related CHD risk. Next, LDL-P should be considered when evaluating abnormal HDL-C and TG values. As discussed previously, progressively greater elevations of LDL-P values are encountered as HDL-C declines below 50 mg/dL and TG rises above 125 mg/dL [1]. As shown in Table 19.5, different clinical considerations are present given the degree to which LDL-P, or the lipid parameter in question, are at or near goal values.

At hospital discharge the patient was appropriately begun on statin therapy. By inhibiting the rate-limiting enzyme (HMG Co-A reductase) involved in cholesterol synthesis, increased numbers of LDL receptors are expressed. LDL particles of all size bind to increasingly expressed receptors resulting in decreased LDL-P. The percent reduction in LDL particle number on statin therapy roughly mirrors the percent reduction in LDL-C for the agent and dosage selected [40–46]. The patient's laboratory values on atorvastatin 20 mg daily showed LDL-C (84 mg/dL) to be at ATP III goal of <100 mg/dL (20th percentile) with continued low HDL-C (27 mg/dL) and unremarkable triglycerides (96 mg/dL). However, LDL-P (1137 nmol/L) remained above a population equivalent goal for high-risk patients (1000 nmol/L) due to continued elevation of small LDL-P (1040 nmol/L) above the 50th percentile (850 nmol/L). To achieve further LDL particle reductions as well as to increase HDL-C, extended release niacin was added to statin therapy. The LDL effects of niacin therapy are usually described as qualitative "shifting" of LDL particles from small to large size, coupled with a modest decrease in LDL-C. The quantitative

NMR measured lipoprotein effects of extended release niacin were reported by Morgan *et al.* [47] in a study of the effects of 1000 mg and 2000 mg dosages of extended release niacin monotherapy. In a dose-related fashion, LDL-P declined 15% and 23%, while small LDL-P decreased 47% and 50% on dosages of 1000 mg and 2000 mg, respectively.

In response to combination, statin plus extended release niacin therapy, repeat laboratory studies showed a slight decrease in LDL-C (79 mg/dL), substantial increase in HDL-C (38 mg/dL), and further reduction of triglycerides (42 mg/dL). Despite the small net decrease in LDL-C (5 mg/dL), the quantitative LDL particle response to this combination was robust. LDL-P decreased from 1137 nmol/L to 905 nmol/L (goal <1000 nmol/L) and small LDL-P decreased from 1040 nmol/L to 120 nmol/L (goal <850 nmol/L). In patients with elevated numbers of small LDL particles, combination of niacin or fibrates with statins usually decrease triglycerides, raises HDL cholesterol, and increases LDL size—causing LDL-P to be decreased more than LDL-C.

Having achieved LDL-C and LDL-P targets, further optimization of HDL-C should be considered. Unlike decreased LDL values, which reach steady state levels within 3 months after institution of therapy, increases in HDL values may take 9 months or more to reach steady state levels. This time to maximum HDL effect is clinically important in gauging therapeutic response, as well as deciding when additional dosage adjustments are needed to achieve additional HDL-C raising.

Case 2

MS is a 46-year-old man with moderate hypertriglyceridemia and a constellation of CHD risk factors consistent with the "metabolic syndrome."

Selected health assessments include:

CHD history	No history of known CHD
Blood pressure	High blood pressure, well-controlled with an angiotensin converting enzyme inhibitor
Cigarette smoking	One pack per day, for the past 30 years
Diabetes mellitus	None
Exercise	Minimal
Past medical history	No history of alcohol intake
Family history	Father with MI at age 61
Medications	ACE inhibitor, aspirin
Height	70 inches (178 cm)
Weight	245 lbs (111 kg)
Body mass index	35 kg/m^2
Waist circumference	41 inches (104 cm)
Blood pressure	110/75 mm Hg
Physical exam	Non-contributory

Blood chemistries	Normal, except mild elevations in liver transaminases
Thyroid blood tests	Normal, including normal thyroid-stimulating hormone
Creatinine blood level	Normal
Urinalysis	Normal with no protein
Fasting blood glucose	112 mg/dL
Hemoglobin A1c	6.0% (normal 4.5–6.3%)
Fasting insulin level	Normal, not elevated
Highly sensitive C-reactive protein	3.6 mg/L (CHD risk = <1.0 low; 1.0–3.0 average; 3.1–10.0 high; >10 mg/L may represent non-cardiovascular inflammation)
Standard lipid profile	Total cholesterol = 240 mg/dL
	LDL cholesterol = 145 mg/dL
	HDL cholesterol = 35 mg/dL
	Triglycerides = 300 mg/dL
Framingham risk score	25% 10-year risk of CHD
NMR lipoprotein values	LDL-P = 2279 nmol/L (Optimal)
	(High-risk goal <1000 nmol/L) (Moderate high-risk goal <1300 nmol/L)
	Small LDL-P = 1918 nmol/L (Low)
	(Moderate- and high-risk goal < 850 nmol/L)
	LDL size = 19.9 nm
	(Pattern B, high metabolic risk)
	Large HDL-P = 3.0 μmol/L
	(High metabolic risk)
	Large VLDL-P = 10.4 nmol/L
	(High metabolic risk)

Discussion of Case 2

Due to the presence of increased waist circumference, elevated fasting glucose, decreased HDL-C, and increased triglycerides, this patient meets the NCEP ATP III definition of the "metabolic syndrome" (Table 19.3), placing him at increased CHD risk. His high risk for CHD is further exacerbated by poor lifestyle habits (particularly cigarette smoking), obesity, and a lack of exercise. This clinical impression is supported by the calculated Framingham risk score, suggesting a very high, 25% risk of a CHD event in 10 years. Given that obesity is at epidemic levels, with more than 1 billion overweight adults, at least 300 million of them obese [13], this presentation is increasingly common. The mild elevations in liver enzymes likely represent hepatic steatosis or "fatty liver," which is also common in patients with this clinical presentation [19, 21] (Fig. 19.8). Additionally, the elevation in CRP reported is expected, given the presence of multiple CHD risk factors, particularly cigarette smoking, obesity, and dyslipidemia [22]. Although the patient's fasting insulin level was within the normal range, approximately 25% of insulin resistant patients do not manifest hyperinsulinemia—an important finding that contributes to questions regarding the utility of the term "metabolic syndrome" [23].

NMR lipoprotein parameters are consistent with values previously discussed for metabolic syndrome patients. At lipoprotein particle level, this patient demonstrates extreme elevations of LDL-P and small LDL-P indicating much greater quantitative LDL-related risk than implied by an LDL-C of 145 mg/dL. Additionally, the patient demonstrates the triad of small LDL particle size, decreased large HDL-P, and increased large VLDL-P, findings that are significantly associated with metabolic syndrome [13] and development of incident type 2 diabetes mellitus [15].

This patient harbors multiple sources of lipoprotein-related CHD risk. As shown in Table 19.5, priorities of therapy should first address reduction of his LDL-related risk followed by efforts to increase HDL-C and reduce TG.

Case 3

AF is a 55-year-old male with a 4-year history of type 2 diabetes mellitus, hypertension, and hypercholesterolemia.

Selected health assessments include:

CHD history	No history of known CHD
Blood pressure	High blood pressure, well-controlled with an angiotensin converting enzyme inhibitor (ACE inhibitor) and thiazide diuretic
Cigarette smoking	No history of tobacco use
Diabetes mellitus	4-year history—diet and oral agent controlled
Exercise	Minimal
Past medical history	Hyperlipidemia (elevated LDL-C and Triglycerides)—4-year history improved on HMG Co-A reductase inhibitor
Family history	Mother nonfatal myocardial infarction (age 54)
	Mother type 2 diabetes mellitus (age 50)
Medications	Simvastatin 20 mg daily, metformin 1000 mg BID, ramipril 10 mg daily, ASA 81 mg daily, hydrochlorothiazide 12.5 mg daily
Height	66 inches
Weight	192 lbs
Body mass index	31 kg/m^2
Waist circumference	41 inches
Blood pressure	124/70 mm Hg
Physical exam	Non-contributory

Blood chemistries	Within normal limits
Thyroid blood tests	Within normal limits
Creatinine blood level	Within normal limits
Urinalysis	Within normal limits, no protein or albumin
Fasting blood glucose	108 mg/dL
Hemoglobin A1c	6.8% (normal 4.5–6.3%)
Fasting insulin level	Not performed.
Highly sensitive C-reactive protein	3.0 mg/L (CHD risk = <1.0 low; 1.0–3.0 average; 3.1–10.0 high; >10 mg/L may represent non-cardiovascular inflammation)
Standard lipid profile	Total cholesterol = 162 mg/dL
	LDL cholesterol = 98 mg/dL
	HDL cholesterol = 43 mg/dL
	Triglycerides = 105 mg/dL
Framingham risk score	CHD risk equivalent (type 2 diabetes mellitus)
NMR lipoprotein values	LDL-P = 1502 nmol/L
	(High-risk goal <1000 nmol/L)
	(Moderate high-risk goal <1300 nmol/L)
	Small LDL-P = 1050 nmol/L
	(Moderate- and high-risk goal <850 nmol/L)
	LDL Size = 20.4 nm
	(Pattern B, high metabolic risk)
	Large HDL-P = 5.2 μmol/L
	(Intermediate metabolic risk)
	Large VLDL-P = 8.5 nmol/L
	(High metabolic risk)

Intervention: Options for therapeutic lifestyle modification and medication adjustments were discussed with the patient. Although he was encouraged to receive dietary counseling, the patient indicated frustration with prior efforts at diet therapy and declined formal dietary instruction. The general tenets of a weight optimization, Step II AHA diet was reviewed in the office. He did agree to undergo treadmill stress testing which revealed no abnormalities. Exercise prescription was generated and the patient agreed to begin a supervised aerobic exercise program. Simvastatin dosage was increased to 40 mg daily.

Patient returned 3 months later having complied with medication, which he tolerated without difficulty. He was noncompliant with dietary recommendations and only intermittently compliant with exercise, which he tolerated without complaints.

Standard lipid profile	Total cholesterol = 124 mg/dL
	LDL cholesterol = 74 mg/dL
	HDL cholesterol = 41 mg/dL
	Triglycerides = 70 mg/dL

NMR lipoprotein values   LDL-P = 999 nmol/L
                         (High-risk goal <1000 nmol/L)
                         (Moderate high-risk goal <1300 nmol/L)
                         Small LDL-P = 850 nmol/L
                         (Moderate- and high-risk goal <850 nmol/L)
                         LDL size = 20.3 nm
                         (Pattern B, high metabolic risk)
                         Large HDL-P = 5.8 μmol/L
                         (Intermediate metabolic risk)
                         Large VLDL-P = 3.2 nmol/L
                         (Intermediate metabolic risk)

Intervention: Due to concerns about potential adverse effects with increasing medication, the patient decided to engage in therapeutic lifestyle changes previously outlined. Medical regimen was continued at previous dosages.

He returned 6 months later having been compliant with diet and exercise recommendations, which he tolerated with complaints. During this period the patient experienced a 16-pound weight loss.

Standard lipid profile   Total cholesterol = 134 mg/dL
                         LDL cholesterol = 74 mg/dL
                         HDL cholesterol = 48 mg/dL
                         Triglycerides = 60 mg/dL
NMR lipoprotein values   LDL-P = 721 nmol/L
                         (High-risk goal <1000 nmol/L)
                         (Moderate high-risk goal <1300 nmol/L)
                         Small LDL-P = 432 nmol/L
                         (Moderate- and high-risk goal <850 nmol/L)
                         LDL Size = 21.2 nm
                         (Pattern A, low metabolic risk)
                         Large HDL-P = 7.2 μmol/L
                         (Intermediate metabolic risk)
                         Large VLDL-P = 0.1 nmol/L
                         (Low metabolic risk)

Discussion of Case 3

Lipoprotein abnormalities encountered in type 2 diabetes mellitus, as well as insulin resistance and the metabolic syndrome, emanate from a combination of large VLDL particle overproduction, impaired VLDL clearance, CETP mediated cholesterol depletion of LDL and HDL particles, and lipase mediated generation of small LDL and small HDL particles, as discussed above. Two consequences flow from this composite lipoprotein abnormality. First, due to variability in the amount of cholesterol carried per particle, the standard lipid panel frequently fails to reflect the magnitude of quantitative lipoprotein abnormalities present. This is of particular clinical significance when attempting to assess LDL-P response to therapy at LDL-C values at or near goal. Second, quantitative lipoprotein abnormalities are easily exacerbated by poor glycemic control, obesity, decreased physical activity, and ineffective diet therapy. In response to unsuccessful therapeutic lifestyle changes, patients often require significantly higher dosages of mono—or combination therapy in efforts to achieve lipoprotein goals. Conversely, successful implementation of diet and exercise often results in significantly less drug therapy to reach lipoprotein targets.

The NCEP designates type 2 diabetes mellitus, regardless of cardiac status, as a CHD risk equivalent state for which an LDL-C goal of <100 mg/dL is recommended [18]. An optional LDL-C target of <70 mg/dL is also advocated for patients judged to be at very high risk [86]. At presentation, laboratory studies showed LDL-C (98 mg/dL) was at NCEP goal with reasonable HDL-C (43 mg/dL) and triglyceride (105 mg/dL) values. Additionally, excellent glycemic control (HbA1C 6.8%) was noted in response to metformin therapy. However, NMR lipoprotein values demonstrated elevated LDL-P (1502 nmol/L) above the population equivalent goal for CHD risk equivalent patients (1000 nmol/L) and increased small LDL-P (1050 nmol/L) above the 50th percentile (850 nmol/L). At a qualitative level, LDL particles were small in size due to differential enrichment in small LDL particle number. With a primary need to lower elevated LDL-P and small LDL-P, the patient was counseled to engage in therapeutic lifestyle changes and simvastatin dosage was increased to 40 mg daily.

In response to increased statin therapy, but without change in lifestyle, repeat laboratory studies showed a decrease in LDL-C (74 mg/dL), a little or no change in HDL-C (41 mg/dL), and reduction of triglycerides (70 mg/dL). NMR lipoprotein testing showed that LDL-P (999 nmol/L) and small LDL-P (850 nmol/L) values were approaching recommended goal levels (1000 nmol/L and 850 nmol/L for LDL-P and small LDL-P, respectively) advocated for CHD risk equivalent patients. Due to the patients continued increased BMI and failure to adopt therapeutic lifestyle measures, dietary therapy continued to represent a significant treatment option.

The ability of non-pharmacologic intervention to limit need for additional medication should not be underestimated. Concerns about potential adverse effects secondary to increasing medication dosage can serve to motivate patients to engage in therapeutic lifestyle changes. In this case, following 6 months of diet and exercise, the patient experienced a 16-pound weight loss. Repeat laboratory studies showed no change in LDL-C (74 mg/dL), increased HDL-C (48 mg/dL), and further reduction of triglycerides (60 mg/dL). Despite no change in LDL-C, the quantitative LDL particle response to therapeutic lifestyle was substantial. LDL-P decreased from 999 nmol/L to 721 nmol/L (goal <1000 nmol/L), while small LDL-P decreased from 850 nmol/L to 432 nmol/L (goal <850 nmol/L). Continued compliance with lifestyle and medication may result in even further improvements over time.

References

1 Otvos JD, Jeyarajah EJ, Cromwell WC. Measurement issues related to lipoprotein hetero-geneity. *Am J Cardiol* 2002;**90**(suppl):22i–29i.

2 Blake GJ, Otvos JD, Rifai N, Ridker PM. LDL particle concentration and size as deter-mined by NMR spectroscopy as predictors of cardiovascular disease in women. *Circulation* 2002;**106**:1930–1937.

3 Mackey RH, Kuller LH, Sutton-Tyrell K, Evans RW, Holubkov R, Matthews KA. Lipopro-tein subclasses and coronary artery calcification in postmenopausal women from the Healthy Women Study. *Am J Cardiol* 2002;**90**(8A):71i–76i.

4 Rosenson RS, Freedman DS, Otvos JD. Relations of lipoprotein subclass levels and LDL size to progression of coronary artery disease in the PLAC I trial. *Am J Cardiol* 2002;**90**:89–94.

5 Kuller L, Arnold A, Tracy R *et al.* NMR spectroscopy of lipoproteins and risk of CHD in the Cardiovascular Health Study. *Arterioscler Thromb Vasc Biol* 2002;**22**:1175–1180.

6 Otvos JD, Collins D, Freedman DS *et al.* LDL and HDL particle subclasses predict coronary events and are changed favorably by gemfibrozil therapy in the Veterans Affairs HDL Intervention Trial (VA-HIT). *Circulation* 2006;**113**:1556–63.

7 Schaefer E, Parise H, Otvos J, McNamara J, D'Agostino R, Wilson P. LDL particle num-ber, size, and subspecies in assessing cardiovascular risk: results from the Framingham Offspring Study. *Circulation* 2004;**110**:III-777.

8 Otvos JD. Measurement of lipoprotein subclass profiles by nuclear magnetic resonance spectroscopy. In: Rifai N, Warnick GR, Dominiczak MH, eds. *Handbook of Lipoprotein Test-ing.* AACC Press, Washington, DC, 2000:609–623.

9 Otvos J, Jeyarajah E, Bennett D. A spectroscopic approach to lipoprotein subclass analysis. *J Clin Ligand Assay* 1996;**19**:184–189.

10 Lounila J, Ala-Korpela M, Jokisaari J. Effects of orientational order and particle size on the NMR line positions of lipoproteins. *Phys Rev* 1994;**72**:4049–4052.

11 Otvos JD. Measurement of lipoprotein subclass profiles by nuclear magnetic resonance spectroscopy. *Clin Lab* 2002;**48**:171–180.

12 Cromwell WC, Otvos JD. Low-density lipoprotein particle number and risk for cardio-vascular disease. *Curr Atheroscler Rep* 2004;**6**:381–387.

13 Garvey WT, Kwon S, Zheng D *et al.* The effects of insulin resistance and type 2 diabetes mellitus on lipoprotein subclass particle size and concentration determined by nuclear magnetic resonance. *Diabetes* 2003;**52**:453–462.

14 Goff DC, D'Agostino RB, Jr, Haffner SM, Otvos JD. Insulin resistance and adiposity in-fluence lipoprotein size and subclass concentrations. Results from the Insulin Resistance Atherosclerosis Study. *Metabolism* 2005;**54**:264–270.

15 Festa A, Williams K, Hanley AJG *et al.* Nuclear magnetic resonance lipoprotein abnor-malities in prediabetic subjects in the Insulin Resistance Atherosclerosis Study (IRAS). *Circulation* 2005;**111**:3465–3472.

16 Otvos J. Measurement of triglyceriderich lipoproteins by nuclear magnetic resonance spectroscopy. *Clin Cardiol* 1999;**22**(6 suppl):II21–II27.

17 Otvos JD. Why cholesterol measurements may be misleading about lipoprotein levels and cardiovascular disease risk—clinical implications of lipoprotein quantification using NMR spectroscopy. *J Lab Med* 2002;**26**:544–550.

18 Executive Summary of the Third Report of the National Cholesterol Education Program (NCEP) Expert Panel on detection, evaluation, and treatment of high blood cholesterol in adults (Adult Treatment Panel III). *JAMA* 2001;**285**:2486–2497.

19 Kathiresan S, Otvos JD, Sullivan LM *et al.* Increased small LDL particle number: a prominent feature of the metabolic syndrome in the Framingham Heart Study. *Circulation* 2006;**113**:20–29.

20 Cromwell WC, Otvos JD. Heterogeneity of low-density lipoprotein particle number in patients with type 2 diabetes mellitus and low-density lipoprotein cholesterol <100 mg/dl. *Am J Cardiol.* 2006 Dec 15;**98**(12):1599–602.

21 Krauss RM. Heterogeneity of plasma low-density lipoproteins and atherosclerosis risk. *Curr Opin Lipidol* 1994;**5**:339–349.

22 Austin MA. Triglyceride, small, dense low-density lipoprotein, and the atherogenic lipoprotein phenotype. *Curr Atheroscler Rep* 2000;**2**:200–207.

23 Berneis KK, Krauss RM. Metabolic origins and clinical significance of LDL heterogeneity. *J Lipid Res* 2002;**43**:1363–1379.

24 Lamarche B, Lemieux I, Despres JP. The small, dense LDL phenotype and the risk of coronary heart disease: epidemiology, pathophysiology, and therapeutic aspects. *Diabetes Metab* 1999;**25**:199–211.

25 McNamara JR, Campos H, Ordovas JM, Peterson J, Wilson PWF, SchaeferEJ. Effect of gender, age, and lipid status on low density lipoprotein subfraction distribution. Results of the Framingham Offspring Study. *Arteriosclerosis* 1987;**7**:483–490.

26 Austin MA, King MC, Vranizan KM, Krauss RM. Atherogenic lipoprotein phenotype: a proposed genetic marker for coronary heart disease risk. *Circulation* 1990;**82**:495–506.

27 Reaven GM, Chen YD, Jeppesen J, Maheux P, Krauss RM. Insulin resistance and hyperinsulinemia in individuals with small, dense low density lipoprotein particles. *J Clin Invest* 1993;**92**:141–146.

28 Sniderman AD, Furberg CD, Keech A *et al.* Apolipoproteins versus lipids as indices of coronary risk and as targets for statin treatment. *Lancet* 2003;**361**:777–780.

29 Ginsberg HN. New perspectives on atherogenesis: role of abnormal triglyceride-rich lipoprotein metabolism. *Circulation* 2002;**106**(16):2137–2142.

30 Ginsberg HN. Hypertriglyceridemia: new insights and new approaches to pharmacologic therapy. *Am J Cardiol* 2001;**87**(10):1174–1180.

31 Ooi TC, Cousins M, Ooi DS *et al.* Postprandial remnant-like lipoproteins in hypertriglyceridemia. *J Clin Endocrinol Metab* 2001;**86**(7):3134–3142.

32 Bays H, Abate N, Chandalia M. Adiposopathy: sick fat causes high blood sugar, high blood pressure, and dyslipidemia. *Future Cardiol* 2005;**1**(1):39–59.

33 Bays H. Adiposopathy, metabolic syndrome, quantum physics, general relativity, chaos and the theory of everything. *Expert Rev Cardiovasc Ther* 2005;**3**(3):393–404.

34 Bays H. Adiposopathy: role of adipocyte factors in a new paradigm. *Expert Rev Cardiovasc Ther* 2005;**3**(2):187–189.

35 Bays H, Mandarino L, DeFronzo RA. Role of the adipocyte, free fatty acids, and ectopic fat in pathogenesis of type 2 diabetes mellitus: peroxisomal proliferator-activated receptor agonists provide a rational therapeutic approach. *J Clin Endocrinol Metab* 2004;**89**(2):463–478.

36 Bays HE, McGovern ME. Once-daily niacin extended release/lovastatin combination tablet has more favorable effects on lipoprotein particle size and subclass distribution than atorvastatin and simvastatin. *Prev Cardiol* 2003;**6**(4):179–188.

37 Bays H, McKenney J, Davidson M. Torcetrapib/atorvastatin combination therapy. *Expert Rev Cardiovasc Ther* 2005;**3**(5):789–820.

38 Bays HE. Extended-release niacin/lovastatin: the first combination product for dyslipidemia. *Expert Rev Cardiovasc Ther* 2004;**2**(4):485–501.

39 Bays H, Stein EA. Pharmacotherapy for dyslipidaemia—current therapies and future agents. *Expert Opin Pharmacother* 2003;**4**(11):1901–1938.

40 McKenney JM, McCormick LS, Schaefer EJ, Black DM, Watkins ML. Effect of niacin and atorvastatin on lipoprotein subclasses in patients with atherogenic dyslipidemia. *Am J Cardiol* 2001;**88**(3):270–274.

41 Soedamah-Muthu SS, Colhoun HM, Thomason MJ *et al.* CARDS Investigators. The effect of atorvastatin on serum lipids, lipoproteins and NMR spectroscopy defined lipoprotein subclasses in type 2 diabetic patients with ischaemic heart disease. *Atherosclerosis* 2003;**167**(2):243–255.

42 Schaefer EJ, McNamara JR, Tayler T *et al.* Effects of atorvastatin on fasting and postprandial lipoprotein subclasses in coronary heart disease patients versus control subjects. *Am J Cardiol* 2002;**90**(7):689–696.

43 Schaefer EJ, McNamara JR, Tayler T *et al.* Comparisons of effects of statins (atorvastatin, fluvastatin, lovastatin, pravastatin, and simvastatin) on fasting and postprandial lipoproteins in patients with coronary heart disease versus control subjects. *Am J Cardiol* 2004;**93**(1):31–39.

44 Miller M, Dolinar C, Cromwell W, Otvos JD. Effectiveness of high doses of simvastatin as monotherapy in mixed hyperlipidemia. *Am J Cardiol* 2001;**87**(2):232–234.

45 Rosenson RS, Otvos JD, Freedman DS. Relations of lipoprotein subclass levels and low-density lipoprotein size to progression of coronary artery disease in the Pravastatin Limitation of Atherosclerosis in the Coronary Arteries (PLAC-I) trial. *Am J Cardiol* 2002;**90**(2):89–94.

46 Rosuvastatin Dose Ranging Study. FDA PI August 2003.

47 Morgan JM, Capuzzi DM, Baksh RI *et al.* Effects of extended-release niacin on lipoprotein subclass distribution. *Am J Cardiol* 2003;**91**(12):1432–1436.

48 Al-Shaer MH. The effects of ezetimibe on the LDL-cholesterol particle number. *Cardiovasc Drugs Ther* 2004;**18**(4):327–328.

49 Pearson TA, Denke MA, McBride PE, Battisti WP, Brady WE, Palmisano J. A community-based, randomized trial of ezetimibe added to statin therapy to attain NCEP ATP III goals for LDL cholesterol in hypercholesterolemic patients: the Ezetimibe Add-On to Statin for Effectiveness (EASE) Trial. *Mayo Clin Proc* 2005;**80**(5):587–595.

50 Ikewaki K, Tohyama J, Nakata Y, Wakikawa T, Kido T, Mochizuki S. Fenofibrate effectively reduces remnants, and small dense LDL, and increases HDL particle number in hypertriglyceridemic men—A nuclear magnetic resonance study. *J Atheroscler Thromb* 2004;**11**:278–285.

51 Steinmetz A, Schwartz T, Hehnke U, Kaffarnik H. Multicenter comparison of micronized fenofibrate and simvastatin in patients with primary type IIA or IIB hyperlipoproteinemia. *J Cardiovasc Pharmacol* 1996;**27**(4):563–570.

52 Bilz S, Wagner S, Schmitz M, Bedynek A, Keller U, Demant T. Effects of atorvastatin versus fenofibrate on apoB-100 and apoA-I kinetics in mixed hyperlipidemia. *J Lipid Res* 2004;**45**(1):174–185.

53 Superko HR, Greenland P, Manchester RA *et al.* Effectiveness of low-dose colestipol therapy in patients with moderate hypercholesterolemia. *Am J Cardiol* 1992;**70**(2):135–40.

54 Rosenson RS. Colesevelam HCl reduces LDL particle number and increases LDL size in hypercholesterolemia. *Atherosclerosis* 2005;[Epub ahead of print].

55 Castelli WP, Garrison RJ, Wilson PW *et al.* Incidence of coronary heart disease and lipoprotein cholesterol levels: the Framingham study. *JAMA* 1986;**256**:2835–2838.

56 Multiple Risk Factor Intervention Trial Research Group. Relationship between baseline risk factors and coronary heart disease and total mortality in the multiple risk factor intervention trial. *Prev Med.* 1986;**15**(3):254–273.

57 Assmann G, Schulte H, von Eckardstein A, Huang Y. High-density lipoprotein cholesterol as a predictor of coronary heart disease risk. The PROCAM experience and pathophysiological implications for reverse cholesterol transport. *Atherosclerosis* 1996;**124**(suppl):S11–S20.

58 Goldbourt U, Yaari JS, Medalie JH. Isolated low HDL cholesterol as a risk factor for coronary heart disease mortality: a 21-year follow-up of 8,000 men. *Arterioscler Thromb Vasc Biol* 1997;**17**:107–113.

59 Genest J, Jr, McNamara JR, Ordovas JM *et al.* Lipoprotein cholesterol, apolipoprotein A-I and B and lipoprotein (a) abnormalities in men with premature coronary artery disease. *J Am Coll Cardiol* 1992;**19**:792–802.

60 Toth PP. High-density lipoprotein and cardiovascular disease. *Circulation* 2004;**109**:1809–1812.

61 Gordon DJ, Probstfield JL, Garrison RJ *et al.* High-density lipoprotein cholesterol and cardiovascular disease: four prospective American studies. *Circulation* 1989;**79**:8–15.

62 Shai I, Rimm EB, Hankinson SE *et al.* Multivariate assessment of lipid parameters as predictors of coronary heart disease among postmenopausal women. Potential implications for clinical guidelines. *Circulation* 2004;**110**:2824–2830.

63 Toth PP. Reverse cholesterol transport: high-density lipoprotein's magnificent mile. *Curr Atheroscler Rep* 2003;**5**:386–393.

64 Eriksson M, Carlson LA, Miettinen TA *et al.* Stimulation of fecal sterol excretion after infusion of recombinant proapolipoprotein A-I. Potential reverse cholesterol transport in humans. *Circulation* 1999;**100**:594–598.

65 Toth, PP. High-density lipoprotein as a therapeutic target: clinical evidence and treatment strategies. *Am J Cardiol* 2005;**96**(suppl):50 K–58 K.

66 Li X-P, Zhao S-P, Zhang XY, Liu L, Gao M, Zhou Q-C. Protective effect of high density lipoprotein on endothelium-dependent vasodilatation. *Int J Cardiol* 2000;**73**:231–236.

67 Barter PJ. Inhibition of endothelial cell adhesion molecule expression by high density lipoproteins. *Clin Exp Pharmacol Physiol* 1997;**24**:286–287.

68 Nofer JR, Levkau B, Wolinska I *et al.* Suppression of endothelial cell apoptosis by high density lipoproteins (HDL) and HDL-associated lysosphingolipids. *J Biol Chem* 2001; **276**:34480–34485.

69 Aviram M, Hardak E, Vaya J *et al.* Human serum paraoxonases (PON1) Q and R selectively decrease lipid peroxides in human coronary and carotid atherosclerotic lesions. *Circulation* 2000;**101**:2510–2517.

70 Toikka J, Ahotupa M, Viikari J *et al.* Constantly low HDL-cholesterol concentration relates to endothelial dysfunction and increased in vivo LDL oxidation in healthy young men. *Atherosclerosis* 1999;**147**:133–138.

71 Nofer JR, Walter M, Kehrel B *et al.* HDL$_3$-mediated inhibition of thrombin-induced platelet aggregation and fibrinogen binding occurs via decreased production of phosphoinositide-derived second messengers 1,2-diacylglycerol and inositol 1,4,5-tris-phosphate. *Arterioscler Thromb Vasc Biol* 1998;**18**:861–869.

72 Viñals M, Martínez-González J, Badimon L. Regulatory effects of HDL on smooth muscle cell prostacyclin release. *Arterioscler Thromb Vasc Biol* 1999;**19**:2405–2411.

73 Sacks FM. The role of high-density lipoprotein (HDL) cholesterol in the prevention and treatment of coronary heart disease: expert group recommendations. *Am J Cardiol* 2002;**90**:139–143.

74 Chapman MJ, Assmann G, Fruchart JC, Shepherd J, Sirtori C. Raising high-density lipoprotein cholesterol with reduction of cardiovascular risk: the role of nicotinic acid—a position

paper developed by the European Consensus Panel on HDL-C. *Curr Med Res Opin.* 2004;**20**(8):1253–1268.

75 Mosca L, Appel LJ, Benjamin EJ *et al*. Evidence-based guidelines for cardiovascular disease prevention in women. *Circulation* 2004;**109**:672–693.

76 American Diabetes Association. Dyslipidemia management in adults with diabetes. *Diabetes Care* 2004;**27**(suppl 1):S68–S71.

77 Toth PP. High-density lipoprotein: epidemiology, metabolism, and antiatherogenic effects. *Disease-a-Month* 2001;**47**(8):365–416.

78 Brooks-Wilson A, Marcil M, Clee SM *et al*. Mutations in ABCA1 In Tangier disease and familial high-density lipoprotein deficiency. *Nat Genet* 1999;**4**:336–345.

79 Salonen JT, Salonen R, Seppanen K, Rauramaa R, Tuomilehto J. HDL, HDL$_2$, and HDL$_3$ subfractions, and the risk of acute myocardial infarction. A prospective population study in eastern Finnish men. *Circulation* 1991;**84**:129–139.

80 Lamarche B, Moorjani S, Cantin B, Dagenais GR, Lupien PJ, Despres JP. Association of HDL$_2$ and HDL$_3$ subfractions with ischemic heart disease in men. Prospective results from the Quebec Cardiovascular Study. *Arterioscler Thromb Vasc Biol* 1997;**17**:1098–1105.

81 Stampfer MJ, Sacks FM, Salvini S, Willett WC, Hennekens CH. A prospective study of cholesterol, apolipoproteins, and the risk of myocardial infarction. *New Engl J Med* 1991;**325**:373–381.

82 Sweetnam PM, Bolton CH, Yarnell JW *et al*. Associations of the HDL$_2$ and HDL$_3$ cholesterol subfractions with the development of ischemic heart disease in British men. The Caerphilly and Speedwell Collaborative Heart Disease Studies. *Circulation* 1994;**90**:769–774.

83 Robins SJ, Collins D, Witters, JT *et al.*, for the VA-HIT Study Group. Relation of gemfibrozil treatment and lipid levels with major coronary events. VA-HIT: a randomized controlled trial. *JAMA* 2001;**106**:1585–1591.

84 Syvanne M, Nieminen MS, Frick MH *et al.*, for the Lopid Coronary Angiofraphy Trial Study Group. Associations between lipoproteins and the progression of coronary and vein-graft atherosclerosis in a controlled trial with gemfibrozil in men with low baseline levels of HDL-C. *Circulation* 1998;**98**:1993–1999.

85 Davidson MH, Toth PP. Comparative effects of lipid-lowering therapies. *Prog Cardiovasc Dis* 2004;**47**:73–104.

86 Grundy SM, Cleeman JI, Merz CN *et al.*, for National Heart, Lung, and Blood Institute; American College of Cardiology Foundation; American Heart Association. Implications of recent clinical trials for the National Cholesterol Education Program Adult Treatment Panel III guidelines. *Circulation* 2004;**110**(2):227–239.

Index